THE AIDS PANDEMIC IN LATIN AMERICA

SHAWN SMALLMAN

THE AIDS PANDEMIC IN LATIN AMERICA

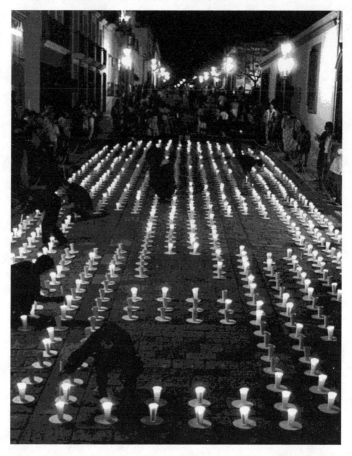

The University of North Carolina Press ■ ■ Chapel Hill

© 2007 The University of North Carolina Press
All rights reserved

Designed by Heidi Perov
Set in Scala and Modula
Manufactured in the United States of America

This book was published with the assistance of the
Anniversary Endowment Fund of the University of North
Carolina Press.

The paper in this book meets the guidelines for permanence and
durability of the Committee on Production Guidelines for Book
Longevity of the Council on Library Resources.

Library of Congress Cataloging-in-Publication Data
Smallman, Shawn C.
    The AIDS pandemic in Latin America / by Shawn Smallman.
    p. ; cm.
    Includes bibliographical references and index.
    ISBN-13: 978-0-8078-3093-2 (cloth : alk. paper)
    ISBN-13: 978-0-8078-5796-0 (pbk. : alk. paper)
    1. AIDS (Disease)—Latin America. I. Title.
    [DNLM: 1. Acquired Immunodeficiency Syndrome—epidemiology—
Latin America. 2. Acquired Immunodeficiency Syndrome—prevention
& control—Latin America. 3. Cultural Characteristics—Latin America.
4. Disease Outbreaks—prevention & control—Latin America. 5. Socioeconomic Factors—Latin America.   WC 503.4
DA15 S635 2007]
RA643.86.L29S634   2007
614.5'993920098—dc22
2006031022

cloth   11 10 09 08 07   5 4 3 2 1
paper   11 10 09 08 07   5 4 3 2 1

To my parents,
Lee and Phyllis Smallman,
*who gave me my love of books
and my memories of the farm*

CONTENTS

ILLUSTRATIONS

ACKNOWLEDGMENTS

This book could not have been completed without the assistance of a large number of people. First I would like to thank my two research assistants in Latin America. In São Paulo, Claudia Carlini arranged interviews with drug users, sex workers, addiction counselors, employees of nongovernmental organizations, and government officials. I could not have found someone with more experience in the field or a stronger work ethic. And we had fun. In Oaxaca City, Liliana Sanchez located my interviewees, identified sources, and accompanied me on my work. She spent a great deal of time with me clarifying points, explaining issues, and discussing HIV/AIDS. On my last night she invited me to a party at her house, and I will long remember how much I enjoyed that evening with her husband, family, and friends. She was as dedicated as she was gracious. To both, I owe a debt of gratitude that I cannot repay.

Within Latin America so many people gave me their time that I cannot possibly list them all. In particular, however, I must thank Bill Wolf of Frente Común in Oaxaca, who helped me to identify many people to interview and with whom I shared long conversations over dinner or Mexican hot chocolate. Paulo Roberto Teixeira graciously took the time to speak with a visiting scholar at length, despite the great demands he faces in his role leading São Paulo's HIV/AIDS program. I also owe a particular debt of gratitude to Gisele Everett and her family (Telma, Caio, Marco, and Simone), who hosted me in São Paulo. Mônica Èboli de Nigris gave me several useful suggestions.

My travels to Cuba, given current travel restrictions in the United States, could not have happened without Cuba AIDS

Project, a nongovernmental organization that brings medical supplies to sanatoriums and health organizations in Cuba. I want to thank the leadership of Cuba AIDS Project, the medical students from the University of Chicago with whom I traveled, my new friend Ananda Kiamsha Madelyn Leeke, and most of all the Cubans living with HIV whom I met on this trip. My experience gave me a great appreciation for the humanitarian work done by Cuba AIDS Project despite difficult political circumstances.

Many undergraduate students worked on this project, in particular finding academic articles on HIV/AIDS in Latin America. Some of these students, such as Lucy Wilkinson, who worked on the Caribbean region, located a vast amount of resources. I would like to thank (in the order in which they worked with me) John McKee, Lucy Wilkinson, M. J. Ruhlman, Leslie Watson, Tanya Feliu, Danika Zundel, Ryan Watson, Ronald Paradis, Melissa Burgess, and Jessica Acee. I also served as the faculty adviser for a McNair Scholar, Lorena Martinez. For her project on HIV/AIDS among the Latin population in the Pacific Northwest she interviewed many Latinos and Latinas and worked with census statistics. Examining her study deepened my own thinking about the role migration plays in the spread of HIV/AIDS in Mexico. Finally, Victoria May Eaton shared with me her undergraduate thesis, "Eso Es Lo Que Me Chinga Más: Social Changes Experienced by HIV-Positive Woman in Oaxaca, Mexico," which she completed at Pacific University in 2005. This document is important because it records the voices of women diagnosed with HIV and their perspective on their own experience.

Much of my fieldwork was funded with support from a Faculty Development Grant at Portland State University (PSU) as well as the Provost's Development Award. When bureaucratic difficulties arose, I received crucial help from Miles Turner and Gil Latz. Without their support, my research in Brazil could not have taken place. As the past director of international studies, I particularly want to know how Miles, who managed the finances of the College of Liberal Arts and Sciences at PSU, could have an office without one piece of paper on the desk and a schedule open to faculty drop-ins. I also want to thank Cynthia Sloan, who teaches Portuguese at PSU, with whom I gossiped in Portuguese at Broadway coffee next to East Hall. This not only helped me to reclaim the language before my fieldwork in São Paulo but also let us discuss campus politics without worrying about being overheard.

I met Paula Anderson when she came to ask me if I would serve on her M.A. thesis in conflict resolution, which would focus on HIV/AIDS and women in Oaxaca. I learned far more from her than she ever did from me. Her photographs appear in this book, as do pictures taken by Jana Kopp, a PSU student who did a by-arrangement with me. Jack Corbett, who has ex- tensive contacts in Oaxaca, put me in touch with Liliana Sanchez and gave me the contacts that enabled me to begin work there. I hope to have the chance to work with Jack in the future, particularly as he combines research on Canada and Latin America, as I wish to do. Henise Telles Ferreira has been a good friend, without whom I would not have met Claudia. Patrice Hudson worked with me in international studies at PSU. The most capable and positive person I know, she solved many problems that made my field-work possible and helped me greatly with my manuscript. Lisa Stensby also helped me with my editing.

Most of all, I wish to thank my wife, Margaret Everett, who supported my travels while I worked on this project, although Paige and Audrey were still small. I look forward to our future fieldwork together in Oaxaca.

INTRODUCTION

I first became interested in HIV/AIDS in Latin America in 1993, when I was living in Rio de Janeiro. That January a friend invited me to visit a rehearsal for a samba school that was preparing for Carnival. We left around midnight and traveled to the club, which was in a large, one-story cinder block building in a tough section of town. There was a person, unconscious or dead, lying in the street near the center. A crowd had gathered around him. Entering the club was like walking into Sodom and Gomorrah. I grew up in a rural area a few miles outside Ancaster, Ontario. It was the kind of place where, when a car drove down the gravel road, my mother might know not only who it was but also where they were going. As a student at Queen's University in Ontario, my experience was not very diverse, nor was I very adventurous. When I entered the club, I tried to hide what I was feeling. I was stunned.

In the back was a large stage where a panel of judges was convening to select the club's beauty mascot. In front a large crowd circulated with transvestites, men in leather clothes out of *Spartacus,* and women in strange lingerie. Gender was indeterminate. People embraced, yelled, groped, necked, primped, and laughed. Suddenly, a roller-skating transvestite with a feather headdress and sequined spandex grabbed my shoulders and asked me to dance. I agreed, as it seemed I should, but someone else more interesting passed by. She rushed off to join him. Soon the beauty contest started, and the crowd grew raucous.

In the midst of this madness, I noticed two men who seemed

out of place. They circulated through the crowd, ignoring the show. Instead they approached people, who grew quiet when they talked with them. This fact alone seemed strange in that wild atmosphere. I grew increasingly curious about these individuals, especially when I noted the respect that the crowd seemed to have for them. After a few minutes they approached a couple next to me. They spoke for a few minutes, and then the men pulled out a string of brightly colored condoms. The music had grown louder, and the crowd was roaring for a beauty queen, who had clearly had extensive surgery. She was spectacular. It was hard to talk. But I approached the two men, introduced myself, and asked what they were doing. Over the screams of the crowd they explained that they were doctors who volunteered to do AIDS education work before Carnival. I said that it seemed a strange time to do such serious work. But they said it was the most important time of the year, and they had to talk to people early in the night. In the background some of the drummers began to warm up. I told the doctors that I had been surprised by the earnestness with which people listened to them, given the mood of the crowd. They agreed that people listened, but they were depressed. The future of HIV in Brazil looked bleak. They did not really think that they were making a difference. They were only doing this out of a sense of obligation; they had to try to do something. I watched as they strode back into the crowd, tapped on revelers' shoulders, and repeated their talk.

The encounter lasted only a few minutes, but it set me on the path to this project. In the years that followed, while pursuing other lines of research as a historian, I maintained my interest in HIV/AIDS and followed trends in Brazil. The doctors were wrong. In the early years of the epidemic there were dire predictions about the disease in Brazil, a country with a reputation for sexual license and Carnival. In truth, there were good reasons to be worried about HIV not only in Brazil but also throughout Latin America: an active sex trade, the large number of men having sex with men, the inability of many wives to negotiate condom use, a significant population injecting drugs, efforts by the Catholic Church to block sex education, and the prejudice that warped the early response to HIV/AIDS. And yet the early predictions that HIV/AIDS would take off exponentially in Brazil were wrong, and the country never suffered from a generalized epidemic. Instead, in the mid-1990s the Brazilian government and nongovernmental organizations (NGOs) collectively fashioned a sophisticated system to provide care and medications to all HIV-positive people. Condom use climbed while prevention efforts paid off. HIV remains a serious challenge, but Brazil has managed to keep the lid on this virus. Not all countries in Latin America have met with such success.

Despite the efforts of people like the doctors that I met that night, more than 2 million people are now infected with HIV in Latin America and the Caribbean. Throughout the region the disease has fractured into a series of subepidemics, each driven by different factors. This book seeks to tell the story of HIV/AIDS in Latin America in a manner that can account for this "mosaic of infections."[1] Why has HIV heavily affected one nation while a neighboring state has been left almost untouched? Countries with some of the highest rates of HIV in Latin America, such as Honduras, are located next to countries with extremely low prevalence, such as Nicaragua. Figures from the Pan American Health Organization (PAHO) suggest that the proportion of people living with HIV infected by injecting drug use is 170 times higher in the Southern Cone than in the Andean nations.[2] Such differences are mystifying, as Latin America is far less diverse than most other major world regions, given the commonalities in its culture, history, language, religion, gender roles, and sexual practices. Moreover, the region shares many of the same risk factors that have driven the epidemic in parts of Africa and Asia. In some countries, such as Haiti, Guyana, and Honduras, the epidemic has reached high levels. Yet for all the suffering this disease has brought the region, Latin America as a whole has not experienced devastation comparable to that which sub-Saharan Africa has already endured, or which may now loom in the future for some Asian countries. Why not? To begin to frame an answer to these questions, my work will draw on multiple disciplines to tell the story of the virus's arrival and spread, with a clear international focus.

As I researched this book and traveled in the region, I was struck by a paradox. HIV is a disease spread by the most personal of behaviors, but it is profoundly influenced by impersonal forces. Throughout my work, I became convinced that the story of HIV/AIDS in Latin America could only be told in a broad international framework that would take into account the sweeping factors shaping the evolution of the epidemic. Patterns of HIV in the slums in Buenos Aries were shaped by the international drug trade. The epidemiology of HIV in rural southern Mexico was influenced by the ebb and flow of migration to the United States. War shaped the progress of

the virus in places as diverse as Nicaragua and Colombia. It is true that factors particular to each country—from the effectiveness of the public health
system to the political will of national leaders—also affected the course of
the epidemic. Still, Paul Farmer's observation from the early years of the
epidemic in Haiti remains true.[3] The history of HIV in Latin America suggests that the disease needs to be understood in relation to international
forces, and the region's experience must be seen in the broadest possible
context.

■ Sexual Culture and Gender Roles in Latin America

Latin America has a social and cultural unity that has shaped the region's
experience of the virus. Latin America is generally considered to be that
area of the Americas south of the United States that was discovered, settled,
and governed by the countries of the Iberian peninsula. The inhabitants of
Latin America speak Spanish and Portuguese, are predominately Catholic,
and have a shared history of colonialism. This description would generally exclude countries such as Belize and Suriname, in which English and
Dutch are the dominant languages. But the Caribbean presents something
of a challenge. Many scholars would not consider Haiti to be part of Latin
America, given its French heritage and language. But Haiti was discovered
and initially governed by Spain, its experience is intimately connected to
that of the Dominican Republic (the two nations share an island), its citizens also speak a Romance language derived from Latin, and the Catholic
Church is a powerful religious force, as in most of Latin America. For the
purposes of this work, therefore, I will treat Haiti as a Latin American country, given that the severe HIV epidemic in that country and the nation's close
ties to the Dominican Republic make it difficult to ignore in this context.
For similar reasons I will also discuss Guyana, an English-speaking country
in South America that is nonetheless culturally part of the Caribbean.

   With this caveat, what is perhaps most striking about this region is its
cultural unity. Linguistically, there are two dominant languages. Despite
the presence of syncretic religions, from candomblé in Rio de Janeiro to
Santeria in Santiago de Cuba, the Catholic Church is the religion of elites
throughout Latin America. Three centuries of Spanish and Portuguese rule
meant that these nations had a shared experience of common institutions.
Economically, all of these countries were shaped by their long experience of

mercantilist policies and colonial rule. How, then, can the diversity of HIV in Latin America be explained?

In the aftermath of HIV there has been extensive research undertaken on attitudes, beliefs, and practices about sexuality throughout the region. This literature has also been enriched by the emergence of feminist authors such as Silvana Paternostro.[4] There are pockets of Latin America that have beliefs about sexuality and gender roles that differ widely from the norm, particularly in areas with strong indigenous heritage, from the isthmus of Oaxaca (where many people believe in a third gender) to remote areas of the Amazon (where sexuality is a central aspect of the mythology and culture of native peoples). Many major cities also have beliefs that are greatly influenced by dominant ideas in the North, from New York to Paris. Nonetheless, there are common themes in gender roles, sexual identity, and idealized sexual practice in Latin America.

Despite significant changes in social practice, extensive research on sexual practices and gender roles in Latin America has found that machismo is alive and well. Husbands are expected to take the dominant role within marriage. Sex outside marriage by men is tolerated, so long as it does not undermine their ability to financially support their family. Men are reluctant to use condoms with stable partners. A man whose wife has an affair loses social status and becomes an object of ridicule. Effeminate behavior is denigrated. Homosexuality is seen as incompatible with being a true man. Risk taking and aggression, particularly within relationships, are an accepted part of a man's role.

This gender role contrasts with *marianismo*, a Mexican term that nonetheless describes a complex of beliefs pertinent to Latin America as a whole. The term describes a power relationship in which the woman is supposed to subordinate her needs to those of the man. A woman is expected to be a virgin at the time of marriage. Women are not required to enjoy sex, particularly after having children. A woman who appeared to enjoy experimenting with different sexual practices would be putting her identity as a good wife and mother at risk. This belief also entails that sexual experimentation by men takes place outside marriage. Men would be afraid to ask their wives to do acts that they perceive as "dirty." Women are expected to tolerate their husbands' affairs, as long as the men are discreet. In contrast, extramarital affairs by women are rejected. Violence against women in this circumstance was not only tolerated historically but even expected. Aspects of this belief endure. Women find it difficult to negotiate condom use, even

5

if they believe that their husbands are being unfaithful to them. Women are supposed to be subservient and to sacrifice themselves for the desires of their husband and family.

6   Homophobia is an aspect of machismo that denigrates all aspects of femininity in a man. Being gay is equated with being passive. This entails a different conception of sexuality. Men are not necessarily thought of as being gay if they assume the dominant role in the sex act. This leads to an alternative identity in which men may be married and not think of themselves as being gay, despite the fact that they may engage in regular sex with other men. This realization led many scholars studying sex roles in Latin America to reject Western conceptions of sexual identity, in which all men having sex with men were defined as homosexual. Instead, a new category was created: men who have sex with men. This identity is particularly important when considering transvestites, who many studies have found play a critical role in Latin American sexual culture. Given the fact that transvestites are associated with femininity and that they also assume the passive role during sexual encounters, men can have sex with transvestites without endangering their masculinity. Many men go to transvestites, who are perceived as "dirty," to request the particular sexual practices they could not ask for within marriage, as their wives are not though of as sexual beings. This reality has made it hard to organize the gay community, as many men having sex with men do not consider themselves to be gay and would be horrified to be described in this manner. I heard this lament from gay leaders from São Paulo to Oaxaca City. Even so, this aspect of sexual culture is changing, particularly in major urban areas.

One cannot discuss gender roles and sexual attitudes in Latin America without referring to the Catholic Church. Of course the Church is not a monolith, and its power varies widely among Latin American nations. In recent years the rapid rise of evangelical Protestant groups, particularly among the poor, has become particularly important, especially in Guatemala. There are also numerous syncretic faiths. Nonetheless, the Church retains considerable influence over social norms in much of Latin America. In general, the Church has opposed sex education and condom use. At times Church leaders have been pragmatic, as will be evident in descriptions of my work in Mexico and Brazil. The Catholic Church has also played a leading role in providing hospice care to persons dying of AIDS. But most of the Church remains faithful to the Vatican's direction, which has led the

Church to fight HIV education campaigns while also limiting the effectiveness of the Church's own programs in these areas. In 1997 the opposition of the Catholic Church halted an HIV education campaign in Guatemala.[5] In the Dominican Republic, an order of nuns (Religiosas Adoratrices) is dedicated to working with prostitutes, but they refuse to mention condoms because of the Vatican's teachings.[6] From Tijuana to Santiago, the Catholic Church and its teachings formed part of the cultural and historical context within which HIV first appeared in Latin America. Because HIV is a sexually transmitted disease, its arrival required people to address many social and moral issues that were more complex than even the virus's biology.

■ The Nature of HIV

HIV stands for Human Immunodeficiency Virus. It is a retrovirus, a class of viruses that were discovered just before HIV itself emerged. But HIV is less a single virus than a family of viruses, each of which is called a clade. The study of these family relationships within HIV is called cladistics, and it can tell us much about the origins and evolution of the disease. There are two main forms of the virus, called HIV-1 and HIV-2. The main family of the virus is HIV-1, which is itself subdivided into a series of different forms named by letters (as well as into three major forms, M, N, and O). The dominant form of the disease in the United States and Europe is HIV 1-B. But HIV 1-C circulates widely in Asia and Africa. In Thailand, HIV 1-E is the main form. The virus can also combine with other forms of itself to form a so-called recombinant virus. The second class of the virus, HIV-2, is mostly found in Western Africa and former Portuguese colonies. It appears to be less contagious than HIV-1 and takes perhaps twice as long to cause illness. New forms also appear, and there are doubtless others that have yet to be identified. Part of the challenge that vaccine developers have faced in dealing with this disease is its diversity.

In some respects, the world was perhaps lucky that HIV was not a more terrible virus. It could have been airborne. Instead, HIV is spread only by contact with blood, semen, and vaginal fluids as well as from mothers to babies, either through infection in the womb or during delivery or through breast-feeding. The virus itself is characterized by a long latency period. One of the terrible realizations that people came to early in the epidemic was that the average latency period could be ten years. This meant that people could be infected for a very long time before they manifested any symptoms. When people are infected, they may briefly have the symptoms of a flulike illness. During this period the level of the virus in their bloodstream soars, before their immune system finally beats back the infection. But HIV is only hiding in the body; it has not disappeared. It is at this point that a person seroconverts—displays antibodies to HIV. The virus then enters a long-term contest with the body that endures for years. What is unusual about this virus is that it does not kill people directly. Instead, it attacks the white blood cells that form part of the body's immune response. With time the level of white blood cells in the blood falls, and when it reaches the level at which opportunistic infections begin to appear, the person is said to have AIDS, which stands for Acquired Immunodeficiency Syndrome. Eventually, the person's white blood cell count collapses, and these opportunistic infections kill the person. There may also be a very small proportion of HIV-positive people who do not progress to AIDS or for whom the process is unusually slow.[7] In Cuba I met a woman who had been HIV-positive for seventeen years but had never been ill and had never taken any medication.

Until 1996 the treatments for HIV were of marginal effectiveness. That year Dr. David Ho and others at the XI International Conference on HIV/AIDS in Vancouver reported that a therapy with three different classes of antiretroviral medications could suppress the virus so effectively that it could not be detected in the blood. This led to a wave of optimism that perhaps people could be cured by means of the therapy. It was later learned that when the treatment was stopped, the virus always returned. Still, the impact of these new medications was dramatic. People on the verge of death recovered. As always, there were problems with these medications, which entailed a complicated regimen and could have painful side effects. People who stopped treatment created an opportunity for the virus to develop resistance. Nor did the medications work for everyone. The existence of treatment may have made some people careless. Finally, in 1996 the cost of a year's treatment could be $10,000 to $15,000 a year. This meant that the treatment might be available for Americans, Canadians, Japanese, or Europeans, but it was not likely to be widely used in the developing world. Or so it seemed.

There is continued progress in developing medications to treat HIV, and someday a cure might be found. But the best long-term hope for containing the virus is a vaccine, even one that is only partially effective. There are currently a broad range of vaccine trials in place, despite a frustrating history of vaccine development.[8] The contributions of the Bill and Melinda Gates Foundation have accelerated this process. But our understanding of this challenge has profoundly changed from the moment the virus was first isolated and people believed that a vaccine would be developed in a few years.[9] The diversity of HIV confounds vaccine developers. A vaccine that worked against HIV 1-B would not necessarily work against HIV 1-C. Would financial incentives lead to the creation of a vaccine that would work only against the dominant strain of the virus in Western Europe and the United States rather than Africa? HIV is also mutable. It evolves. While this characteristic is familiar to everyone who receives a yearly flu shot, it remains a key challenge to all vaccine efforts. Scientists must target sites that are in common across many strains of the virus and that are slow to change. Work is advancing, but it is technically challenging. A vaccine might emerge sometime in the next decade, but no one I have spoken with in the field believes that the breakthrough is imminent.

■ Origins

If we are to understand HIV, we need to know where the disease came from. At this point, our knowledge is limited. AIDS first came to public attention on June 5, 1981, when the Centers for Disease Control (CDC) published an article titled "Pneumocystis Pneumonia—Los Angeles" in the *Morbidity and Mortality Weekly Report*. In dry medical language the report described how five men, all homosexuals, had fallen ill with similar symptoms. Doctors in New York had witnessed the same phenomenon and published their own observations a few months later.[10] These initial reports helped to define the perception of HIV (as the virus would later come to be known) for the first decade of the epidemic. HIV was viewed as a disease of gay, promiscuous men and drug users. Internationally, the disease was viewed as a problem of the United States that was unlikely to spread as widely in other nations. Accordingly, the first few cases in each country were almost inevitably surrounded by fear and discrimination. In late 1983 a French team led by Luc Montagnier isolated the retrovirus that caused the condition.[11] This development helped to limit the initial hysteria around the disease, although people still feared that it might be spread by casual contact or even mosquitoes. But the question remained: Where had this disease come from?

As Edward Hooper has described (his work is among the best on the early history of the epidemic), early accounts to explain the emergence of the virus were filled with strange ideas that blamed everything from "kinky stuff with monkeys" to "swine fever and voodoo rites."[12] Further research clarified that HIV is close cousin to similar retroviruses (SIV, or Simian Immunodeficiency Virus) found in chimpanzees, sooty mangabeys, and other primates. While SIV was not identical to HIV, the paternity of HIV was clear. But how and when had it crossed into people? As Alan Fleming has argued, it is clear that HIV did not exist in Africa before the late 1800s, when the slave trade had ended, or it would have been brought to the Americas during this massive population movement.[13] We also know that blood drawn from an unknown man in Kinshasa in 1959 was subsequently found to contain HIV by multiple tests.[14] The question is why did SIV emerge at this particular point in time?

Some scholars, such as Mirko Grmek, have argued that HIV may have long been present in rural areas of Africa but that it was unable to spread until urbanization, modern roads, and social changes in the 1960s gave it this opportunity.[15] But many medical historians are skeptical of this explanation, given the population displacements that accompanied colonization and the widespread presence of Europeans in Africa by the late 1800s.[16] Another possibility was that the introduction of modern medicine into Africa had itself led to the emergence of HIV. According to this argument, in the past people may have been infected with SIV through bites from primates such as sooty mangabeys or blood that entered hands cut while preparing primates for food. But these were so-called dead-end infections that could not spread from person to person. What led the virus to adapt to its new host was its rapid transmission from one individual to another on dirty needles introduced by missionaries and doctors.[17]

Other authors, of which the most important is Edward Hooper, have argued that modern medicine led to the appearance of HIV by means of a polio vaccine that was developed from primate tissue contaminated with SIV. Although Hooper's book, *The River*, is a masterpiece of research, this theory has a number of problems. Among the most important issues is that recent work on the rate at which HIV has changed genetically suggests that the virus emerged in people during the 1930s.[18] In addition, the vaccine was tested on multiple continents, but HIV first emerged in Africa, where SIV is indigenous. This is a striking coincidence. While modern medicine may have led to the spread of HIV, the emerging consensus seems to be that the polio vaccine itself was not responsible.[19]

Whatever factors led to the emergence of HIV, it is becoming clear that SIV has entered human hosts many times. Indeed, this process is still ongoing. One team of researchers has identified Liberians who have been infected with SIV recently. It is not known how this disease will affect them.[20] This process of repeated infection likely helps to explain the staggering diversity of the virus. It also suggests that there was no single introduction of this virus into humanity. In other words, if we could travel back in time, we might not be able to identify a single "source" person for the HIV epidemic whom we could isolate to stop the disease's emergence.[21] There are many possible explanations for why in the 1960s and early 1970s the virus became capable of effective human-to-human transmission.[22] Perhaps the increased capture of primates for Western medical researchers, which led to different species of African primates being housed together in close quarters, created new opportunities for the virus to spread among different species. Or maybe the growth of the bush meat trade increased significantly the number of people handling meat from primates. Perhaps the introduction of blood transfusions or the use of contaminated needles provided new ways for the virus to be transferred.[23] It may be that all these factors shaped the emergence of different clades of the virus.

Although a great deal of work has been done on the earliest history of HIV, many mysteries remain.[24] For example, HIV I-B is the dominant form of the virus in most of the developed world, including Europe and North America. But this strain is found only rarely in Africa. Why would this clade nearly die out in its homeland when it proved so efficient at human-to-human transmission that it has become the dominant form of the disease in the developed world? For some of these questions there is so little data that the truth may not ever be uncovered. But the disease has left traces of its earliest presence. The genetic diversity of HIV isolates taken from the Democratic Republic of the Congo strongly suggests that this country may have been the original home of HIV-I. This argument is strengthened by HIV-positive samples of blood from Kinshasa in the 1970s.[25] HIV-2 most likely emerged in Western Africa, perhaps in Guinea-Bissau, which had the highest rate of HIV-2 in the world in the 1990s.[26] But tracing the exact moment when HIV left its hearth is difficult.

■ From Africa to Latin America

The first clinical cases of HIV appear in the African medical record in the 1960s, and the disease next entered Europe. The first case of HIV outside Africa proved to be a dead end, however, because the HIV-positive Norwegian sailor infected only his wife and child. A few cases then began to appear in Europe in 1976, generally among African immigrants or returning expatriates, but these cases did not seem to start a wider epidemic, for reasons that are unknown. The disease then appeared in Haiti and the United States in 1978, although no one yet knew enough to identify AIDS as a syndrome.[27] It is unclear if HIV was brought to Haiti by technicians returning from Africa or by sex tourists from the United States. HIV appeared in both Haiti and the United States at virtually the same moment, so there is no clear way to know which nation was the source of the infection.

It is clear that both air travel and contact with Africa were important in the early history of the epidemic. For example, in 1984 two of the first cases of HIV in Colombia were men from Zaire, friends who both worked for "an airline that covered African routes."[28] In the United States, Randy Shilts made famous the case of Gaetan Dugas, a Canadian air steward known as "Patient Zero," who had sex with many of the first men to die of HIV.[29] In Cuba, many of the first cases of HIV were among soldiers returning from that country's wars in Africa.[30] Yet in the early 1980s this fact was largely overlooked, because it was in the United States that AIDS was first described as a disease entity and large numbers of cases were first reported. This fact shaped the international perception of HIV. Not until 1986 did people realize that there was a widespread heterosexual epidemic in sub-Saharan Africa. Early evidence of this heterosexual epidemic was often disbelieved. People found it difficult to think of HIV as anything but a gay disease.

HIV appeared in Latin America in an era when there was considerable anti-Americanism because of President Ronald Reagan's policies in Central America. Accordingly, AIDS became a powerful symbol of the cultural dangers posed by American beliefs. HIV was emblematic of the perceived social breakdown, urban decay, and moral corruption of the American people. Fidel Castro was unusual in publicly blaming the appearance of HIV on the United States; this idea became a recurring element in his speeches, as his words from September 1988 suggest: "Who brought AIDS to Latin America? Who was the great AIDS vector in the Third World? Why are there countries like the Dominican Republic, with 40,000 carriers of the virus, and Haiti, and other countries of South and Central America—high rates in Mexico and Brazil and other countries? Who brought it? The United States, that's a fact."[31] In a more subtle fashion, this perspective shaped many early media accounts of HIV in Latin America. The underlying message was reassuring: this illness would not spread in Latin America as it had in the United States, because Latin Americans had moral values different from those of their northern neighbors. The statement of one Chilean authority was typical: "Homosexual Chileans—said the then chief of the Programs Department of the Ministry of Health—are not so promiscuous as in the United States. Besides, here there are few intravenous (IV) drugs users. All this leads us to think that the situation in Chile is going to be different."[32] Health officials proclaimed that their populations did not need to fear HIV, as they lacked U.S. vices (Cuba), had a greater history of exposure to bacteria (Mexico), or were geographically isolated by the Andes (Chile).[33] In Latin America people initially viewed HIV as an exotic illness of urban, U.S. gays.

When the first cases of HIV did appear in Latin America, the reaction was often one of hysteria. In Chile the second patient to appear with AIDS was kept in isolation, and the newspapers issued daily updates on the state of his health. The hospital workers were happy when he finally went home.[34] In Colombia a doctor later recalled that he repeatedly washed a telephone that an early HIV patient used in such harsh disinfectant that it was destroyed.[35] Such fear was often accompanied by ostracism. In Brazil one homosexual was forced to leave a town in the northeast after people said they saw him "touching several fruits at the open-air market."[36] Another "domestic servant of a homosexual was 'accused' of having AIDS and then of spreading her virus by mixing her blood in the children's ketchup in supermarkets."[37] Some aspects of the depiction of HIV were surprising. The association of the disease with the United States meant that it was seen as a disease of the rich, and the Brazilian media asked if the nation was "sophisticated" enough to be vulnerable. From this perspective, the arrival of the disease was taken as a sign that Brazil was "civilized."[38]

The fact that HIV initially affected urban, well-educated, gay men in Latin America meant that the disease seemed isolated from the general population in 1981–83. Between 1984 and 1986 the sex ratio of those infected began to change quickly, and there was a rapid rise in the number of women infected. Within the region the number of AIDS cases increased exponentially. After 1986 it was also apparent that there was a heterosexual epidemic in Africa, which made it clear that the disease could no longer be thought of only as a "pink plague." Yet the disease received less attention than these factors might suggest (despite exceptions such as Cuba) because

of homophobia, the stigma associated with "risk groups," the belief that the general population was not threatened, and the reality that other diseases (tuberculosis, malaria, and diarrhea) killed more people.

Beginning in the late 1980s the situation began to change quickly. Governments in Latin America began to address the epidemic with a new level of seriousness. Part of the reason for this shift was the fact that the sheer number of cases had become so large that the illness had to be faced. The African example, where HIV had spread with striking rapidity in Uganda, also weighed on the minds of national leaders. But equally important, the gay community organized, following the example of its European and North American counterparts. HIV emerged in Latin America as military rule was ending and civil society was challenging old political structures. A plethora of NGOs appeared that received a steady stream of funding from international agencies. These NGOs did critical work, lobbying for the human rights of people living with HIV, supporting free testing for HIV, demanding that the blood supply be cleaned up, and pushing for HIV education programs. Despite these political advances, however, the news on the medical front remained bleak into the 1990s.

■ Triple Therapy: The Rules Change

The medical outlook changed in 1996 when Western researchers announced at an international conference on HIV in Vancouver that a "triple cocktail" of three medications could reduce the level of the virus in the blood to undetectable levels. The medicines proved to have a dramatic effect on life expectancy and morbidity, despite treatment failures, side effects, and resistant strains. The question was who would have access to this life-saving treatment? It seemed that the world would be divided into two blocs, North and South, given the great expense of these drugs. The ground was set for a massive struggle. On one side were pharmaceutical companies, the U.S. government, and the World Trade Organization (WTO). On the other side were developing countries, NGOs, and people with HIV. At issue was the question of intellectual property. Could poor countries produce generic copies of these medications for their populations, given that they faced a health emergency? NGOS pointed out that these medications were often developed with public funds and that only a fraction of the drug companies' profits came from developing countries. Multinational pharmaceutical companies argued that they needed an incentive to invest millions of dollars in research, which they would do if they could profit from their work. The U.S. government initially backed the companies' argument and sought to use the TRIPS (Trade-Related Aspects of Intellectual Property) provision of the new WTO to impose its will. Brazil quickly moved to the forefront of this struggle.

By the turn of the millennium it was clear that the South was winning this contest. The United States was losing its will for the fight. The cost of treatment plummeted in places such as Brazil, which as early as 1996 had begun to provide antiretrovirals free to anyone living with HIV. The impact on the health of this population was so immense that the Brazilian government saved money because these people were no longer lingering and dying in public hospitals. Moreover, individuals now had an incentive to be tested, and they were less infectious while on treatment.[39] The Brazilian example helped to move forward an international effort in which other Latin American countries also participated. There was a palpable sense of hope.

Sadly, the appearance of triple therapy has not stopped the progression of the global pandemic. There have been appalling failures such as South Africa, where the government of Thabo Mbeki has listened to radical AIDS dissidents who do not believe that the disease is caused by HIV.[40] His government has fought providing the new medications at every step. Other nations such as Uganda and Thailand have successfully lowered their national prevalence of HIV.[41] Still, there are reasons to believe that these nations could backslide because of complacency. And most AIDS educators and scholars worry about the course of the epidemic in Asia, which they fear could indicate the epidemic's future.

■ HIV/AIDS Globally

According to the United Nations Program on HIV/AIDS (UNAIDS), as of 2005 more than 40 million people globally are living with HIV. The number is expected to climb to over 100 million by 2010. Between 20 million and 30 million people have already died of AIDS. These figures will be long surpassed by the time many people read these words. Africa remains the continent most affected by the virus, with 25 million people now living with the disease south of the Sahara.[42] In southern Africa, where the epidemic has been particularly severe, there are countries such as Botswana and Swaziland where the HIV prevalence among adults is approaching 40 percent. In some urban areas the prevalence is significantly higher. The majority of the people living with the disease in this region are women. It is difficult to imagine what the impact of these deaths will be in coming years. Reporters in this area of Africa describe hospitals almost emptied of doctors and nurses because they have died of AIDS, orphans that are eking out a living after all their adult family members have died, and grave diggers who are beginning to stack coffins because cemeteries are running out of space.[43] In Botswana, in the space of a decade the life expectancy has dropped from seventy-two to thirty-nine years, which is widely described as the most stunning decline known for any country in modern times.[44] But such figures mask the particular impact that HIV has on subgroups within African societies. In some militaries in southern Africa more than half of all troops are HIV-positive. Individual units have been found with HIV rates approaching 90 percent.[45] In Africa, where the epidemic first emerged, it is difficult to comprehend the impact of HIV on particular communities, much less major countries. Now other regions face similar challenges.

The disease threatens the future success of important states. Some authors have suggested that HIV will even shape the global balance of power in coming decades by reducing the population and economic growth of key countries. In particular, authors such as Nicholas Eberstadt point to Russia, where HIV threatens to undermine the demographic and financial basis of the nation's strength to such a degree that the country might not remain a great power.[46] Although HIV is spreading more rapidly in Russia than in any other major European or Asian nation, other key countries are also affected. India has probably outstripped South Africa to become the country with the largest number of people living with HIV. China is finally addressing HIV in a serious manner, but in Henan province there may be hundreds of thousands of people who were infected during corrupt blood-selling (plasmapheresis) schemes in which local government officials participated. In Southeast Asia, Myanmar has become a center for the creation and diffusion of new strains of HIV that spread throughout Asia with human trafficking and the heroin trade.[47] The story of HIV is not over. Unless there is a dramatic breakthrough, everything that humanity has witnessed so far is only a preview.

Thus Latin America's experience with the disease is so important. The region, and Brazil in particular, has provided a model for how developing countries may create a system to provide care to all people living with HIV. Before Brazil sought and succeeded in this effort, almost all analysts be- lieved that such a policy was impossible. The region also provides important insights into a variety of key problems: Does war accelerate the spread of the virus, or in some cases does it actually constrain it? What is the association between HIV and poverty? How do the flows of international migration shape the diffusion of the virus? How have different nations balanced the public's need to control the virus's spread with the human rights of individuals? What have been the costs of these choices? What role has the international drug trade played in the diffusion of the epidemic? Why did the epidemic reach high levels in some countries, while neighboring states escaped this suffering? And given the severity of the HIV/AIDS epidemic in much of the world, why has Latin America's experience not been worse? A discussion of HIV/AIDS in Latin America can provide insight into these issues, as the greatest pandemic in centuries continues to unfold.

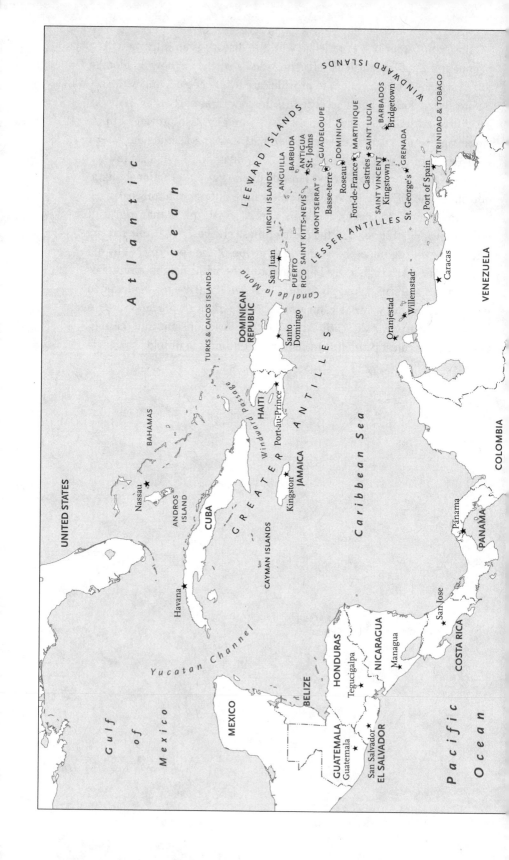

1

THE CARIBBEAN
CUBA AND HAITI

For twenty-eight-year-old Noremia Duarte Perez the worst
part about being HIV-positive wasn't the illness but, rather,
that she was separated from her son. The state had confined
her to a sanatorium, and HIV-children could not be with their
parents. Noremia's family found it difficult to deal with the boy's
questions. Clara Perez, Noremia's mother, had worked hard to
prepare him for his trip to the sanatorium: "The first time he
visited his mother he asked why he couldn't live with her since
she had such a nice little house? I drilled into him that she was
living at a school and that children couldn't live there." Noremia's
illness devastated Clara Perez: "For several weeks I was sick. I
had to see a psychologist since I was feeling suicidal." But she had
rallied because she believed she had to be strong for her daughter.
Noremia knew how difficult her situation was for her family, but
she carried a double burden in that she not only had to live with
the disease but also had to keep secret the fact that she had
deliberately injected HIV-positive blood: "My mother is terribly
shaken too, but I've never told her about the self-injection. No-
one would ever forgive me for that. I mean I have a child." Her
father still thought that her fiancé hadn't told her that he was
HIV-positive. Noremia herself couldn't understand why she had
done something that brought such suffering on her family: "I
regret it terribly. I'd like to beat myself black and blue for what
I did." And she worried endlessly about her son and how he

would deal with his mother's illness and what she should tell him, because she had seen what this information could do to other children: "At the home, I have a girl friend with a nine year old boy. She told him that he had the disease and he tried to hang himself."[1] Somehow both Noremia and her friend—whose son survived—continued and tried hard to make a good life for their families.

Noremia and her friend weren't alone. Throughout Cuba between 1989 and 1992 perhaps more than 200 people deliberately injected themselves with the virus. Some of them, like Mercedes, had seemed almost desperate to become infected: "I injected myself with blood eight times. I didn't test positive. One day Ivan and I got into an argument and broke up temporarily. When I saw him again he told me that he injected himself. One month later Ivan was positive and I was still negative. Then he gave me a shot of his blood and one week later I was positive. I was confined to the sanatorium."[2] Like Noremia, Mercedes lamented her decision.

Early in my reading on HIV/AIDS in Latin America I came across a book by Marcos Cueto that referred to "a mosaic of infections" in the region.[3] I loved this phrase, which captured the fractured nature of the epidemic. But certainly in no part of Latin America would this description be more apt than in the Caribbean. It is typical for works addressing the Caribbean to begin with a sentence such as "To construct a coherent overview of the Caribbean is extremely difficult because of the region's profound geographical and cultural diversity."[4] This diversity is reflected in the varied presentations of the HIV/AIDS epidemic: from Puerto Rico, where the disease is often spread by IV drug users and where shooting gallery owners announce that their needles are "almost new," to Haiti, which has a widespread epidemic driven by unprotected heterosexual sex, to Cuba, where a quarantine and education program have managed to contain the epidemic, which is becoming increasingly focused in the homosexual community.[5]

With its hundreds of islands, contested history, and cultural complexity, this region does not fit neatly into a history that focuses solely on Latin America. But it was here that a widespread heterosexual epidemic was first discovered outside Africa, and some countries now have HIV-positive rates that are surpassed only in Africa itself. Unless current trends are reversed, in the future AIDS may sharply decrease life expectancy in the region and lead to a corresponding rise in child mortality.[6] Ties of trade, tourism, and migration link the region to the rest of the Americas. Any consideration of HIV in Latin America must address the Caribbean. This chapter will focus on two countries in particular: Haiti, which has the highest HIV-positive rate in the Americas, and Cuba, which has the lowest. Despite the obvious differences between the two countries, the perception and response to the epidemic in each was shaped by its relationship to the United States as well as its particular political culture. Thus the region demonstrates the extent to which international context and local culture continue to shape the development of this epidemic.

■ Haiti

During the early years of the HIV/AIDS epidemic, Haiti was depicted abroad as a barbaric land where inhuman rituals might have introduced the virus into people. These beliefs in turn reflected long-held stereotypes of Haiti not only in the United States but also in the West. It might seem surprising that such a small country—one-third of the island of Hispaniola, which it shares with the Dominican Republic—once caused fear throughout the Western hemisphere. Today the island has more than 7 million people inhabiting an area the size of a small New England state. The majority of Haitians live either in a single city (Port-au-Prince) and its suburbs or in rural communities straining under the weight of land shortages, high unemployment, and environmental degradation.[7] Yet this small nation once terrified elites in the Americas, who constructed an image of Haiti that has influenced popular perceptions of this country until the present.

Haiti won its freedom in an uprising that began as a slave rebellion in 1791 and continued as a war for independence until 1804, when the nation escaped from the control of European powers under the leadership of Jean-Jacques Dessalines. Haitian independence terrified national leaders from Brazil to the United States, where plantation owners feared that this example might inspire their own slaves to rebellion. Worried that if Haiti proved to be an economic and political success then the entire model of slavery in the Western Hemisphere would be threatened, the United States withheld diplomatic recognition from Haiti for fifty years.[8] Accordingly, Haiti was isolated from birth and was generally depicted in the United States and Europe as a place of cannibalism and voodoo.

Haiti faced immense challenges after defeating France militarily as well as repelling invading forces from both Spain and Britain. The plantation agricultural system collapsed as freed slaves refused to work the land for others. The island had been left without any administrative structure, and there were bitter divisions within Haitian society between a mulatto class that looked to French culture for its legitimacy and a black underclass that resented the mulattos' power. These tensions exacerbated the political chaos (captured by Alejo Carpentier in his novel *The Kingdom of This World* [1949; first English trans., 1957]). The nation, already devastated by the wars for independence, was further damaged by civil wars as contending groups contested for the presidency. In 1915 the United States invaded Haiti to restore order, in accordance with the Roosevelt Doctrine. Although the United States fought and won a guerrilla war, in the long term the intervention failed to bring enduring political stability to Haiti.

In editorial cartoons in American newspapers in the early twentieth century, Haiti was inevitably depicted as a small black child engaged in some act of violence or rebellion, often with a knife in hand. In one image, published in the *Detroit Journal* in 1908, a small black child labeled "government" cowered in terror before an alligator named "revolution" while Uncle Sam looked on from a distance.[9] The message in these cartoons was clear: only the United States could save the island from disaster. But U.S. leaders did not hide their belief that Haiti's fundamental problem was the racial makeup of its population. After the United States had invaded in 1915, the new Haitian "president was barred from entering the U.S. Officers' Club in Port-au-Prince because he was black."[10] The head of the U.S. military forces occupying Haiti also made his attitude toward the president clear: "Once he forced the refined head of government to sleep on the floor while he, the major, occupied the only bed in the room at the quarters where they put up during a tour of the country."[11] While ostensibly the U.S. intervention took place to bring stability to Haiti, many American leaders harbored serious doubts that Haiti could ever govern itself.[12]

These attitudes influenced the U.S. approach to governing Haiti and, after the United States withdrew from the island in 1934, perhaps encouraged the United States to tolerate Haitian dictators. For nearly two decades the Haitian political system seemed to function, but after Francois "Papa Doc" Duvalier seized power in 1957, the island descended into a reign of terror. Papa Doc based his rule on an informal police force, the Tontons Macoutes (the term means "bogeymen"), who protected his regime with force. Despite the corruption and brutality of Duvalier's rule, the United States accepted it because of Haiti's staunchly anti-Communist position during the Cold War. When Francois Duvalier died in 1971, his son came to power in a rule that echoed his father's but lacked his political savvy. It was under the rule of "Little Doc" that AIDS came to Haiti. When Jean-Claude Duvalier fled Haiti in 1986, a military junta seized power, which led to political unrest and brutal repression that badly hampered basic social services on the island. Haitian migrants had been trying to leave the island for decades before this, but the ongoing violence and economic chaos led waves of refugees to take boats to try to reach Florida. In the United States this created a backlash, as people denounced the "economic" migrants who were shown on television landing on the beaches. This history, which created not only an exoticized image of Haiti but also a widespread fear that the United States would be swamped by illegal Haitian immigrants, underlay what can only be described as a hysterical U.S. reaction to the discovery of AIDS in Haiti.[13]

■ Fear and Hysteria: The Arrival of AIDS in Haiti

AIDS seems to have come to Haiti about the same time that it arrived in the United States, based on some possible early cases that scholars have uncovered. Two doctors at Toronto General Hospital first reported one early case, a Canadian woman who had spent twenty years in Haiti working as a nun. She had left the order in 1972 to begin working with prostitutes in the capital, which she continued until 1979. Sometime during this period (perhaps in 1976) she had a single sexual encounter. She then fell ill with a series of opportunistic infections and died in Montreal in 1981 of what was later diagnosed as AIDS. A few Western visitors also may have subsequently acquired the virus through sex or blood transfusions during their time in Haiti in 1978, although this is controversial.[14] Retrospective tests on blood samples taken from 191 people in Haiti during 1977–79 failed to find any instances of HIV, so the disease was certainly not widespread.[15] Nonetheless, it remains possible that HIV was first introduced to the island by 1976/1977, around the time it first arrived in New York and Los Angeles. The two earliest cases of AIDS in Haiti date from 1978 and 1979, and the number increased sharply after 1980.[16] The existence of AIDS in Haiti, however, did not draw any international attention until cases appeared among Haitian emigrants to the United States in the 1980s.

On July 9, 1982, *Morbidity and Mortality Weekly Report* (the same journal that had first described a new disorder in gay men a year earlier) published an article titled "Opportunistic Infections and Kaposi's Sarcoma among Haitians in the United States." The report described how Haitian patients in Miami had died of strange infections that seemed similar to those reported earlier in the gay community. Many of these people were recent arrivals (fleeing the political violence and extreme poverty of Haiti) who already held a marginal position in American society. By September 1982, when *Morbidity and Mortality Weekly Report* published an article titled "Update on Acquired Immune Deficiency Syndrome (AIDS)—United States," Haitians were noted as a category of people with the disease. By March 1983 the CDC referred to four groups that were at risk for AIDS, of which one was Haitians.[17] The majority of the HIV-positive Haitians denied being homosexual, which set off a firestorm of media attention.

With Haiti's popular association with voodoo rituals, extreme poverty, and social chaos, most Americans found the country to be a believable source for this frightening new disease. Because most early Haitian AIDS patients denied they were infected through gay sex, doctors wondered if the disease could be spread by mosquitoes or by voodoo rituals or if it began with an outbreak of swine fever in Haitian pigs.[18] William Greenfield suggested in the *Journal of the American Medical Association* in 1986 that voodoo priests acquired the disease while processing corpses to make poison, which would explain the appearance of the disease in Haiti's heterosexual community: "In his book on the pharmacologic basis of zombiism, E. W. Davis of Harvard reports on a voodoo priest and his acolytes processing a relatively fresh cadaver for inclusion in a sorcerer's poison. Their manner of handling human brain and other tissues could easily result in autoinoculation with infectious viral particles, which is similar to suspected modes of transmission of Kuru."[19] Another author speculated about rituals involving female menstrual blood.[20] Jacques Leibowitch (whose book was introduced by Robert Gallo, the codiscoverer of HIV) described how the Canadian ex-nun might have become infected by an insect: "What about AIDS transmission in Haiti? Was Sister Y., whom we have already described, a late victim of her own humanly fall or was she stricken by a divine scourge? Bitten by a bedbug in one of those dubious hotels which her vocation obliged her to visit?"[21] Dr. George Hensley had another theory for how AIDS was spread: "'I personally believe that it's a water-borne disease. Believe me,' says Hensley, 'the water supply of Haiti is badly contaminated.'"[22]

Americans had more reason to be fearful of Haitians in May 1983 when Dr. James Oleske reported that AIDS cases had been found among children in New Jersey. Anthony Fauci, the head of the National Institute of Health, commented on this report: "The finding of AIDS in infants and children who are household contacts of patients with AIDS or persons with risks for AIDS has enormous implications with regard to ultimate transmissibility of this syndrome. . . . If routine close contact can spread the disease, AIDS takes on an entirely new dimension."[23] In August a letter to the editor in the *Lancet* made the tie between this "discovery" and the spread of HIV in Haiti: "Though the cause of AIDS remains elusive, evidence points to a transmissible but unidentified virus transmitted by blood, bodily secretions, and intense exposure in a household where members share common kitchens and bathrooms. The filth and squalor of Port-au-Prince would seem a perfect medium for the transmission of such a disease."[24] It is ironic that the author of this comment was writing a letter to denounce discrimination against Haitians based on fear of AIDS. It soon became clear that HIV could be spread from mother to child during pregnancy and birth, but for Haiti—and the Haitian community in the United States—the damage was lasting.

Given this climate, it is probably not surprising that the Haitian tourism industry collapsed: "The impact on Haitian tourism was instantaneous. Visitors fell away from 75,000 in the winter season of 1981/2 to a mere 10,000 the following year."[25] The Haitian government responded by arresting gay men, who would "be jailed for six months and then spend an additional six months in rehabilitation."[26] The Haitian government also raided gay bars and institutions and expelled all foreigners who owned businesses that catered to a gay clientele. These desperate measures did not lead to the return of North American and European tourists, a grave economic blow to the island.[27] As Edward Hooper points out, in the 1990s there "was only one cruise line (running both gay and straight vacations) still calling at Haiti, and only at Labadie, a 260 acre 'private tropical paradise' on the northwest coast. Disembarking passengers were not told that they were entering Haiti, nor was this fact mentioned in the glossy brochures."[28] The depiction of Haiti as a possible home to the virus had widespread economic and social repercussions.

The effect on the Haitian community in the United States also proved devastating. One Haitian said that his wife did not speak creole at the laundromat because other people would be afraid to use their washer.[29] It became much more difficult for Haitians to find work: "On several occasions we have received phone calls from prospective employers of Haitians asking if it was safe to employ them."[30] Haitian businesses were devastated and children traumatized.[31] Even non-Haitians were affected by the discrimination: "I stepped off a plane from Port-au-Prince the other day, and the immigration officer at Kennedy Airport refused to touch my passport. Because I had been to Haiti, he was afraid he might catch AIDS from me."[32]

While medical authors often said that they empathized with the Haitian community, they were unwilling to reconsider the description of Haitians as a group peculiarly at risk for the disease: "It is perhaps understandable that members of a particular national or ethnic group wish not to be stigmatized as potential carriers of any disease. Although we can all sympathize with the plight of Haitians, or, for that matter, anyone who suffers discrimination as a result of being considered capable of transmitting AIDS, it is impossible to deny that Haitians in this country have had a vastly greater incidence of AIDS than almost any other identifiable group."[33] But Haitian doctors argued that this was not the case: "Haitians made up only 6% of the total 1,220 reported AIDS cases, and any other U.S. ethnic group could have made up a similar or greater percentage of the total."[34] In fact, the HIV seropositive rate in rural Haiti remained relatively low until the late 1980s (comparable to figures for New York City), including in comparison with other Caribbean and Latin American nations such as Bermuda and French Guiana.[35] Haitian doctors also did not think that there was any evidence for a different mode of transmission among Haitians—especially since 88 percent of the initially reported cases were among men, over half of whom had lived or traveled outside Haiti. Careful medical research later disproved the idea that AIDS was likely to have been present in Haiti before 1976, as well as the idea that this was where AIDS had originated.[36] Haiti had long been a travel site for sex tours of gay men from the United States and Europe looking for economically desperate people to sell themselves.[37] But until 1983, most works continued to state that the means of transmission among Haitians was unknown, an interpretation that the CDC supported.[38]

This process of labeling led Haitian activists in the United States to claim that the CDC's action was based on stereotypes rather than science, an accusation that the CDC resented: "'It's really insulting for people to say that we're making mistakes because we don't know how to do epidemiology,' Harold Jaffe bristles. 'I wouldn't go into an operating room and tell someone how much anesthesia to use, and I don't see where they get the idea that it's any different in my discipline.'"[39] It would be the careful epidemiological work of Haitian physicians that ultimately revealed that the risk factors for Haitian AIDS patients were the same as those for patients in the West. Indeed, although HIV spread very quickly among Haiti's urban poor, the initial profile of HIV for reported cases in Haiti looked much the same as that in the United States and Europe. In retrospect, it was unsurprising that Haitian AIDS patients in the United States had been unwilling to discuss their sexual histories with U.S. doctors. When re-interviewed, a number of these original male patients acknowledged that they had sex with men. When Haitian doctors looked at unexpected risk factors, they found a link with the injection of medications rather than with voodoo rituals.[40] With the realization in late 1984 that HIV was readily transmitted through heterosexual sex, and that many of the early cases involved men having sex with men, the mystery evaporated. In 1985 the CDC stopped listing Haitians as a separate category of people at risk for HIV/AIDS, although the Food and Drug Administration still banned Haitians who had come to the United States after 1977 from donating blood. Indeed, in 1990 the administration banned all Haitians from donating blood, a move that created an uproar in the Haitian community and which was quickly overturned.[41]

Doctors' letters to medical journals and journalists' reports perhaps revealed more about the stereotypes of Haiti in the West than about the island itself. Most of these ideas for the possible introduction of HIV into people were absurd, in particular the urban legend in the United States that Haitians had acquired HIV from sex with primates in "monkey brothels." As the distinguished Haitian epidemiologist Jean William Pape commented, "The value of this hypothesis may be judged from the fact that there have never been monkeys in Haiti, either in the wild or in captivity."[42] But many Americans and Europeans had formed an enduring association between Haiti and AIDS. I remember seeing a *Saturday Night Live* skit some years ago that was an ad for "Bad Idea" jeans. In the skit people would describe something stupid that they had done, after which the ominous voice of an announcer would intone, "Bad idea!" One of the characters said to his friends, "I thought about using protection, but then I realized: when will I be in Haiti again?"[43] AIDS caused widespread suffering because of economic deprivation and social discrimination years before it began to cause widespread illness on the island.

Haiti needed significant outside aid to deal with HIV/AIDS during its early history. HIV arrived in a nation with an extremely weak public health system, a poor doctor/patient ratio in rural areas, a widespread tuberculosis epidemic, scant government resources, and political chaos. According to

Renée Sabatier's calculations, in the late 1980s only Uganda had a poorer index of funds on a per capita basis to deal with HIV/AIDS than did Haiti.[44] All these problems were exacerbated by a political coup in September 1991.[45] The disease first appeared in Port-au-Prince, particularly in the poor community of Carrefour, which was known as a center for prostitution (by the end of the 1980s perhaps half of the capital's female prostitutes were infected).[46] Although initially concentrated among men having sex with men (often tourists), it rapidly made the jump to the heterosexual population, and "by 1986 homosexuals or bisexuals accounted for only 7% of male Haitian AIDS cases, and 40% of total cases were women."[47] Women living in Haiti's urban slums were especially hard hit. One study found that in Cité Soleil, a slum-city of more than 100,000 people bordering the capital, the HIV-positive rate among pregnant women "increased from 8.9% in 1986 to 9.9% in 1987 and 10.3% in 1988."[48] While this study was focused on a specific community, what was striking was its finding that of 533 mothers who had been bled in 1982, 7.8 percent tested positive for HIV-1.[49] Although these women were not identified in early reports on the disease, obviously HIV-1 had moved among women in this community with stunning speed. This was probably due to the fact that the majority of the initial Haitian HIV infections occurred among bisexual men who might have sex with male tourists for money but whose preferred sexual partners were women. In some impoverished suburbs, many women turned to prostitution to survive or relied on serial relationships with a male provider. By the early 1990s HIV had become a disease that infected far more women than men in Haiti, and it gradually spread from the city into the countryside.[50]

One important issue is how rural Haitians reacted to and understood the appearance of this new disease. We have a historical record of this process because of the work of Paul Farmer, a Harvard faculty member who is both a physician and an anthropologist. He worked and studied in a rural Haitian community called Do Kay during the latter half of the 1980s, during which he followed the lives of three people who contracted the virus in this community. Each of them had lived in the capital, where they had probably been infected, a typical pattern in the early course of the disease. In 1983 the townspeople viewed HIV as a "city sickness," but this changed by 1987 as HIV/AIDS made inroads into all sections of the country. As in the United States, Haitians struggled to understand this strange new disorder. Some people in Do Kay viewed the disease through the lens of their African-based religion, in which AIDS could be a "sent-sickness" caused by jealous rivals.

When Manno, a schoolteacher, fell ill with AIDS, people believed that he had been hexed because he beat a student with a hose in a dispute over a pigsty. Other people, however, viewed the disease as a natural disorder, much like tuberculosis. Nor were these two views necessarily exclusive, as Farmer found: some cases of HIV might be caused by magic; others, by natural means such as sex, although the latter view became more powerful with time.[51] There was one other important question that people in Do Kay raised: Had the United States introduced this disease to Haiti?

While Americans viewed Haitians through racist and stereotyped imagery as the home of AIDS, Farmer found that Haitians viewed the United States through the lens of conspiracy theories in which their powerful neighbor created the disease to maintain its power and exterminate the poor. Some Haitians feared the return of the Tontons Macoutes, who were believed to be acquiring the medical knowledge abroad to spread such diseases. Haitian teenagers in the United States also believed that AIDS had been deliberately introduced into their community. While the beliefs themselves were not accurate, Farmer argued that they were comprehensible within the context of what Haitians had experienced, both within their country and living abroad.[52] Such beliefs allowed people facing discrimination and suffering to reverse the blame and anger they experienced back upon the powerful. Throughout the developing world, and in particular in Latin America, many groups have blamed the United States and the West for the creation of this disease, particularly during the early years of the epidemic.[53] In this sense, AIDS provided an outline of how people in the region perceived their nations' relationship with the United States, and the structures of power that shaped their collective experience. These myths have faded with the passage of time and with promises for funding from the United States to fight HIV/AIDS.

Despite the promise of new resources, however, significant problems continue to exist in fighting the spread of HIV/AIDS in Haiti. One study of condom usage among men in Haiti found that in Cité Soliel, despite the fact that the men knew that using a condom could prevent sexually transmitted diseases, "only one out of twenty were currently using condoms and fewer than one half (43 percent) had ever used them."[54] A similar problem exists in the countryside, where one study found that in the Artibonite Valley in 2000 perhaps 4 percent of the adult population was HIV-positive, but fewer than 20 percent of women said that they felt vulnerable to HIV infection.[55] Prostitution, particularly among children, remains a serious problem, given

Haiti's economic deprivation.[56] Finally, people with AIDS face heartbreaking discrimination, even from their own families, in part because of a popular understanding that AIDS may be sent as a punishment for a sin. In his experience in Do Kay, Paul Farmer found that patients did not face the revulsion that people with HIV/AIDS faced during the early history of the epidemic in the United States.[57] Yet other accounts have described how people with HIV have faced brutal treatment in rural communities, where some families forced their HIV-positive children to sleep outside the house, stopped feeding ill family members, or abused them.[58] Education remains a significant challenge, not only in Haiti but also throughout the Caribbean, including the other half of Hispaniola.

It is impossible to discuss the AIDS epidemic in Haiti without considering the Dominican Republic, with which Haiti is tied not only by geography but also by history. Together the two countries have between 80 and 85 percent of the Caribbean's HIV/AIDS cases.[59] The Dominican Republic had also been affected by AIDS from the earliest years of the epidemic, when a young Dominican woman in the spring of 1979 came to Mount Sinai hospital with what would later be diagnosed as AIDS.[60] Still, the Dominican Republic received less attention than Haiti as a home of the epidemic, and in 1983 many epidemiologists were confused by the appearance of a radically lower rate of HIV-positive infection on the Dominican side of the island.[61] In fact, the Dominican Republic quickly developed a significant rate of HIV infection, which reached more than 2.5 percent of the adult population by 1999.

Within the Dominican Republic, the islands' epidemic was largely blamed on visiting Haitians who worked as migrant laborers in rural communities, known as *bateyes*, based on sugarcane production. This perception continued a long tradition in which Dominicans have denigrated their Haitian neighbors, an attitude rooted in Haiti's occupation of the Dominican Republic from 1822 to 1844 and a subsequent border dispute between the two countries. Dominicans, who are generally wealthier and perceive themselves as being whiter, have a long history of resentment toward their neighbors. To promote a sense of national unity, Dominican leaders have contrasted (to paraphrase Dominican researchers) the "Christian, white, Spanish" culture of the Dominican Republic with the "voodoo, black, African" nature of Haiti, despite the very similar origins and heritage of the people of both islands. In 1937 the Dominican dictator Rafael Trujillo manipulated these sentiments to launch a brutal massacre of Haitian laborers living in a disputed border area, during which perhaps 20,000 Haitians were either killed or expelled.[62]

Haitian cane cutters have continued to face intense discrimination into the contemporary period, although Dominicans continue to hire them because their labor is much cheaper than that of Dominican workers. The per capita income in the Dominican Republic in 1998 was nearly six times that of Haiti. Poor Haitians can more easily walk through the mountains to the Dominican Republic or take a short trip by sea to favored beaches on Hispaniola than risk the trip to Florida. Most of them come to the Dominican Republic intending to stay. This itinerant population of mostly young men, most of whom were separated from their families, has had a significantly higher rate of HIV infection than the general population. Within the bateyes, the HIV infection rate is much higher among Haitian workers than among their Dominican counterparts. But this emphasis may also distract attention within the Dominican Republic from the fact that the HIV/AIDS rate is also particularly high in tourist areas, especially in the north around Puerto Plata. The Haitian laborers, who speak creole, have not been reached by AIDS education programs that function in Spanish, and they have only the most minimal of social services. Many of them are in the Dominican Republic illegally. They are not covered by Dominican labor codes and fear deportation if they come into contact with the state. Women in the bateyes seem to be particularly vulnerable: they are less likely to speak Spanish than their male counterparts, know less about HIV transmission than Dominican women, and have higher HIV rates than women in Haiti. When asked about the human rights of HIV-positive people living in the bateyes, one informant told his interviewers, "The right that they have is to die, because they don't have other options in their bateye."[63] Even now, people living in the bateyes and dying of AIDS refuse even to name their illness out of fear. Any effort to address HIV in either nation will have to deal with the situation in the bateyes. As the study of López Severino and her colleagues argues, fighting AIDS in the Dominican Republic will entail not only HIV/AIDS education but also language training, social work, and the defense of basic human rights.[64]

Despite the staggering extent of AIDS in Haiti and the Dominican Republic, there are reasons for hope. Haiti's religious diversity may make AIDS prevention efforts more acceptable to many Haitians. Doctors from the Hospital Albert Schweitzer reached out not only to Haitian churches but also to local voodoo leaders, who began to incorporate AIDS prevention messages into their religious events: "In several instances, the 'loas' or voodoo spirits told stories about people with AIDS during the ceremony and warned people to protect themselves from AIDS."[65] In the early 1990s the U.S. Agency for International Development (USAID) realized that voodoo priests represented a potential resource in the fight against AIDS, so it helped to finance safe-sex training of these leaders. The irony may be that some of the same voodoo leaders whose rituals were stigmatized early in the epidemic as a possible origin for AIDS are now referring people for HIV testing, advocating safe sex, handing out condoms, and promoting abstinence as part of a broader effort to limit the spread of this disease.[66] From the start of the epidemic, the social and medical perception of HIV/AIDS in Haiti was shaped by beliefs not only on the island but also in the United States. As Paul Farmer has argued, the cultural practices of the Haitian people do not represent an obstacle to the implementation of an effective HIV/AIDS reduction program.

■ Other Caribbean Countries

Indeed, the cultural and religious obstacles to HIV/AIDS prevention in Haiti are much the same as in other parts of Latin America, where traditional Catholic practices and teachings have hampered efforts to fight the disease. In the Dominican Republic, for example, an order of nuns (Religiosas Adoratrices) is dedicated to working with prostitutes, but the sisters refuse to mention condoms because of the Vatican's teachings.[67] Other churches elsewhere in the Caribbean have adopted similar policies: "The Bahamas Christian Council has come out against a proposal to give prison inmates condoms to control the spread of HIV. The council, comprised of all Christian denominations in Nassau, Bahamas, has a list of alternatives for the government to consider. The council recommended that Her Majesty's Prison hire more social workers and appoint an assistant chaplain to give prisoners spiritual guidance."[68] In Jamaica, when the government proposed handing out condoms to prisoners and guards, riots left six people dead. Both inmates and guards had been enraged by the implication that they were homosexuals.[69] The religious obstacles to HIV/AIDS prevention programs are not unique to Haiti. While significant, other cultural issues—such as the stereotypical images of Haitians in the Dominican Republic and the West—are probably more important.

New resources are being brought to bear on these challenges in the Caribbean. Guyana is an English-speaking country of 861,000 people on the north coast of South America, between Venezuela and Suriname. Although geographically part of the South American continent, culturally and politically the country clearly forms part of the Caribbean. Guyana has one of the highest rates of HIV/AIDS in the Americas, although the exact figure is debated. According to UNAIDS the national prevalence of HIV was 2.5 percent in 2003.[70] That same year, however, Guyana's minister of health suggested that 5.5 percent of the population was HIV-positive and that even this figure "might well reflect significant underreporting of those affected by HIV/AIDS. The prevalence rates of 45 percent and 29 percent among sex workers and persons with sexually transmitted infections are not unlike prevalence rates seen in many African countries."[71] It is clear that the rate is quite high in the context of the Americas and that good surveillance is not currently in place, as "HIV information is limited outside the country's cities, making it difficult to gauge the actual extent of the epidemic."[72]

Given the seriousness of the epidemic and the lack of a good monitoring system, Guyana was chosen as part of President George W. Bush's Emergency Plan for AIDS Relief, which has promised to make US$15 billion available over five years to those countries most affected by HIV/AIDS. There are fifteen countries selected to be part of this plan, "which collectively represent 50 percent of HIV infections worldwide."[73] This program is making significant amounts of money available in Guyana to fight the epidemic: "Under the Emergency Plan, Guyana received more than $12 million in Fiscal Year (FY) 2004 and nearly $19.4 in FY2005 to support a comprehensive HIV/AIDS prevention, treatment and care program. In FY2006, the United States plans to provide approximately $21.7 million to support Guyana's fight against HIV/AIDS."[74] There are some concerns about how these funds are being used. The U.S.-funded program emphasizes abstinence and fidelity over safe sex. According to the U.S. State Department, under the Emergency Plan 155,500 people had been reached with "programs that promote Abstinence and/or Being Faithful in FY2005," while the number of people reached by "prevention activities that promote Condoms and related prevention services" that year was 35,200.[75] The emphasis on the U.S.-funded program is clear. It does not, however, address the Guyanese concerns, as expressed by Health Minister Leslie Ramsammy, who called for debt relief and low-cost generic drugs to fight HIV.[76] But other sources of funding are also becoming available.

In March 2004 Guyana negotiated a loan agreement with the World Bank that promises to make US$10 million available to that country and which should transform that nation's surveillance for the disease. The proposal notes that this "project will complement the Guyana government's own funding and already secured or expected funds from the Canadian International Development Agency (CIDC); the United States government through the Centers for Disease Control (CDC) and USAID; the United Nations Program on HIV/AIDS (UNAIDS); the Global Fund; the Inter-American Development Bank; and the Pan-American Health Organization/World Health Organization (PAHO/WHO)."[77] Guyana will continue to face serious challenges fighting its HIV epidemic, but new funds should greatly increase the state's capacity to address the problem.

Similar funds are also becoming available to fight HIV/AIDS elsewhere in the Caribbean. The World Bank has approved significant loans for the Dominican Republic, Barbados, Jamaica, and Grenada to fight HIV/AIDS, and money is becoming available through the Global Fund, which in 2003 released $48 million for AIDS treatment in the Dominican Republic and an even larger amount for Haiti ($66.7 million over five years).[78] Thanks to the work of Paul Farmer and others, it is also becoming clear that fighting HIV/AIDS may be far less expensive than once thought, even in such a resource-poor country as Haiti. Farmer's Haitian center, Clinique Bon Saveur, began an HIV treatment effort that sharply decreased mother-child transmission of the virus and offered antiretroviral treatment in a poor rural area of Haiti. Meanwhile, Gheskio now provides antiretroviral drugs to about 2,000 people, and "plans to extend this treatment to 25,000 people over the next five years."[79] There is hope that the percentage of people in Haiti who are HIV-positive may be falling.

While still small steps, these efforts suggest that if political will can be found in the international community, the region's AIDS problem can be addressed with a scale of resources that may be manageable. But any such effort will need to be comprehensive. Dominican leaders, therefore, are unhappy that President Bush's promise of funds to fight HIV/AIDS will flow to Haiti but not to their country.[80] Given labor flows throughout the Caribbean, networks of sex work and tourism, and the ease with which HIV can move through populations, a holistic approach is needed to address the disease. This will be difficult, given the fractured experience of HIV in the region, not only epidemiologically but also politically. No country more embodies the problem of political and cultural isolation than Cuba, the sole remaining dictatorship in Latin America, which has survived a forty-year embargo by the United States.

■ Cuba and the United States

Cuba's experience with HIV/AIDS is profoundly different from that of Haiti, with which it is often compared, and inevitably controversial. In the United States any discussion of Cuba becomes politicized, and this is certainly true regarding HIV/AIDS. Scholars and public health specialists find it difficult to discuss the Cuban government's response to the epidemic without in some way passing judgment on the Castro regime, a fact that has encouraged impassioned opinions but has complicated scholarship. Still, Cuba merits study because its experience is so different that it stands out not only in the Americas but also in the world. Cuba has been nearly unique in originally adopting a policy of forcible quarantine, in having large numbers of people deliberately inject themselves with HIV, and in having an epidemic in which men are increasingly targeted by the virus. It has also proven impressively successful at containing the spread of the disease. To understand both the evolution of the AIDS epidemic in Cuba and the state's response to this health crisis, it is critical to understand both the island's history and the Cuban revolution.

The fact that Cuba, the largest island in the Caribbean, lies only 112 miles from Florida has shaped its political experience ever since the late nineteenth century. The last Spanish colony in the New World to gain its independence, Cuba fought for ten years (1868–78) to break away from Spain, only to be crushed by greater Spanish resources. This did not end the aspirations of the Cuban people, however, who began yet another struggle in 1895 using guerrilla tactics. When the United States finally intervened in 1898 (after the famous explosion of the U.S. warship the *Maine*), the island found that it had gained its independence from Spain only to be dominated by a new master.

Cuba became an American protectorate. It was not alone. Both Puerto Rico and the Philippines were brought under American rule, and U.S. economic influence waxed in Central America. Theodore Roosevelt announced the Roosevelt Corollary to the Monroe Doctrine, which said that the United States would intervene in any Latin American country where chaos might invite a European invasion. The United States fostered the uprising that created Panama in order to gain the treaty right for a canal. From Haiti to Nicaragua, the marines invaded to impose an American order. From this perspective, Cuba was only one part of an emerging American empire, formalized by law. Under the terms of the Platt Amendment to Cuba's constitution, the United States had the right to intervene in key aspects of Cuba's affairs and to send in troops to enforce its will.

The decades that followed saw rapid economic growth (also characterized by great inequality and dependence on the United States) and political weakness. The association of the island's leadership with the United States served to undermine Cuba's legitimacy. Cuban nationalists resented the repeated dispatch of the marines to support U.S.-backed rulers, while Cuba's economic reliance on sugar created an impoverished and underemployed rural class. By the 1950s it was clear to disinterested observers that the island was headed toward a crisis. Cubans lamented the fact that their capital had become synonymous with moral corruption. Student groups were becoming increasingly radical. And on July 26, 1953, an outspoken son of Spanish immigrants, at the head of a motley army of middle-class youth, led an assault on army barracks at Moncada.

The attack was a disaster. Many of the young assailants were killed, and Fidel Castro received a lengthy prison sentence, but not before he made a stirring speech, "History will absolve me," which denounced Cuba's corrupt political system. After spending nineteenth months in prison, Castro traveled to Mexico, where he plotted revolution. In 1956 he returned to Cuba with eighty-two followers who set out in a ship called the *Granma*. After a disastrous landing, the twelve men still free or alive fled under Castro's leadership to the mountains, where the weakness of their forces at first compelled them to focus as much on survival as on overthrowing the government. In the cities, however, an escalating campaign of armed resistance brought the regime of Fulgencio Batista to the brink, while Castro continued to attract followers. In June 1959 Batista's government collapsed, and Castro came down from the mountains with his revolutionaries.

Once in power, Castro began a series of reform measures—confiscating estates and key industries—that led him into a cycle of confrontation with the United States. When U.S. companies refused to process Soviet oil, Cuba nationalized them, only to have President Dwight Eisenhower suspend all sugar imports from the island. The crisis that followed led the United States to enact an economic embargo of the island that has been upheld by every successive presidential administration. In April 1961 President John F. Kennedy launched a failed invasion of Cuba at the Bay of Pigs, which would be followed by unsuccessful attempts by the CIA to assassinate Castro. In December 1961 Castro declared himself a Communist (whether from conviction or necessity), and the following year saw the world brought to the brink of nuclear war by the Cuban missile crisis after Castro agreed to accept nuclear missiles from the Soviet Union. Cuba found that it had once again become a client of a major power as the price of its independence. The United States and Cuba were locked into an adversarial relationship that has shaped all aspects of the island's politics for more than forty years. While this contest challenged Cuba, it also proved to be an important tool in legitimating Castro's rule among the population and winning international support.[81]

The United States failed to overthrow the new government in part because the superpower had misjudged the strength of Castro's support. There is no question that many Cubans were impressed by the revolution's achievements. In the years following the revolution Castro poured funds into education and began a literacy campaign in the countryside that had a profound impact on the lives of many rural people. His government fought racism, improved the status of women, guaranteed access to basic food supplies, sought to ensure full employment, and subsidized housing. But no aspect of the revolution has done as much to ensure its legitimacy as Castro's commitment to health care.

As Julie Feinsilver has argued in her careful study of the Cuban health care system, even after the revolution Cuba measured its success in terms of how the United States perceived it. Castro believed that Cuba was in a competition with the United States in which Cuba could attain a symbolic victory by becoming a "world medical power." This meant that Cuban authorities viewed health care as an important field of political struggle.

The central metaphor of Cuba's anti-imperialist struggle as recounted in this analysis is that of health. The health of the individual is a metaphor for and symbol for the health of the "body politic," and in which the achievement of the status of "world medical power" is synonymous with victory over the imperialists. Medical doctors are the protagonists in this war both at home and abroad. They are warriors in the battle against disease, which is largely considered a legacy of imperialism and underdevelopment. Cuba, a David fighting Goliath (the United States), seeks to slay the giant in the battle for international prestige in health care.[82]

Only in this context is it possible to understand the capital and energy that Cuba has poured into health care, with impressive results.

Despite immense challenges, including the early flight of nearly half of Cuba's doctors after the revolution, Cuba has managed to create an integrated national health plan that provides a high level of service for free to all Cubans. No rural area in Cuba is too remote for patients to receive care. Cuba eliminated many infectious diseases, such as polio, and its immunization rates were good even for the First World. Cuba's life expectancy and infant mortality rates also compared favorably with those of many developed countries. The country made these achievements while still sending many doctors abroad to gain international support. Cuba also created an impressive research establishment, and it counted on biomedical exports to create much needed hard currency. Knowing the importance that Cuba places on its health care system, and the fact that it uses this system to compete politically with the United States, is key to understanding Cuba's response to the emergence of HIV/AIDS.

■ Cuba and AIDS

Doctors in the United States first reported a strange cluster of illnesses, which would later be called AIDS, in July 1981. The medical community did not become aware of the existence of a widespread epidemic among heterosexuals in Africa until 1986. Accordingly, in the early years of the epidemic in Latin America people initially viewed the illness as a U.S. and gay disease. It served as a symbol for weaknesses of U.S. society and was seen to represent the social breakdown, lack of family unity, frequent drug use, and poor moral values of the American people. Accordingly, AIDS became a powerful symbol to counter the political power of the United States and to warn against the cultural dangers posed by American beliefs. This reaction to the disease was neither new (many previous epidemics have been blamed on outsiders) nor confined to Latin America. But it was an especially powerful rhetorical device in Cuba, given that nation's long equation of American moral corruption with physical illness. In the 1980s, therefore, the Cuban state built on common Latin American attitudes to denounce the United States for inflicting AIDS upon the region, as Fidel Castro stated in a September 1988 speech: "Who brought AIDS to Latin America? Who was the great AIDS vector in the Third World? Why are there countries like the Dominican Republic, with 40,000 carriers of the virus, and Haiti, and other countries of South and Central America—high rates in Mexico and Brazil and other countries? Who brought it? The United States, that's a fact."[83]

As well as describing AIDS as an American disease, Cubans also associated the affliction with gay promiscuity. For example, the Cuban government announced that the first person to die of AIDS in Cuba was a "theater designer who became infected on a New York visit, an account that plays into the stereotypes of theater people in Cuba."[84] As Ian Lumsden has noted, this information was misleading because Cuba was unusual in that the epidemic in its early years was dominated by heterosexuals.[85] To some extent Cuba may have been shielded early in the AIDS epidemic because of its isolation from the United States. But Cuba also had significant exchange programs with other countries and welcomed large numbers of students from African nations where the virus was present early in the pandemic: "Of primary concern were the more than 380,000 Cubans who had traveled abroad, as soldiers in Africa, or as advisers, diplomats, or participants in cultural exchange programs."[86] It would be a mistake to view Cuba as having been internationally isolated. Cuba had sought to support revolutionary regimes by military force, and many Cubans had done military service in Ethiopia and Angola. Fifty-six of the early HIV cases were among soldiers returning from service in Africa, and most early infections were among people who had contracted the disease abroad, almost none of whom had ever been to the United States.[87] But the Cuban government portrayed the AIDS as a symbol of Western capitalist corruption. Accordingly, Cuban leaders perceived HIV/AIDS as a test of the Cuban revolutionary state, which would enable the government to demonstrate its superiority over wealthier governments, which nonetheless lacked a commitment to the well-being of their populace.

Cuba's response to the epidemic was energetic. In 1983 the government seized and destroyed all imported blood in the country, even though the 22,000 containers of foreign blood represented a great deal of money.[88] By this means Cuban hemophiliacs escaped the disaster that swept away many of their counterparts in Japan, France, Brazil, and the United States. But the core of the Cuban response to the epidemic was mass HIV testing.

When commercial tests for HIV antibodies became available in 1985, the government started to test all Cubans who had been out of the country since 1981. Among those found seropositive were a large number of Cuban soldiers, "internationalists" returning from Africa. By June, 1986 testing had been extended to all blood donors and to those whose work involved extensive travel, such as tourist and resort and airline workers, fishermen, and sailors. When the first Cuban diagnostic kits became available in 1987, HIV screening was extended to all pregnant women, all those with sexually trans-mitted diseases, and all inpatients and prisoners. Later, entire neigh-bourhoods in tourist locations, such as Old Havana were screened. In 1985 a special group was set up to trace and test, regularly and repeatedly, the sexual partners of all seropositive persons. For every seropositive there is a confidential sexual contact tree that traces the spread of HIV infection through sexual partners, all of whom are contacted and screened.[89]

By 1989 the government had tested more than 75 percent of the popula-tion over age fifteen for HIV.[90] This figure continued to increase: "By April 1991, 9,771,691 people, almost the entire population had been tested."[91]

The most controversial aspect of this policy was the government quar-antine in sanatoriums of people who tested HIV-positive. The first sanato-rium to be constructed was Los Cocos in Santiago de las Vega, just outside Havana. Since it opened in 1986, it has evolved to become the flagship of the Cuban sanatorium system and the one designed for foreign visitors to tour.[92] It remains the largest and most important sanatorium in Cuba. Other sanatoriums were constructed throughout Cuba, and by the early 1990s one existed in every province. These sanatoriums soon attracted in-ternational attention because of human rights concerns. On one hand, pa-tients in the sanatoriums received free medical care, access to medications, additional food rations, their salaries, and living conditions that were better than those available to Cubans living outside. On the other hand, this policy confined HIV-positive Cubans who were often otherwise healthy, who could not pass on the disease except with intimate contact, and who had no clear date for their release except upon their death.

In practice, many HIV-positive Cubans found it impossible to say no when asked to enter the sanatoriums during the 1980s.[93] While these fa-cilities with their small cabanas and manicured lawns appeared attractive,

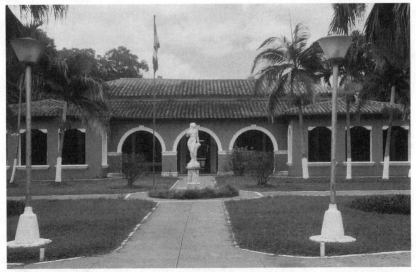

The entrance to Los Cocos, the main HIV/AIDS sanatorium in Cuba. Photo by
Shawn Smallman.

they initially had guards, gates, and in some cases fences topped by barbed
wire. This was especially true for the sanatoriums created for people who
had fled from a facility in the past.[94] Even Los Cocos, which later became
the showcase sanatorium to which all foreign visitors would be brought, at
first had an aura of a prison. Los Cocos was first created in what had been
a rest and recreation center for military officers. According to a subdirector
at the clinic, the Cuban government originally turned to Los Cocos when
creating a sanatorium because many of the early cases of HIV were among
returning soldiers. But this also meant that the sanatorium "was adminis-
tered until 1989 by MINFAR, the Ministry of Defense."[95]

Family members and friends could visit patients at Los Cocos and other
sanatoriums. The residents also could leave the facilities on trips to educational events, and trusted residents could obtain weekend passes. HIV-
positive couples could enter the sanatoriums, but not married couples in
which only one member was HIV-positive; HIV-positive parents could not
bring their uninfected children into the sanatoriums. One woman commented that the most difficult part of being in a sanatorium had been being
removed from her nine-year-old son.[96] Cuba was nearly unique internationally in adopting this policy, which reflected a number of distinct aspects of
Cuban society and Cuba's perception of itself.

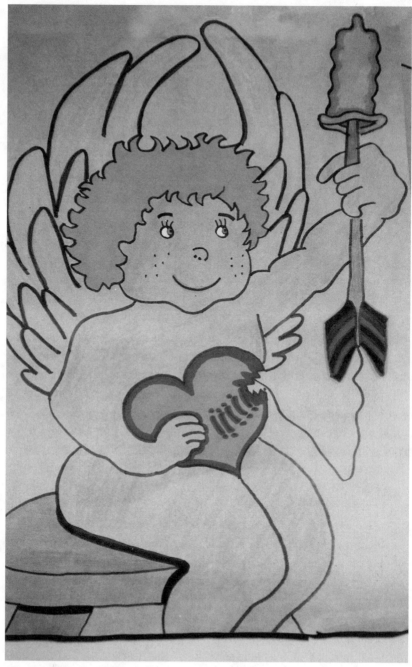

A homemade HIV/AIDS education poster at Los Cocos sanatorium, Cuba.
Photo by Shawn Smallman.

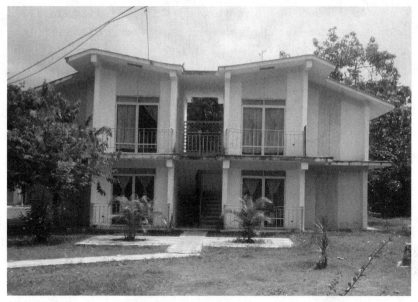

A two-family home at Los Cocos sanatorium, Cuba. Photo by Shawn Smallman.

The country took immense pride in its international reputation in the field of public health. Cuba had invested both energy and capital in its public health infrastructure and probably was the only country in Latin America that had the resources to carry out mass testing. The Cuban government argued that this policy actually benefited internees, who received education, security, and free medical care. The Cuban government has also stated that it has not treated HIV/AIDS any differently than other communicable diseases. When I toured Los Cocos on June 17, 2004, our guide told us that as of June 1, 2004, Cuba had detected 5,514 cases (4,386 among men, 1,128 among women). Thus Cuba had the lowest HIV rate in the Americas, a fact that gave the sanatorium staff immense pride. The Cuban government contrasted its success with the failure of other Caribbean nations to control the epidemic and the national disaster that swept across Haiti.

Critics of the program have said that Cuba adopted this policy in part because of the widespread homophobia in Cuban political culture, particularly among the revolutionary leadership, which equated homosexuality with psychiatric illness as well as capitalist decadence. After the revolution Cuba adopted policies to reeducate its homosexual population. In 1965 the Cuban government created Military Units to Aid Production (UMAP).

These camps included many people whom the Cuban state deemed unfit for military service, but in particular young men who appeared effeminate. Although many people in Cuban society had to do hard labor as a revolu-

tionary obligation, the conditions in these camps were terrible. One Cuban writer described the actions of one young man on a truck being sent to do forced labor for UMAP: "Well, one of those sitting at the back suddenly jumped down and ran past the truck carrying them (UMAP members) and threw himself in front of it. He wanted to kill himself. That is how desperate he was, and no one can deny it, for I was one of the ones who took him to the hospital at El Ciego de Ávila. He was fortunate—he tore up an eyebrow, scraped his face and lost a four tooth plate. He was out of his mind with desperation."[97]

While these camps were phased out by 1969, government legislation and policies in the 1970s sought to exclude gays from all branches of employment (such as schools) where they might come into contact with youth. All centers for gay organization or pride were repressed by the police. Homosexuals were banned from the Communist Party. As the work of Ian Lumsden and Marvin Leiner has shown, the situation for gays improved markedly in the 1980s and 1990s. As Leiner also notes, there is hypocrisy in some conservative denunciations of Cuba's treatment of gays when the criticism comes from those who have not advocated gay rights in other situations.[98] It is also true that there was considerable public support for the quarantine policy, including among homosexuals, in large part because the Cuban people were accustomed to thinking that social duties took precedence over individual rights.[99] Still, the early reaction to the epidemic was shaped not only by the Cuban government's profound commitment to health but also by the disease's association with homosexuality, even though this was misleading in the Cuban context. In the long run, however, the Cuban government has probably continued to maintain the sanatoriums because of the priority it places on public health, its privileging of social responsibilities over individual rights, and its vision of health care as a forum for international competition.

People who have questioned Cuba's policy of mass quarantine have also argued that this policy represents a violation of human rights that could only take place in a dictatorship that represses public dissent. Advocacy on behalf of HIV-positive Cubans has been politically dangerous: "Those in Cuba who have questioned the quarantine policy are labeled 'enemies of the revolution,' thus effectively excluding the possibility of public advocacy for . . . people in quarantine and for their families."[100] Nor have their been political organizations capable of challenging the Cuban state on this issue, because the Cuban state defines them as threats to national security: "Organizations such as gay rights groups are seen in terms of their potential for CIA infiltration."[101] All these factors, but in particular the equation of political organization with pro-U.S. sympathies, bolstered the Cuban government's quarantine policy. As a result, the Cuban people never had the opportunity for a national discussion about this issue, which might have created more public awareness of HIV.

Since HIV-positive people were removed from society, they became invisible. People sent to the sanatoriums could decide whether or not to tell their employers and family what was happening: "For persons who do not want to inform others, health officials provide elaborate and apparently effective alibis so that the persons' absence from their jobs and neighborhoods is not attributed to their HIV status."[102] This shielded HIV-positive people from discrimination, but it also left them in a position (common to their counterparts in most countries during the early years of the epidemic) in which they were excluded from society and terrified that their secret might be discovered.

> Salvador Rodriguez Garcia, 20, says doctors have attended him in body suits because they know so little about HIV and AIDS. Garcia says he was expelled from nursing school when he was diagnosed HIV positive. When he tried to return, the police were waiting. "It's an injustice," he says. In Cuba, anyone who tests HIV positive gets a special ID card indicating they have a fatal illness. The card allows bearers to quickly reach the front of the bus or grab a seat in a crowded room. Garcia says that he and his friends once used the ID card to enter an ice cream line, which is usually very long. When they were allowed to move to the front, a worker shouted out that they had AIDS and that's why they were in the front. That was the last time Garcia and his friends used the card.[103]

While isolating HIV-positive Cubans protected them from discrimination, it also served the government's political interests by keeping these people from participating in discussions involving HIV/AIDS policy. By this means, the government retained its privileged position so that the state alone could define Cuba's response to the epidemic.

As late as 1989 some authors argued that the Cuban government was concealing the true number of HIV-positive people on the island. By the early 1990s, however, it had become clear that the Cuban statistics for the total number of individuals with HIV/AIDS were accurate.[104] At this time scholars began to wonder about some of the unintended consequences of the Cuban approach to controlling the spread of HIV. Given the strength of the public health system, the political system for mass mobilization, the government control over mass media, and the high level of literacy, Cuba had the resources to mount an effective AIDS education campaign. But as Leiner has stressed, the government did not place its emphasis on education in the struggle against HIV/AIDS.[105] This would begin to change in the 1990s, but in general safe sex has not proved to be a powerful message in Cuba. Condom usage rates are low, not only because they can be difficult to obtain, but also because Cubans perceive their risk of contracting HIV to be low, as the following story from one sanatorium resident indicates:

> This woman had a weekend pass and enjoyed her freedom to visit a nightclub. There were two young men at the next table. One of them was telling the other, "You know, you have to be really careful on Sundays, because that's when they let the 'siderosos' out." I turned around and must have glared at him, because he said somewhat defensively, "Excuse me Ma'am, but it's true. You should be careful too." "I don't have to be careful," I told him, "because I already have AIDS." The young man said, "Señora, you shouldn't joke about things like that."[106]

Although health care leaders worry that this attitude might lead some individuals to have unprotected sex with tourists or with people who had not yet tested positive, Cuba's HIV rates have remained low until the present. In the end, Cuba began to change its quarantine policy in the 1990s not because it failed to control HIV but rather because of economic and political pressures.

■ Rethinking Quarantine

In 1991 the Soviet Union collapsed and Cuba lost its major source of aid and trade. Cuba had already dealt with serious economic problems in the 1980s: the shortage of housing, the lack of parts for machinery, and the dearth of consumer supplies. The situation, however, became far worse in the early 1990s, which Castro termed "the Special Period in Times of Peace." Statistically, Cuba entered a decline at least as sharp as that which the United States experienced during the Great Depression: "Between 1990 and 1993 the gross domestic product (GDP) fell by roughly 35 percent, exports by 80 percent, and imports by roughly 75 percent."[107] Water was rationed in Havana, and the city began to have rolling blackouts. Oil became difficult to obtain, and food rations were cut so sharply that perhaps 50,000 people suffered in an outbreak of blindness likely caused by a vitamin deficiency.[108] Large numbers of people began to move from the cities to the countryside to become farmers because they lacked jobs and the government ration did not provide enough food: "The unemployed population grew from 7.9 percent in 1989 to 34 percent in 1993."[109] People in the countryside stopped using tractors, for which there was no fuel, and returned to using oxen, while city residents turned from cars to bicycles. These cuts had a heavy impact even in such a privileged area as health care. After 1991 doctors were encouraged to rely on herbal medicine, as drugs became increasingly difficult to obtain.[110] The number of surgeries performed dropped shortly.[111] Alma Guillermoprieto described how one woman left a hospital after an operation without any medication: "There are no painkillers for minor surgery at Havana's largest and most modern hospital."[112] Health education campaigns had to be curtailed because it was difficult to obtain paper for brochures or posters. This was true even for efforts to fight AIDS, which Cuba considered to be a priority: "The dissemination of any research findings related to HIV/AIDS and other medical, nursing, and/or public health issues is limited, however, as nearly all medical and nursing journals ceased publication in 1992, due to the shortage of paper."[113]

I toured a maternity hospital in Havana in June 2004 that took in women whose pregnancies were deemed to be high risk because of multiple factors: anemia, poor nutrition, a negative family situation, or residence in an apartment building without a working elevator. The women would stay in the home until their thirty-sixth week, when they would return to their community to give birth. The center had been impressively successful in cutting the rate of miscarriage and stillbirth. But I was struck by the laboratory, in which the equipment was for the most part pre-electronic. The library for the four doctors on staff also impressed me. It had only two small shelves of books, 95 percent of which had been donated and most of which were out of date. Although doctors did have access to a medical information system online, obviously they would have difficulty staying up-to-date in the latest developments in their field. Doctor's salaries were also quite low. One doctor I met in Cuba received $25 a month. When I commented that at least he did not pay much in terms of his bills, he commented that his electric bill was $20 a month. Like everyone else, many doctors began to turn to other means to survive in this difficult economic situation, which put further pressure on the system.

All these problems were exacerbated by the Cuban Democracy Act of October 1992, which tightened restrictions on U.S. trade to Cuba and prohibited foreign ships from first calling on Cuba and then the United States. U.S. economic restrictions only mounted throughout the 1990s, in particular with the passage of the Helms-Burton Act in 1996, which enabled foreign companies to be brought to court in the United States if they did business with Cuban entities created from properties that the government expropriated from U.S. owners. While this measure created outrage in Europe and Canada, it also made foreign companies much more reluctant to invest in and trade with Cuba.

In this environment, the policy of HIV quarantine became problematic. Some aspects of the sanatoriums had begun to change already. For example, when Dr. Jorge Pérez Ávila became the director of the Los Cocos sanatorium in 1989, he allowed people to work within the sanatorium. But larger forces accelerated this process of change in the facilities. Tourism became increasingly important to providing the government foreign exchange, and with the tourists came prostitution, especially after the government permitted its citizens to hold foreign currency in 1993.[114] Many women formed short-lived relationships with visiting tourists in which money was exchanged, although it was not always an obvious payment for sex. The *jinteras* were common sights in hotels and restaurants with their foreign boyfriends, and this became a much-discussed phenomenon. But other women practiced more traditional sex work; the family I stayed with in Cuba was very concerned that I be prepared to deal with aggressive prostitutes when I walked Havana's famed Malecón, even though I was walking with a female friend. Many sex workers did not use condoms with their foreign customers: "An 18 year old sex worker here says that over the last two years, the foreign tourists she services have used condoms 'maybe four times at the most.'"[115] The Cuban government could not afford to offend visiting tourists by mandating that they submit to HIV tests.[116] This made education increasingly important in fighting the disease. At the same time, the sanatorium project was relatively expensive ($24,000 a year) on a per capita basis.[117] Such expenses were more difficult to continue in Cuba's new economic climate. In 1992, therefore, the Cuban government began to relax its sanatorium policy. At first it allowed people to leave the clinic without chaperones, and ultimately HIV-positive people could return to their communities, after careful screening by the staff of the sanatoriums.[118] While most HIV-positive people remained in confinement, a significant minority of sanatorium residents left. The government carefully screened individuals returning to the community; any resident who had criticized government policy on AIDS was unlikely to be released.[119]

The Cuban government's decision to relax the sanatorium policy was especially important as Cuba's quarantine program attracted increasing international attention. Some scholars worried that mistaken test results might lead to the incarceration of HIV-negative people, despite a careful program of checks that made this unlikely.[120] Political activists, some of whom had long sympathized with the Cuban revolution, argued against the Cuban policy of quarantine.[121] Cuba was not isolated because of this issue. Cuba's long record in public health, its success containing HIV, and the terrible spread of HIV in Africa and Haiti meant that Cuba retained considerable support internationally in public health and academic communities.[122] Still, in the early 1990s Cuba's sanatoriums attracted increasing international attention.

In October 1992, for example, Timothy Martins, a student at John Marshall Law School, and Mark Woods, a faculty member, traveled to Cuba to take part in the First International Conference on AIDS. They produced a video on Cuban AIDS policy in which Martins clearly expressed reservations, despite his efforts to appear balanced. In the video several sanatorium residents criticized their internment: "I would give up one year of my life to have my liberty again." Another person said, "We shouldn't be here. We haven't broken any laws. We should be in our homes."[123] At the same time, other interviewees defended the sanatorium system and denounced its negative portrayal abroad. And in his narration, Martins noted a division within those interned within the sanatorium. People interred for less than a year generally resented the loss of their liberty, while those confined for three years or more seemed resigned to their fate.[124] Such materials increased the pressure on the Cuban government, which badly wished to defend its progressive international image.

■ Rockers and Freaks: Self-Injection with HIV

Defending its image became an even higher priority for the government because of surprising events within Cuba. A small subculture of rock music
fans (called *roqueros* or *frikas*) had entered into frequent conflict with government authorities over issues such as military service, dress codes, and
work. Beginning in 1989 people as young as fifteen began to deliberately
inject themselves with HIV-positive blood as an act of political protest. From
the Cuban city of Pinar del Rio this movement quickly spread to surrounding areas and Havana. By 1992 perhaps more than 200 individuals had
deliberately infected themselves with HIV.[125] At first some of these people
concealed that they had injected HIV-positive blood, for fear of being sent
to prison rather than the sanatoriums, but as increasing numbers came
into the sanatoriums, authorities realized what was happening.[126] This presented the Cuban government with both a moral and a political crisis.

When word first reached Cuban health officials, there was a widespread
feeling of shock, as Dr. Jorge Pérez Ávila (at the time the head of the Los
Cocos sanatorium) described: "I talked to various government officials—to
journalists too. The officials didn't believe it at first. At first, I didn't believe
what I was being told. I couldn't grasp that anyone would 'self-inject' himself with someone's blood that way, of an unknown blood type. To me, it
sounded like murder."[127] It may be that Cuban health officials were reluctant to inform Fidel Castro himself about the phenomenon, as he claimed
that he first heard the news from a Catholic priest. Carlos Manuel de Cés-
pedes himself had talked to many of these young people in a vain effort
to persuade them not to inject the virus: "I once met Dr. Fidel Castro at a
dinner. It was early in this phenomenon, and I informed him (about it).
'I know you're an honest man, who doesn't lie,' he said. 'If you say you
know young people who've done this, I know it's true. But I've never had an
inkling of it.'"[128]

The government never viewed this movement as a serious political challenge and has generally not denied that this phenomenon took place.[129]
Many of the young people who injected themselves with HIV were perceived by the government to be antisocial, which meant that government
officials had little sympathy for them. One Cuban doctor working in the
sanatoriums made this clear to reporter Scott Malcomson, who described
the conversation in the *New York Times Magazine*: "According to one doctor
in Havana's flagship sanatorium, the dead and dying rockers are no great

loss because they wouldn't have contributed much to society anyway."[130] Still, this situation was politically embarrassing for Cuba. No Cuban newspapers or television news accounts covered the story, even to try to warn other youth against taking this step. By 1994, however, foreign reporters and Cuban dissidents made it impossible to further conceal this problem outside the country.

In 1994 Vladimir Ceballos produced a documentary titled *Maldita Sea Tu Nombre, Libertad (Cursed Be Your Name, Liberty)*. This would not be the only documentary on the Cuban roquero movement, but it probably led to the initial discovery of this story by U.S. and European media. Both *Newsweek* and the *New York Times Magazine* published articles by reporters who interviewed some of these people the same year.[131] Ceballos was a roquero from Pinar del Rio who had many friends who had injected the virus. The film begins with a dedication: "To Papo, my brother, who offered me his blood to escape from this world." Ceballos and a friend, Carlos Zequeira, videotaped interviews with their HIV-positive friends who had been released from the sanatorium "over a long weekend when the rockers had passes to attend a local baseball game."[132] When they could not show the film in Cuba, Ceballos and Zequeira sought political asylum in the United States.

The film was shot outdoors, and at times the sound quality is poor. It consists of a series of interviews with the roqueros in which they describe how they injected themselves with HIV, and their subsequent thoughts on their decision. With its descriptions of police brutality and reflections on death, the film is painful to watch. The roqueros describe the rise of this phenomenon, which they understood would confuse anyone outside their world: "Look Vladi, the problem we had with this AIDS thing was more than anything the rise of a fever that we had among us in the years of '90 and '91. But all that is due to the repression that existed against us. . . . The most outstanding thing of all is that this was done completely voluntarily."[133] The film is especially convincing because the sanatorium patients give their names and describe their life histories in detail.

> I decided to get HIV. That way they couldn't force me to work. . . . I
> went to Santa Clara for the first festival of rock. When we were coming back, we went by Los Cocos Sanatorium. And there myself and
> Ramon Pereza, who's now dead, "el Bruja" as we called him, injected
> ourselves with Juan Miguel Garcia's blood, the son of the director of
> education, who's now also dead. Orlirio was also with us. That's how

it all went. Until today there still continue to appear new people who injected themselves. Almost all the patient population here infected themselves with a syringe through direct contact. Since we injected ourselves the sale of syringes in pharmacies has been prohibited. And then, Vladi, like me many get HIV. Now almost all of them are dead.

Other rockers described the emotional impact that having several of their friends infected and dying had on them.

Some of these cases were a tragic result of Cuba's policy of separating couples by sending HIV-positive partners to the sanatorium. Spouses and lovers injected themselves with HIV in order to join their loved ones. This was the case with Raysa Valdes, who was desperate to join Orlirio, an HIV-positive rocker confined to the sanatorium: "Then I chose to get HIV. He is already dead. He never wanted to involve me but I wanted to do it. I went to where he was so that he would inject me in October 1991. He didn't want to do it but I was under the effects of the drug called 'droom.' With 'droom' you lose your mind, you don't know what you are doing but you know. Do you understand me? I insisted so much that he did it." Raysa was not the only one who performed the injection under the influence, and some self-injectors were IV drug users. But other people decided to inject HIV only after long and careful thought.

Juan Miguel Guiterrez, a twenty-two-year-old man from Pinar del Rio who had been invited to inject HIV-positive blood by his friends spent months thinking about the decision. He seemed to be at pains to describe the careful reflection that went into his decision:

I was thinking about injecting myself too. I was analyzing everything. I met a friend who is actually in jail because he had sexual relations with a girl. She knew he was infected but she still wanted to be with him, because she was in love with him. And because of that the authorities punished him. Before that he gave his blood to another friend in front of me. He asked me why I didn't shoot his blood. I said I was thinking about it and said not yet. Five months later I received a citation to begin my military service. I had problems with my parents who were divorced but still lived together. . . . I decided to change my life. I injected myself with contaminated blood. Three months later the symptoms began to show.

Juan Miguel Guiterrez then had sex with an HIV-positive woman to try to conceal how he had acquired the disease, so that he would not go to jail. Most of the roqueros feared going to jail far more than AIDS itself. Only HIV-positive people who had acquired the disease in a socially acceptable manner made it into the sanatoriums. Those who had acquired HIV through injection or sex with a partner they knew was HIV-positive were often sent to jail, where the conditions were widely perceived as being unbearable.

Most of the rockers interviewed said that they had been forced to take this step because of state repression, as Jorge Alberto Suarez Prieto described: "It's very bad. The government is very bad. I do not wish to die because no one wants death, but if I were healthy at this moment I would not be in Cuba. I would be with my family in Miami, Puerto Rico, or another country." The rockers also seemed to realize that to outsiders their decision would appear bizarre, and they regretted their choice, especially the women like Mercedes: "I think few young people would come up with a stupidity like that. At the very least I, today, regret having injected myself." They also believed that their protest had failed to sway the government, as Mercedes also commented: "It is as if I don't exist. We didn't even achieve our objective because even now we are discriminated against."

The roqueros did manage, however, to gain a brief period of media attention after Ceballos's documentary appeared. For example, in October 1994 Maggie O'Kane, a reporter for the *Guardian*, published one of the first articles on this issue. Traveling to Cuba, she had met a young HIV-positive woman named Dania who described her experience in what became a powerful piece of reporting. As recounted by O'Kane, Dania had met her husband during a taxi ride the same year that he returned from serving as a soldier in Angola. Luis Alberto Benitus did not tell her that he was HIV-positive, and they began a physical relationship. Then he disappeared into the sanatoriums, from which he sent her a message apologizing for not having told her the truth, saying that he loved her, and inviting her to join him. What happened next is as remarkable as it is disturbing: "On the evening of June 4, 1991, Dania climbed on to a wooden egg box and scrambled over the two-metre-high concrete fence into the garden of Los Cocos sanatorium and her terrestrial paradise."[134] Her cousin helped her to go over the wall.

Once inside, she described being stunned by the material goods that the residents had access to: color television and ice cream. Somehow, she claimed, Luis had managed to hide her from the authorities. But she soon faced pressure to inject HIV-positive blood. Unlike most of the roqueros, she did so only under intense pressure:

54

> I said that I didn't want to. He said that it was because I didn't
> love him—that I was really a whore. There were six of us in the
> house and two of his friends were saying, go on—you have it any-
> way—it would be great here. So one night before supper he said,
> do you want to or not? I started to cry and he got up and went to his
> friend and got a syringe. His friend drew out his blood and then
> one of his two friends gave it to me. I don't remember their names—
> they are both dead now. I felt weak afterwards and was shaking
> but he held me and said it would be fine, that he loved me
> and would take care of me.

When O'Kane interviewed Dania, Luis was in prison for having left the sanatorium to have sex with another woman. This may not have been a bad development for Dania, because Luis beat her.

O'Kane also interviewed the man who founded the first AIDS sanatorium, Hector Terry, who defended Cuba's AIDS policy. He blamed the self-injection phenomenon on drugs: "'Yes,' he says, 'we have patients who admit to having voluntarily inoculated themselves with the AIDS virus, but believe many of them were taking drugs or were under the influence of alcohol at the time.'" He also argued that the roqueros lacked any political motivation for their activity: "At least in the Sixties the hippies had an ideology, a philosophy. The problem with the Frikas is that they didn't have any."

The following year, 1995, Bengt Norborg and Bo Sand produced *Socialism or Death*, a second documentary that contained interviews with HIV-positive Cubans who had deliberately infected themselves with the disease. Unlike Ceballos, Norborg included extensive interviews with the parents of the self-injectors. Niurka Rojas had decided to have unprotected sex with her husband after she learned that he was HIV-positive, so that she could be with him. Her mother, Bernadina Rojas, described the impact that her daughter's infection had on her and on Niurka's father: "My husband cried a lot and lay awake nights when he thought about her problems. Both of us just cried nights. He'd look at me and say 'Quiet, Tete. Don't torment her.'"[135] The mother of Juan Luis Perez, Teresa Arencibia, said that she spent three months in the hospital after receiving the news.

Some of the self-injectors had been able to leave the sanatoriums and live with their families, as Rolando Pareda's mother described: "Here, he can live his usual life, as though he weren't sick at all. Here he doesn't have to have separate plates, towels, and sheets. And I feel better just seeing him." Other self-injectors preferred to live in the sanatoriums, as Juan Luis Perez described: "Life in the hospice is laid back. It's no prison like people say, but it is shut in, small, and awfully boring." Niurka Rojas also had a positive vision of the sanatoriums: "I'm almost always here. I don't want to leave. Sure it's awfully boring here but I still prefer to stay. I've adjusted to the hospice life."

The documentary also contained interviews with government officials such as Rolando Piloto, the head of the Pinar del Rio sanatorium. He was at pains to emphasize that self-injection was in no way a political protest: "Most of our patients have an unfavorable family situation. These young people lead rather unsettled lives. They have no parental control; most have no schooling. This is a social refuge for them, not a protest against the state." But this depiction of the roqueros was somewhat contradicted by a youth expert, Maria Gattorno: "The rockers are from the whole city and largely fit the patterns. They include good kids, 'normal' kids and worse. Students, working youth and some do nothing at all."

This documentary did not end the publicity given to the self-injection movement. In 1996 Leon Ichaso released his fictional work *Bitter Sugar/ Azucar Amarga*. In a harsh look at postrevolutionary Cuba, Gustavo, the lead character of the film, is a Communist who aspires to study engineering in Czechoslovakia. His family and new girlfriend, however, suffer bitter experiences that lead Gustavo to rethink his beliefs. In a crucial scene, Gustavo's brother Bobby deliberately injects HIV-positive blood with his friends while being filmed, an act portrayed in this movie as being expressly political: "I'm injecting myself with AIDS blood. With blood tainted with the AIDS virus. Because if I have to choose between 'Socialism and Death' I'll take death."[136] Some of Bobby's words and actions are clearly drawn from Ceballos's video. In a final scene Gustavo visits his brother at the sanatorium, where Bobby leads him to a river, wraps himself in an American flag, and immerses himself in a small waterfall. This dramatic imagery was a careful re-creation of the closing imagery of *Maldita Sea Tu Nombre, Libertad*, and even the music was identical (the film acknowledged Vladimir Ceballos in the credits). This account mixed fiction with actual events to use the issue of self-injection to criticize the Cuban government.

In the end, judging the self-injection movement is difficult. It seems insufficient to dismiss this problem as unrelated to Cuba's political structure because Cuba is the only country in the world that had this systemic problem. Disaffected youth exist in many countries, including nations with extremely repressive regimes. Something particular to Cuba led to this disaster.[137] At the same time, this form of protest is abhorrent to most observers. Perhaps this is why even critics of Cuba failed to seize upon this issue to attack the regime; they did not want to be in the position of defending the self-injectors, some of whom used IV drugs or encouraged their partners to infect themselves. It may seem strange, therefore, that the story of Reinaldo Arenas gained considerable attention. An HIV-positive gay Cuban writer who fled Cuba in 1980 (when Castro's government permitted many homosexuals to leave), his work has been widely read, and his memoir, *Before Night Falls*, was made into a feature film in 2000. But Arenas was likely a more attractive symbol than the self-injectors not only because he possessed an articulate ideological argument that they lacked but, more importantly, because he had not deliberately acquired HIV.

Self-destruction is an old form of political protest, familiar to most Americans from the period of the Vietnam War, when people immolated themselves to protest U.S. involvement in the conflict. To many people that act, too, seemed incomprehensible, but in that situation it was impossible to fathom the motives of these people because after the act they were gone.[138] The roqueros differed because they committed a self-destructive act but then lived to describe their motivation, as the character Bobby expressed in *Bitter Sugar* while talking to his family in the sanatorium: "It's so strange, having committed suicide yet being here talking to you, talking to my friends."[139] To must observers the justifications that they gave—separation from spouses, constant police repression, anger at the state, or family problems—must seem inadequate for such a horrific act. Perhaps all acts of self-destruction as protest are doomed to failure because of the distaste with which most observers must view them.[140] The roqueros also were unusual dissidents in that their protest was not public but, rather, took place in the quiet rooms of the sanatoriums and on urban rooftops. Because of this fact (and because the Cuban government never publicized this problem), in Cuba there is no popular awareness of this history. As a form of political protest, then, its impact on Cuba has been minimal, except on the sanatorium system itself.

There are still HIV-positive roqueros in Cuba. I had the opportunity to meet one. Our conversation took place in the presence of an interpreter. I did not ask him how he acquired HIV, nor did we discuss anything that might be politically sensitive in any way. When he had first tested HIV-positive, he had asked to go to the sanatorium in Santa Clara, which at the time was largely made up of roqueros. He spent years in this sanatorium, which he found incredibly boring despite the endless planned activities. As he put it, "All the time in the world to do nothing, you understand."[141] With the end of the old regime in the sanatoriums he had moved out, and he was much happier living in his own house. He now plays bass guitar in a punk rock band, which usually performs either in his house or at a friend's place. He also has a job working at a local cultural center. I asked him if many of his roquero friends lived outside the sanatoriums too. He paused, looked uncomfortable, and said a few did, but many were dead now. His wife had been too ill to meet us that day; she was in the hospital. The change in the sanatorium system had come in time to give the roqueros back a measure of freedom, but I doubt that it will be much longer until their story will only be history, rather than lived memory.

■ Cuba Alters Its HIV/AIDS Policy

Even before the release of Vladimir Ceballos's documentary, the Cuban government probably realized that it was only a matter of time before the phenomenon of deliberate self-infection with HIV received international attention.[142] The Cuban regime's fear that these revelations might jeopardize Cuba's international political support likely encouraged the state to begin liberalizing the sanatoriums early in the 1990s as a way of defusing this issue. But another key pressure was the growing power of the gay movement internationally during the 1990s. The Cuban epidemic was unique in Latin America in that it became increasingly focused in the homosexual community with time.[143] In June 2004, 5,514 cases of HIV had been detected in Cuba. Of these, 3,792 were among men having sex with men.[144] While many other nations in the hemisphere had historically had policies equally as homophobic as Cuba's, this trend made quarantine politically costly, especially as the literary work of Reinaldo Arenas attracted attention. And as tourism became a growing threat as a means to spread HIV, the Cuban government realized it needed to rethink its policies.[145]

By the late 1990s the Cuban government was placing much greater emphasis on preventing AIDS through education. The government had never ignored education, but it was originally a less important facet of the government's program than the sanatoriums. In 1996 Doctors without Borders traveled to Cuba and advised the Ministry of Health on AIDS education programs and supplied education materials. In 1998 Cuba founded the National Center for the Prevention of STDs and HIV. This organization had a phone line, ran workshops for youth, and organized a trailer covered with flowers that drove through the countryside giving out AIDS information.[146] The sanatorium residents themselves began to play a larger role in AIDS education: "One result of the new environment of the sanatoriums created by Dr. Pérez is the Grupo de Prevencion del SIDA (GPSIDA), an informal, officially authorized group of HIV-positive people, health professionals, and social scientists that has was formed at the initiative of HIV-positive sanatorium residents. GPSIDA has the mission of supporting HIV-positive people in their daily lives and of educating the community at large about the experience of HIV-positive people as well as about modes of transmission and prevention of HIV infection."[147] I have had an opportunity to speak with members of the Grupo de Prevencion de SIDA in Cienfuegos, a city about a three-hour drive from Havana. Its members traveled to schools and other locations to give talks, handed out condoms, and worked to raise awareness of AIDS. The people I spoke with took pride both in their work and in Cuba's low HIV rate.

There are a few other AIDS organizations in Cuba. For example, Father Fernando de la Vega runs a support group at the Montserrate Church in Old Havana. The church has HIV/AIDS support groups that meet on Wednesday and Thursday nights. The Wednesday group is made up of married couples and their children, twenty-six people in total. In general both members of the couple have HIV, but the children do not.[148] The Thursday group has perhaps eighty people, according to Father Fernando, most of whom are men who had sex with men (although there were also three women present when I attended a Thursday meeting). According to Father Fernando most of the members of the Thursday group are not from Havana. Most are men who grew up in interior cities, which they had to leave when it became obvious that they were gay. They arrived in Havana without any family to support them. They lived among themselves, and many were homeless. Father Fernando did not have good statistics on them. But he believed that most of these men did not work either for reasons of health or because they did not want to. They were economically vulnerable. Father Fernando tried to reestablish contact with the men's families, in some cases even after the men had died.[149]

While the state funds the medical care of these patients, the church provides a safe space for them to have a dinner, after which they attend a meeting at which a psychologist is present. The church has two doctors who talk
to the patients, and once a month the church hands out a small bag with
hygiene items and similar supplies. But the key component of what this
group offers is support. One of the most important rules for the group is
that no issues of religion or politics can be discussed, because either could
divide the group. Father Fernando also requires "appropriate dress," as the
meeting is in a church, which he says means that "if your name is Juan, you
come dressed as Juan."[150] The group's work is accepted by the government.
When I attended a meeting as a member of Cuba AIDS Project (CAP), Dr.
Jorge Pérez Ávila answered questions from the group members.

The work of this group is significant, but there are limits to its efforts.
The group does not have an outreach or prevention effort. And Father Fernando says that most of his fellow priests do not want to do this work. Like
all NGOs, this group also had internal political issues. It operated with the
support of CAP, a U.S.-based NGO with a humanitarian license from the
State Department that helped people living with AIDS in Cuba. This support
had been critical for the development of Father Fernando's group. When
CAP first began to talk with Father Fernando, the priest could not even pay
the electric bill to keep the lights on at night. In 2004 CAP was sending
roughly $1,000 a month to the church, most of which went for food.[151]

Through CAP, I visited Cuba in 2004. The night that I attended the Thursday meeting, the head of CAP, Dr. Byron Barksdale, handed out new rules
to the group. Some individuals within this bloc wanted to break away from
the leadership of Father Fernando and create their own organization, with
support from CAP. But Dr. Barksdale was against this because he was concerned that it might raise questions about CAP's State Department license.
And it was much more difficult to deal with many different splinter groups
instead of one united organization. Besides, Father Fernando had originally
approached CAP for support, and it was his church. As Dr. Barksdale told
me, "You have to dance with the person who brought you."[152] Dr. Barksdale
spoke to the group about CAP's decision, which sparked a heated discussion. There were perhaps seventy men in the room, most of whom were
flamboyantly gay. One of the men had such a feminine energy that, despite
his muscular build, I had to look at him twice to make sure that he was not
a woman. This person asked Dr. Barksdale if these rules were intended only
for Father Fernando's group, or for his group as well. But in the end the

men had to accept the new rules (for example, members of the group had to prove to Father Fernando that they were HIV-positive), which were intended to strengthen Father Fernando's authority. CAP's financial power left the members without any real alternative to following Father Fernando's lead.

What struck me most about the group members was their optimism. Given their health issues, discrimination, and often homelessness, I had imagined people who would be overwhelmed by their difficulties. Instead, they were the most enthusiastic, outgoing group I have ever met. I have a photo of myself with them, and in it six men are hugging me and one another while mugging for the camera. They had a thousand questions for me and other members of CAP, and I spoke with some of the patients during and after the meeting. In general, they believed that the government gave them good treatment for their HIV, and they were grateful because they knew that some treatment was not free in other countries. One group member, a nurse, was taking part in an experimental therapeutic AIDS vaccine test run by Dr. Jorge Pérez Ávila through the Instituto Pedro Kourí (the leading medical research organization in Cuba). I later asked Dr. Pérez about this vaccine, and he tried to minimize expectations for it. But these people were aware that they had good opportunities for treatment. They were not absorbed in self-pity. One man approached me after the evening meeting and said that there was something else that he needed, which he hoped that I could obtain for him. I explained that CAP had done its best to bring useful supplies and medications, but that if something else was required, I would pass on word for the next group that came to the church. He told me, "I have a poodle. And I cannot get combs, I cannot get shampoo, and I cannot get clippers anywhere in Havana."[153] He was so insistent and believed that it was so important, that I promised to pass on this information. Despite all the problems this man had, he was worried about his poodle.

The emergence of NGOs such as CAP, and their links to foreign organizations, represented an important change in Cuba's AIDS program, which has continued to evolve. In 2001 Cuba began synthesizing drugs against HIV, both protease inhibitors and reverse transcription medications. According to Cuban health authorities, careful studies at the Instituto Pedro Kourí have established the bioequivalence of these generic medications to the brand-name drugs. This development has had a major impact on both mortality and morbidity, including at Los Cocos. Patients do not automatically start drugs when they test HIV-positive. Instead, the medications are begun based on the patient's viral load. Before these drugs were introduced, perhaps fifteen patients would die in an average year at Los Cocos. In 2001 the sanatorium had eight deaths; in 2002, four deaths; and in 2003, two deaths. And the sanatorium's administration believes that one of the two deaths in 2003 was attributable to an error in sanatorium policy. The patient had been secretly disposing of medication while telling the nurses that he or she was taking it. The doctors realized the truth only when it was too late. The sanatorium used to have two wards for severe cases. Now they only have one. According to doctors treating AIDS patients with whom I spoke at Instituto Pedro Kourí, drug resistance is not yet a problem, in part because these medications have only been available for such a short time. As elsewhere in Latin America, the introduction of these drugs has changed the expectations for patients with HIV/AIDS. The average age of people living with HIV is rising now, with the twenty- to twenty-five-year-old age range being especially important.[154]

The second major change in Cuban policy is that, in theory, no one remains a full-time patient in the sanatoriums any longer. I toured Los Cocos sanatorium in June 2004. At the opening lecture our guide, a subdirector and psychologist at the institution, explained that an individual's stay in a sanatorium is now limited to three months. During that time patients go through a training program on living with HIV. They have their weekends off, when they can return to their communities. They receive 100 percent of their pay while in training, and their jobs are protected. If they have no activities to do, they are given work at the sanatorium. Most people undergo the training for six to eight weeks before returning to their homes. Some, however, would remain in the sanatorium, which would function as a day hospital. In other words, they would spend their days in the community but return to the sanatorium at night. As of June 2004, 5,514 people had tested positive for HIV, of whom 2,385 had developed AIDS and 1,152 had died. There were 2,482 people in the outpatient system who lived in the local community and received care at a local clinic. The remaining 1,880 were either in the sanatoriums doing their initial training or they were in day hospitals.[155] My own experience in Cuba confirmed the strong shift away from the sanatorium system. I spoke with many HIV-positive patients who had spent time in the sanatoriums, some from the very early years of the epidemic, who now lived in the community.

When I visited Los Cocos, our guide stressed that AIDS patients do not face great discrimination in Cuba. He told my group (CAP members, most of whom were medical students from the University of Chicago) that he had worked at the sanatorium since 1988. During that time he had witnessed an annual march on December 16–17 during which perhaps a million Cubans pass by the sanatorium on their way from the Church of St. Lazarus. He said that he had never heard one unkind word shouted against the people in the sanatorium, never one voice of rejection. Instead, he said that people called out, "I will ask St. Lazarus to help you." The staff had a problem with people trying to pass patients bottles of rum through the fence.

Los Cocos is divided into small communities. The houses range from small structures that reminded me of retirement trailers in Florida to large, two-story homes. There were two people in each home, which often led to conflicts, because the first person arriving in the home usually considered himself or herself the owner of it. While there was a fence around the property, it was so low that a child could have climbed over it. I toured the art facility, where some students purchased small objects that people in the sanatorium had made. The funds generated from these sales went into a communal pot to provide necessary items for residents. We were also introduced to a number of patients, including one nurse who has been HIV-positive for seventeen years but has never had a symptom and whose CD-4 cell count was good. We were not allowed to go to the houses to talk to the patients on our own because, we were told, this was not a zoo in which the patients were shown off for tourists.

Our guide, Rodrigo, was very concerned about the sanatorium's image in the United States. During the tour, one CAP member (a medical student from the University of Chicago) had asked Rodrigo if there was any punishment for not taking part in the mandatory training period at the sanatorium. Rodrigo had said no. The student then told Rodrigo that this is not what one HIV-positive person had told him. This person had claimed that people who did not choose to go into the sanatorium were jailed. Rodrigo said that he did not want to say that patients were lying, but he had been working at the sanatorium for sixteen years and knew that this was not true. Rodrigo then told us that one time a visiting North American had asked to see the concentration camps. This had bothered Rodrigo a great deal. So he did not tell the man where he was taking him, but he brought him to Los Cocos. They spent forty minutes wandering around the sanatorium without the North American knowing where they were. When Rodrigo finally told him, the visitor refused to believe it. He thought it was a Potemkin village created to be shown to foreigners. With great emotion Rodrigo told us that if he was going to lie, it was going to be about something important. Our guide was a charming and articulate person who spoke on this point with great conviction.

I left the sanatorium impressed with the level of care, the availability of the medications, and the dedication of the staff. Patients had strolled the grounds in casual clothes. I was perhaps most struck by the quiet of the space. I had certainly not seen a jail. I commented on this to another patient I met later who had spent months in Los Cocos. He said that Los Cocos was a very good place to be, which is why the government usually sent foreigners there, but there were other facilities that were not so good. There was one place, he said, where HIV-positive people were kept hand-cuffed to the walls in terrible conditions, because the government believed that they were practicing unsafe sex. I was shocked and asked him what this place was called. He said "La Serena" in San José. I have no idea what to make of this information. I cannot find this place on a map. According to the Cuban government, there are no HIV-positive people in the prison system, and no one is restrained in this manner.[156] Was this only a rumor that circulated among people living with HIV? I had no means to test the truth of what he had told me, and I remembered the passion with which the guide at Los Cocos had spoken.

I had also heard allegations that the government had used repression to suppress health information in the past, as in the case of Dr. Dessi Mendoza Rivero, who practiced in Santiago. He was sentenced in June 1997 to eight years in jail for "enemy propaganda" because he had given foreign reporters statistics on a dengue outbreak. Alma Guillermoprieto suggests that he received this sentence even though his data on the epidemic was in accord with that from other sources: "This despite the fact that information on the epidemic that was essentially in agreement with Dr. Mendoza's figures was published by the official newspaper, *Sierra Maestra*, one month after his arrest."[157] Guillermoprieto also did her own research to try to judge the seriousness of the dengue outbreak: "I talked to a woman who lives in Santiago and whose husband was hospitalized during the epidemic. She says that the resources of the very large general hospital in Santiago were stretched so thin at the height of it that many dengue victims had to lie on cots on the lawns of the hospital grounds awaiting treatment. One morning when she arrived to visit her husband, she found him in a state of great agitation. He begged her to take him away. 'The young man in the bed on the other side of the aisle died last night; I don't want to die here,' he said."[158] If large numbers of Cubans suffered during this outbreak, it seems strange that the Cuban government would try to conceal it, because the illness would be public knowledge. But Dr. Mendoza Rivero was not one of the prisoners released during the Pope's visit in January 1998, which suggests that the Cuban government views his case as a priority. If the apparent facts in this case are true, it might suggest that the Cuban government does try to suppress negative health information.

When I went to Cuba, I thought that after I had a firsthand opportunity to tour hospitals, speak to government officials, visit the sanatoriums, meet patients, and see the work of AIDS organizations, I would be better able to evaluate Cuba's AIDS program. In the end, I left unsure how to judge what I had seen and heard. It was very difficult to find sustained time to speak to people with HIV in an unsupervised manner. Historians have always argued that it is increasingly difficult to write history the closer in time you are to an event, and I am aware of the limitations my own study faces in this regard. I doubt that anyone will be able to make a comprehensive assessment of Cuba's program for many years.

There is no question, however, that the program has changed immensely from its inception. This change did not take place overnight. Until the late 1990s most HIV-positive people decided to remain in the sanatoriums, perhaps because of the psychological screening they had to go through to be permitted to leave, or because of the material hardships they faced outside.[159] But by 2004, at least in theory, the old system had been entirely replaced. The quarantine regime did enable the Cuban government to restrict the AIDS epidemic to very low levels, although at a high cost in human rights. The challenge will be to continue this success into the new era. Given the excellent education system, strong public health infrastructure, and government pride in Cuba's public health system, Cuba will continue to have the basis for an effective response to the epidemic.

■ An International Perspective

What is striking about Cuba's policy to control AIDS is the extent to which it has been shaped by international factors. The first reported cases were among soldiers returning from Africa. Because of Cuba's pride in its international reputation in the field of public health, its equation of disease with foreign corruption, and its distrust of NGOs because of their possible links to foreign countries, the government adopted a policy of quarantine to control AIDS. With the collapse of the Soviet Union, the dollarization of the Cuban economy, the rising importance of international tourism, and the concomitant growth of the sex trade, this policy became problematic. At the same time, international publicity around the roqueros and the growing power of the gay movement in North America and Europe made this policy politically costly. Cuba needed its international allies in the progressive movement. Still, the program has been altered but not abandoned; the current system is a curious hybrid that has embraced mass education without abandoning mass testing. Cuba continues to put a priority on providing care for its HIV-positive population despite significant challenges, including a U.S. embargo that makes it difficult for the government to obtain access to appropriate medications.[160] This concern has helped Cuba to retain the support of international figures in the field of public health.[161] This international community remains divided by philosophical questions that entail balancing the desire for social justice with the importance of individual human rights.

The most important fact legitimating the Cuban approach to controlling HIV/AIDS was the social disaster experienced by some neighboring islands, such as Haiti. Scholars of AIDS frequently contrast the experience of the two islands.[162] If adopting this policy has prevented such a widespread epidemic, then it is hard to argue that this policy was illegitimate. Yet it may be that Cuba could have done equally well controlling HIV by other means. Given its high ratio of doctors to citizens, its strong mechanisms for mass education, and its excellent literacy rate, in many respects Cuba would seem to be the ideal country to follow the Dutch model to contain HIV, based on education, free testing, and community outreach.[163] At the same time, this would have enabled Cuba to defend the human rights of HIV-positive people and perhaps could have avoided the disaster of self-injection, which in the early 1990s accounted for a significant proportion of HIV-positive people in the country. Fortunately, Cuba's AIDS policy has undergone impressive changes since 1993. In July 2004 Cuba announced that it would sell antiretroviral drugs to its Caribbean neighbors at low prices, while also training medical personnel to treat AIDS. This measure was welcomed by its neighbors and marked the shift in the international perception of AIDS policy in Cuba—from a policy that violated international human rights law to a program that helped to improve Cuba's image with its neighbors.[164]

The idea that international factors have shaped the spread of AIDS in the Caribbean is nothing new. In his classic work, *AIDS and Accusation: Haiti and the Geography of Blame*, Paul Farmer noted that in the 1980s ranking Caribbean countries by either reported cases of AIDS or their trade with the United States created the same order.[165] Farmer's point was that Haiti was not isolated and that its experience with AIDS could be explained as much by its engagement in the international economy as by exoticized images of Haitian voodoo. From the perspective of more than a decade later, what is striking is how many aspects of AIDS in the Caribbean have been influenced by international factors, such as sex tourism from Europe and America, the policies of development agencies and the United States, labor migration between the islands and abroad, and developmental issues that have weakened both some Caribbean states and their ability to provide public health services.

International relations shaped the experience of AIDS in Haiti and Cuba. Early in the epidemic widespread stereotypes of Haiti affected how people viewed the appearance of AIDS there, so that the economy was devastated long before large numbers of people began to die of AIDS. While the initial hysteria has waned, now discrimination is facilitating the spread of disease among transborder labor migrants. Haitians working in Dominican bateyes have proved to be vulnerable to HIV infection not only because of their poverty but also because of a variety of factors related to discrimination: the construction of Haitian and Dominican identities, the political discourses that Dominican leaders have adopted, the perception of race on both sides of the border, and the manner in which religious differences have been portrayed in the two countries. Similarly, Cuba's response to the epidemic, and how that response has been interpreted internationally, has been shaped not only by Cuba's efforts to gain international legitimacy through developing its health care system but also by the sad history of U.S.-Cuban relations. The remarkable characteristic of AIDS is that a disease driven by personal behavior reflects complex international issues, from the economic issues shaping poverty to the cultural beliefs that define prejudice.

2

BRAZIL

Pai Laercio Zaniquelli looked calmly into the camera and
explained how it had happened. A high priest of candomblé,
he had decided to take in HIV-positive children abandoned by
their parents in São Paulo during the early 1990s. To this end,
he had transformed his terreiro into a well-cared-for orphanage, Children of Oxum, which had a sleeping space filled with
cribs, medical equipment such as nebulizers, a kitchen, and even
an outdoor playground. He told the story of one child who had
come to his center. After Flávia's mother had died, her father and
she had lived on the streets, where he had sexually abused her.
When SOS children had brought her to Zaniquelli, she had been
"covered with sores, bruises, cigarette burns. So it was torture for
her."[1] With support from Zaniquelli and his followers she had
thrived in a clean, safe location where she had been treated with
love. But many of the center's neighbors had not been excited at
the transformation of a religious center into an AIDS orphanage:
"When the house first opened, there was a lot of discrimination.
The people around here used to say that the mosquitoes were
going to bite the children and spread AIDS to the whole town. I
was coming back from a meeting of CRTA when four cars stopped
me. There were five people in each car, twenty total. They beat
me until I had a broken collarbone and two broken ribs. They
said I had spoiled the city by keeping children with AIDS. This
was really, really hard. You can't forget something like that. But
I didn't give up. I said to myself 'You are ignorant, not me. I
will prove that you are the ignorant one and I am not. And I
will continue.'" The center had not only endured; it had thrived.

Indeed, on the day the filmmakers came, the center was having a feast to honor Oxum, an Afro-Brazilian goddess. The audience, white and black, watched as Pai Laercio Zaniquelli spooned out food in bowls that followers then carried to the congregation. Normally, the center was only used as an orphanage, so this festival was especially significant. Zaniquelli, clothed in the flowing white dress of his goddess, Oxum, then danced before the congregation to the music of drums. His faith was at the root of his work, Zaniquelli explained: "Oxum is the one who procreates, who shelters, soothes. That is why I like children so much. I protect the children. I actually think it is not me but her, because she is so much of what I am."

In November 2003 both South Africa and China announced that they would make antiretroviral medications available for people with HIV. For both nations this decision represented a major step forward by governments whose AIDS policies had often been marked by denial or apathy. South African president Thabo Mbeki had for years been influenced by extreme dissidents who denied that HIV caused the disease. While his government fought against the use of these medications, the HIV rate in the country steadily increased until the nation had more HIV-positive people than any other on the planet. In China hundreds of thousands of people, many in Henan province, were infected in a blood-purchasing program run by local government officials. In some cases, according to allegations, blood was taken from poor villagers, the valuable components were removed, and then the remaining blood was returned to them so that they could donate more frequently. The contaminated equipment was reused. In some villages virtually the entire adult population was infected with HIV. When the villagers demanded care and sought outside help, they were beaten and terrorized by the police, while the national government exerted every effort to conceal the tragedy.

For both nations, therefore, the decision to provide free medications was a major step forward. In an opinion piece published in the *Wall Street Journal*, former U.S. president Bill Clinton lauded President Mbeki for his cabinet's new policy and asserted that South Africa's "experience will provide valuable lessons—even a model—for other large nations like India and China, once they embark along this very important path."[2] In fact both nation's programs faced significant technical and administrative challenges. The South African system of public health clinics was weak, and nearly two-thirds of the funds in the government's plan were dedicated to creating infrastructure, not medicines.[3] As former president Clinton noted, the provision of such medications entailed a complex medical support system to guarantee proper delivery. What could happen without the existence of this structure became clear from the start in Henan province. Without adequate follow-up and counseling, many people proved incapable of maintaining the drug regimen required to safeguard their health and to prevent the emergence of drug-resistant strains.[4] Much more work remains to enable both countries to deliver properly the required medications to the correct people.

So far in 2006 only one large developing country has met the challenges of providing medications free to all HIV-positive people, and in so doing it has changed the terms of the debate concerning AIDS treatment because of the magnitude of its success. When the Brazilian government decided to make highly active antiretroviral therapy (HAART, the so-called drug cocktail) available to all HIV-positive people within reach of federal clinics, the results included "halving the mortality rate, cutting the HIV/AIDS hospitalization rate by 80% and sharply reducing mother-to-child transmission."[5] It is difficult to overstate the size of the challenge that the Brazilians had to overcome in order to implement this policy.

To support the provision of medications, Brazilians created a structure to test for HIV viral load, CD-4 cell counts, and viral resistance. A network of dispensaries had to be created and maintained. Doctors had to supervise the patients and ensure that they complied with their regimens. Most of all, the government had to obtain the necessary medications, most of which were extremely expensive. This was a seemingly impossible task for a developing country that already had a significant HIV-positive population. Yet Brazil succeeded. Moreover, the program proved to be cost-effective because fewer AIDS patients entered public hospitals. People now had an incentive to be tested for HIV, because they knew that they would receive care. Thus the number of people who knew their HIV status increased, and the medical system had opportunities to educate those who were HIV-positive. Patients receiving these medications complied with their drug regimens as well as their U.S. counterparts did, and the spread of viral resistance was minimized. Lastly, people on regular treatment were less contagious, which also helped to contain the virus. Together with the aggressive education efforts of both the Brazilian government and NGOs, Brazil has not only limited the spread of the virus but also maintained the program through changes in administration as well as financial crises.[6]

Many aspects of Brazilian society and culture combined to create this impressive public health care achievement: the process of democratization that began in 1985, the 1988 constitution that made health a basic right for all, the flourishing of civil society that created hundreds of NGOs dedicated to fighting AIDS, the ability of elites to create a consensus around this program, the tacit agreement with the Catholic Church, and the openness of Brazil's sexual culture. Yet this story also cannot be understood outside an international context, for it is a history of the contradictions and complexities of globalization. On one hand, the Brazilian government faced intense opposition to its efforts to break international patents in order to make generic medications affordable for AIDS patients. This drew the country into a confrontation with not only major pharmaceutical companies but also the United States. Yet the Brazilian program was also funded by three successive loans from the World Bank (which itself claimed that making free drugs available to HIV-positive people was not fiscally sound), which allowed the Brazilians to purchase the necessary health infrastructure to create their policy. International factors continue to influence the program. Indeed, part of the reason that this policy has endured through political and monetary crises is the international attention that it has drawn. Brazil has now integrated its HIV/AIDS program into its foreign policy and views it as one means whereby a developing country can provide meaningful aid to its counterparts. In December 2003 the WHO promoted a new initiative, "Three by Five," to place 3 million people on antiretroviral medications internationally by 2005.[7] When the target date arrived, it was clear that the WHO had not met its goal, largely because of a lack of international will. But without the Brazilian example, it is doubtful that the WHO would have even had enough confidence in the feasibility of this program to have launched it.

■ Brazil's Background

Although Brazil is the largest and most populous nation in Latin America, it plays a small role in the American consciousness of the region, compared with nations such as Mexico or Cuba. Yet Brazil, with its immense size (the fifth largest country in the world, it occupies roughly half of South America), painful history of slavery, and powerful economy, is in some respects the Latin American country that most resembles the United States. Brazil has more than 180 million people. The state of São Paulo alone has more than three times the population of Guatemala, the largest state in

Central America. The Brazilian economy dominates the entire continent, as it is larger than that of every other Spanish-speaking country in South America combined. Yet Brazil also perhaps has the greatest income inequality in the world and immense social misery that is obvious to anyone who spends time traveling in the country. A Portuguese-speaking country in a region Americans associate with Spanish, a developing country that exports sophisticated aircraft, a country marked by military rule now governed by a party of the left, Brazil has great economic and political influence on its neighbors.

This has been particularly true in the area of HIV/AIDS policy. Early in the epidemic, international experts made dire predictions for the future of HIV in Brazil. These warnings perhaps accorded with the sexualized and exotic imagery surrounding Brazil in the West, where Brazil is associated with bikinis, the beaches of Ipanema, and the revelry of Carnival.[8] But given the underfunding of the public health system, the active and open sex trade, and the large populations of men having sex with men, there seemed to be good reason for these predictions. Brazil has a serious problem with HIV/AIDS, but it has escaped the dire future forecast for it in some of the early predictions, for reasons that are intimately associated with its political history since the mid-1980s.

In 1964 the Brazilian military seized power and began a period of military rule marked by political terror and economic growth. By the 1980s, however, the economic miracle was over and the military was losing legitimacy. Facing growing pressure from civil society and losing confidence in its own ability to govern, the military returned power to civilians in 1985, while making it clear that no revenge on the institution would be tolerated. HIV arrived in Brazil precisely when Brazilian society underwent an opening. Brazilian efforts to control the disease have succeeded in part because of the broad network of NGOs that have rallied to lobby for HIV-positive people and to provide aid when the government did not.

■ The Early Response to AIDS in Brazil

As authors such as Jane Galvão have argued, an awareness of AIDS emerged in Brazil before the disease did. The Brazilian media did not report the first diagnosis of AIDS in Brazil until 1983, although in retrospect there had been earlier cases in the country.[9] By the time the first cases had appeared, the disease had already received extensive coverage as a disorder of the First World, where it was depicted as an affliction of urban, gay, well-to-do men. The association of the disease with the United States meant that it was seen as an illness of the rich, and the media asked if Brazil was "sophisticated" enough to be vulnerable. From this perspective, its arrival was taken as a sign that Brazil was "civilized."[10] This perception would change quickly after 1986 as it became clear that there was a significant heterosexual epidemic in Africa. AIDS then quickly came to be associated with poverty and blackness, so that the depiction of the disease was associated with ideas about race. But the original perception of the disease may help to explain the initially slow response of Brazilian authorities.

The government at first failed to make the disease a national priority, in large part because it was perceived as being confined to an isolated group:

> The association of AIDS with privilege at the beginning of the epidemic had two repercussions. On the one hand, it was used as an excuse for the government's lack of attention to the disease, as the government could claim that AIDS affected a very small minority (the "First World Within"), who could afford their own health care abroad and that it should use its resources for the massive endemic diseases, such as malaria and tuberculosis, that were affecting the deprived in massive numbers. In a page-length article that appeared in the daily O Globo on September 8, 1985, Health Minister Carlos Santana declared that even though his office was taking a series of measures against AIDS, this disease could not really be considered a priority.[11]

Herbert Daniel and other activists argued that the government perceived AIDS as "an epidemic of 'minorities,' almost a problem of a few rich and well-provided-for homosexuals."[12] For this reason the government effort appeared to lack energy. It is also true that the Brazilian government faced a major financial crisis in the early 1980s, and it was unwilling to commit significant resources to fight AIDS.[13] By many measures, the Brazilian government's response was weaker than Cuba's. For example, the Brazilian government failed to protect the blood supply, which caused a catastrophe for Brazilian hemophiliacs.[14]

Brazilian gay organizations had historically been weak, in part because Brazilians perceived sexual identity differently than their North American counterparts did. In Brazil, the active male partner was not perceived as being gay, so there were considerable numbers of men having sex with

men who did not associate themselves with a gay identity.[15] Such perceptions made rallying this community to deal with the epidemic difficult. In
the early years, the majority of AIDS cases were in the major urban centers of São Paulo and Rio de Janeiro, among men having sex with men.
AIDS activists such as Herbert Daniel (who died of the disease in 1992) believed that discrimination contributed to the government's indifference to
the spread of the epidemic. While his statements might have exaggerated
the government's laxity, they accurately reflect how activists perceived the
government's attitude in the early 1990s.

> To this day the government has taken no action on the epidemic,
> continuing the five-year record of inaction and indifference of the
> previous administration. There is today absolutely no national pro-
> gram for controlling the epidemic. The service set up by the previ-
> ous administration in the Ministry of Health in 1986, when there
> were already more than 1000 reported cases of AIDS, was a symbolic
> gesture. And so it remains. The idea that AIDS is inevitable, almost a
> kind of price to be paid for the modernity of our cities, the idea that
> it is not quite a Brazilian disease but something foreign or strange,
> has remained almost unchanged from the view that prevailed at that
> nearly forgotten time when AIDS arrived in Brazil.[16]

The Ministry of Health was perceived as considering AIDS a less important disorder than the other serious infectious diseases that plagued Brazil.
The Brazilian minister of health, Carlos Sant'Anna, said that with AIDS "we
are discussing a disease which is preoccupying, but not a priority."[17] The
anger generated by this perception of government apathy, and numerous
examples of discrimination against the HIV-positive, contributed to the for-
mation of gay organizations.

■ Discrimination and Vulnerable Groups

The early history of HIV in Brazil was also marked by extreme discrimination against people with HIV. Flávio Braune Wiik has described the story
of a Xokleng couple in the state of Santa Catarina, in the Brazilian south,
who tested positive for HIV in 1988.[18] Antonio (Wiik changed the names to
protect their families) had met Joanna in a brothel. The couple decided to
live together, and Antonio had brought Joanna to live with him in his na-

tive village. She felt ill for months and finally sought medical help, and she tested positive for HIV. At this point, doctors decided to test Antonio, who was told that he was also positive. Joanna's health quickly deteriorated, and she died soon afterward. Antonio, who was free of any symptoms, returned to his home village.

When the news that a Brazilian native was HIV-positive was first reported, it created national news, perhaps because of the juxtaposition between the popular perception of AIDS as a foreign disease confined to a wealthy minority in urban centers and the reality that a common Brazilian native could be infected. The result was a disaster not only for Antonio but also for the roughly 900 Xokleng. The media descended on Antonio's home village to interview surprised natives. The resulting coverage sometimes had a cruelly mocking tone, and Wiik says that the Xokleng reacted with "panic and fury" to the journalists, government officials, and doctors who came to the village.[19] Antonio faced death threats. His family fell apart, and his parents separated: "The mother and siblings moved to a favela of an industrial city in Santa Catarina. His father returned to his community of origin."[20] The Xokleng perceived AIDS as a *zug-kongó*, a disease like the many others that had been brought to their people by whites; they were badly frightened by the idea that AIDS might repeat the devastation that other Old World diseases had wrought on their people. Their cosmology allowed them to understand contagion, but in their belief system infection also had to be intentional. The person deliberately transmitted the infection under the effect of the illness. As a result, Antonio found that those close to him would no longer share food or drink with him, participate in social activities, or allow him to work on group projects.[21] Antonio died after a short time. The government had tested thirty-five Xokleng for HIV. Ten years later no one had returned to the village to inform the Xokleng of the results.[22]

If this was the discrimination faced by a person who had acquired HIV through heterosexual sex with a loved partner, one can imagine the opprobrium that faced some of the other groups that were vulnerable to HIV early in the epidemic: drug users, prison inmates, sex workers, and transvestites. The Brazilian response to the epidemic was initially slow, in part because of the discrimination that groups such as drug users faced. The large slums surrounding Brazil's industrialized cities have proved to be a major breeding ground for drug use, in particular cocaine injection. This has facilitated the spread of a host of diseases within the community of intravenous drug users (IDUS), from malaria—which has reappeared in major Brazilian cities among drug users who acquire the disease through contaminated syringes—to Chagas's disease. With the U.S. crackdown on the cocaine trade in the Andean region, processing centers and distribution routes shifted into Brazil. Injecting cocaine as a practice began in São Paulo and Rio de Janeiro and spread to the south and the Amazon, especially along the transshipment routes.[23]

Drauzio Varella is a medical doctor who worked in the largest Brazilian prison, located in São Paulo, and wrote a best-selling account of his experiences, *Estação Carandiru*. In this work, he described his experience watching men injecting cocaine in a ritual called a *baque*. Four men sat around a small table in a hotel. Each had arrived with a small packet of cocaine and a syringe. The IDUs preferred the fine needles used by diabetics, as they were less likely to leave marks on their arms. They also made other preparations: "They placed three glass cups in the middle of the table: one empty, another filled with tap water, and a third with boiled water; between them a well-washed soup spoon."[24] One of the men would partially fill a syringe with boiled water and then mix this water with cocaine in the spoon, from which he would then draw the mixture back into the syringe. He would inject one of his partners with the cocaine—but only perhaps a quarter of the dose at a time. Then he would withdraw an equal amount of blood and reinject it into the vein, a process that he repeated several times over "two or three minutes."[25] Then it was the next person's turn. The ensuing high was ephemeral, and in a very short time the person injected wanted to repeat the experience. So the ritual continued with increasing fervor as the men became more and more desperate to be injected.

What most disturbed Varella was the potential to spread HIV. The men cleaned their syringes between uses from water in the full cup, which they would then discharge into the vacant cup on the table: "In the end, the cup initially full of tap water was almost dry and the other, empty at the start, contained a pink solution of dangerous blood. It was a party of HIV. Although each had brought his own syringe, only one person in the rotation had to be infected to spread the virus in the washing water for the syringes and, as well, to contaminate the spoon that they all used. Perhaps because of this later I had met so many ex-users with AIDS that swore never to have shared needles."[26] By the end of the experience the men were in no state to care about the risks from HIV. Varella saw one man reach out to the cup filled with contaminated water and blood and lift it to his mouth.

"Don't drink this!" I yelled.

He didn't understand and began to drink the liquid thick with blood. Before I managed to seize him by the arm, he drank at least half the cup:

"Look what you are drinking, man, this is pure blood!"

"Man! I didn't notice, I thought that it was water."[27]

IDUs have continued to be critical to the expansion of the HIV epidemic in Brazil: "The proportion of IDUs as an HIV exposure category increased from approximately 4% at the beginning of the epidemic to approximately 25% currently."[28] While public health officials noted with concern the spread of HIV among IDUs, their challenge in the 1980s was to make Brazilians care about a community that seemed to care so little about its own health.

Transvestites were another outcast group that was greatly affected by HIV. Since the 1970s, transvestites have become increasingly accepted in Brazil in specific social situations. Some of them (such as Roberta Close) are sufficiently famous to draw media attention.[29] Their attendance has become expected at certain social events, such as the practices held for the drum wings of Carnival blocs, which in the weeks before Carnival are much in demand both by tourists and the Brazilian elite. In the atmosphere of abandon and frivolity reigning at these events, transvestites are common in the crowd, where they flirt with good-natured visitors and tourists. There is no social embarrassment at interacting with these transvestites—if asked, for example, to dance with a roller-skating drag queen—and in my experience the most absurd suggestions are met with amusement. Some of the "transvestites" may, in fact, be heterosexuals who are role-playing as part of Carnival. As Richard Parker has noted, "No symbolic form dominates the symbolism of the festival as completely as tranvestism."[30] What is remarkable about Carnival is that it inverts the regular order, so that the transvestites who are normally marginalized become chic.[31] Yet this atmosphere of acceptance belies the real experience of most transvestites, whose lives are very different from those of the small minority who have become national icons.

Brazil has a significant problem with street children, a large percentage of whom, both male and female, become involved with the sex trade over time. For males, there are two possible gender roles that they can take during prostitution (although all roles are fluid, as Parker stresses). One role is that of a *michê*, a very masculine man who engages in sex for money and who usually takes the dominant role in sexual encounters.[32] Many of these young men do not consider themselves to be gay, and they often have girlfriends who are unaware of their career. The other role for youths involved in prostitution is that of transvestite. Transvestites generally come from the poorest class of Brazilian society. They may begin to display feminine characteristics at a young age, which exposes them to both mockery and violence. For their safety they migrate to the major cities, where they often enter sex work to support themselves. Their partners are Brazilian men who usually do not consider themselves to be homosexual and who generally want to assume the dominant role during sex. The transvestites do not consider themselves to be gay but, rather, a third gender, a fact that has been taken into account during HIV/AIDS education efforts.[33]

The violence and discrimination that they faced made transvestites a difficult group with which to do outreach during the early years of the HIV/AIDS epidemic. Most did not work through advertisements or brothels but, rather, on the street. When I lived in Rio de Janeiro in 1992–93, my apartment was on Rua Hermengildo de Barros in Glória, a neighborhood next to the downtown. One night as walked back to my apartment from a movie in nearby Cinelandia, I was startled when a group of tall women began calling out to me. Only when one of them lifted her dress to a passing car to reveal her penis did I understand their gender. These sex workers were a fixture in the neighborhood on Friday and Saturday nights, when they worked the traffic on the main thoroughfare through Glória. In Brazilian society the distinction between house and street has been filled with cultural meaning, and the street is traditionally perceived as dirty, dangerous, and violent.[34] The fact that transvestites have generally worked on street corners and solicited sex from men in passing cars has placed them on the lowest rung of the sex trade.

Brazilians remain fascinated by a minority of successful transvestites who have undergone extensive surgery to appear more feminine. But the means that most transvestites have to use to alter their bodies has also reinforced negative imagery around this group:

> It was reported that the great majority of transvestites in Rio de Janeiro undergo silicone injections to shape their bodies. These "beauty treatments," as the clients referred to them, are done by other "experienced" transvestites who are too old to support themselves as street prostitutes. The injection equipment was typically

shared by several transvestites, with less than adequate cleaning between each use. Industrial quality silicone was most commonly used because it could be purchased by the gallon at a relatively cheap price. Numerous injections, sometimes more than seventy punctures, were required to accomplish each individual body shape. Since this was a painful process, it was common for transvestites to be under the influence of alcohol and/or drugs during the process. The injected silicone had a tendency to dislodge after a few months, and thus, new injections were required periodically to reshape certain parts of the body. Moreover, infections were common after such procedures and often plastic surgery was the only recourse to remove the dislodged silicone.[35]

The popular awareness of these procedures and how they were accomplished also meant that transvestites as a class were perceived as dirty, and there was little sympathy for this group during the early history of the HIV epidemic.

Brazilian sex workers, homosexuals, street children, drug users, and prisoners all faced severe discrimination if not outright violence. The street children in particular were vulnerable to periodic sweeps by death squads paid for by merchants and often manned by off-duty police officers.[36] As long as politicians and policy makers perceived the epidemic as being confined to clearly defined groups who engaged in high-risk behaviors, health authorities found little support. Brazilian health workers badly wanted to work within these communities, but during the early history of the epidemic there was a lack of high-level commitment to this effort. Because transvestites generally did not use condoms and had little choice in this decision, they were both vulnerable to and a means for HIV transmission. Transvestites were at the bottom of the social hierarchy involved in prostitution, they engaged in the highest-risk sexual acts, and their HIV rates were among the highest in Brazil—sometimes over 70 percent.[37] As many of their partners considered themselves heterosexuals—and many might have been married—these sexual encounters served as an important bridge for HIV to enter both the heterosexual and the female populations.[38] Only if the HIV/AIDS prevention effort was inclusive—and showed a true commitment to human rights—could this issue be addressed.

Given the discrimination and governmental apathy that first characterized the Brazilian response to the epidemic, what is stunning is the speed with which the Brazilian government changed course and began to devote both energy and attention to HIV/AIDS. Two domestic factors help to explain this transformation. The first is the evolution of the disease that largely affected clearly identified risk groups, generally located in major urban centers, to a disease that heavily affected women, was mainly spread through heterosexual sex, affected all geographical regions, and took a heavy toll on the poor. The second factor, as numerous scholars have stressed, was the astounding political organization that took place within affected communities, which rallied together to fight AIDS. In 1989, Brazilian NGOs devoted to fighting AIDS held their first national conference in Belo Horizonte, Minas Gerais.[39] In the five years that followed, a broad array of organizations appeared representing women, Afro-Brazilians, urban youth, transvestites, sex workers, homosexuals, and others.

■ The Changing Character of the Epidemic

In the early history of HIV in Brazil the disease was largely confined to the main cities of the southeast—São Paulo and Rio de Janeiro—and to men: "In 1984, 71% of the notified cases were in male homosexuals and bisexuals."[40] Hemophiliacs were also devastated by the disease at the onset of the epidemic, as were people who received blood transfusions. The disease also entered the IDU population in the mid-1980s, particularly in the center and southeast of the country.[41] But the disease did not remain confined to clearly identifiable subgroups for long, and heterosexual transmission became increasingly important to the HIV/AIDS epidemic in Brazil. With time the ratio of men to women with HIV fell, from "24:1 in 1985, to 6:1 in 1990, reaching 2:1 since 1997."[42] By the mid-1990s most people with HIV/AIDS were infected through unprotected heterosexual sex, although the homosexual community continued to be heavily affected by HIV/AIDS. From the major cities the disease gradually moved to the main centers in each state and, from there, to the majority of Brazilian municipalities. The disease traveled along the Amazon's highways, where it was carried by poor gold miners called *garimpeiros*.[43] By the early 1990s HIV existed in every part of Brazil.[44] As Brazilian epidemiologists have argued, it perhaps would be inaccurate to describe HIV/AIDS in Brazil as an increasingly rural phenomenon. While its geographic spread widened, the majority of cases still occurred in the cities. Indeed, the majority of HIV/AIDS cases remained in two states: São Paulo had 47 percent of the cases in 2000, while Rio de Janeiro had 15 percent.[45] But HIV/AIDS was no longer confined either regionally or in terms of the population it affected.

The disease gradually fractured into what Ana Maria de Brito and her collaborators called "a true mosaic of regional subepidemics."[46] In some areas, such as the northeast, the disease's transmission was dominated by heterosexual sex, while in other areas drug users were much more important to HIV transmission.[47] The disease also crossed class lines. While HIV/AIDS had initially been associated with wealth, by 1989–96 the majority of cases among males occurred in men with a low level of schooling. This trend may have taken place in part because most IDUs have a low level of education.[48] The only good news was that although the disease moved at a very rapid rate early in the epidemic, the rate of its growth slowed with time—from 36 percent a year from 1987 to 1989, to 12 percent a year from 1990–92 to 1993–96. The drop has been most dramatic in the major cities, while the rate of increase has remained relatively higher in the smaller cities. Only in the south did the rate at which HIV/AIDS increased remain high.[49] From 1985 to 1995 the character of the epidemic changed profoundly, as it was no longer confined to high-risk groups in urban areas or the subgroups that faced such intense discrimination when HIV/AIDS first appeared.

This shift would not become clear overnight, but by the late 1980s public health workers knew that the character of the epidemic was changing. In 1986 the international community had become aware that there was a significant HIV/AIDS epidemic in Africa, where the main form of transmission appeared to be unprotected heterosexual sex. This changed the perception of AIDS in Brazil, which in the early years of the epidemic had been associated with urbanity and modernity and now became associated with poverty and blackness. Between 1985 and 1986 the total number of AIDS cases in Brazil more than doubled and, for the first time, reached into the thousands.[50] It also became clear in the late 1980s that the disease was spreading through unprotected heterosexual sex in a rapid manner.[51] Brazilian epidemiologists became increasingly dissatisfied with Western models for treating the disease. North American constructions of sexual identity were not applicable in the Brazilian context.[52] There was a terrifying problem with the blood supply, as private companies paid donors for their blood and largely ignored government regulations that required testing for infectious diseases.[53] The continued spread of the epidemic seemed to require a wholesale rethinking of the governmental and societal response to the epidemic at the most profound level, from policy to outreach and from research to education. At the same time, Brazilian political leaders became aware of the international attention to their national epidemic, and of accounts in the international media that portrayed the government's response as apathetic and ineffective.[54]

■ NGOs and the Public Health System

This international pressure was matched within the country by the vocal protests of a rapidly growing network of NGOs dedicated to the issue of AIDS, most of which originally came from the homosexual community. The first of these organizations was Grupo de Apoio à Prevenção à AIDS, which was founded in 1985. By the late 1980s several other major AIDS organizations had emerged, such as Grupo Pela Vidda, which Herbert Daniel helped to found in May 1989. Some of these organizations were dedicated to policy making or education, while others sought to work more directly with people who had HIV. For example, in São Paulo the transvestite Brenda Lee (her real name was Cícero Caetano Leonardo) was outraged by the lack of care available for HIV-positive transvestites. She spent her time at the Hospital do Emílio Ribas, where she advocated for HIV-positive people lost in the system. In 1985 she converted her "rooming-house for transvestites, the 'Palace of the Princesses,' in the Bela Vista neighborhood, into an improvised hospital."[55] This center took in both transvestites and gay men who had nowhere else to turn, and it survived her murder in 1996. Her organization was only one of numerous organizations that appeared on the scene during this period.

This trend rapidly changed both the governmental and the societal response to AIDS.[56] In his periodization of the AIDS epidemic in Brazil, Parker characterized the years from 1986 to 1990 as a time of growing power for these NGOs, which lobbied for the legal and human rights of people with HIV/AIDS.[57] As Parker and Cristiana Bastos have both emphasized, this was a period when Brazilian civil society was still recovering from the painful legacy of twenty-one years of military rule.[58] After the return to democracy, a host of civil organizations formed to take advantage of new political opportunities and to reclaim a popular voice in governmental policies. The initial AIDS organizations fit into this model, as people living within the gay community rallied to force the government to make AIDS a priority.

These groups were fortunate to find an internationally receptive climate, and funding from abroad proved critical to the survival and growth of many. The number of international organizations that supported grassroots efforts sometimes seemed overwhelming. One expert, Jane Galvão, referred to "organizations such as the Ford Foundation and Inter American Foundation of the United States, Catholic Fund for Overseas Development (CAFOD), of England, Misereor, of Germany, Diakonia, of Sweden, among others."[59] Sometimes it seemed as if one NGO might have alliances with all of the above, as suggested by Bastos's description of one of the best-known Brazilian organizations, the Associação Brasileira Interdisciplinar de AIDS (ABIA):

> Some local organizations excelled at being cosmopolitan: ABIA, from Rio, maintained a constant exchange with major international NGOs, the GPA, USAID's AIDSCOM (which later merged with AIDS-TECH to form AIDSCAP), and major American foundations such as the Ford Foundation and the MacArthur Foundation. ABIA stood out in several international settings: it was central in ICASO in the Latin American Network of AIDS-NGOs; it had formed a partnership with AHRTAG (Appropriate Health Resources and Technologies Action Group) in the publication of *Ação Anti-AIDS*, or *AIDS Action*; and it was represented at a higher level of the Global AIDS Policies Coalition.[60]

This confluence between the grassroots organization and the funding and expertise that the international community offered permitted NGOs to quickly become so powerful in the struggle against AIDS in Brazil. In turn, these organizations supported an invigorated public health response to the disease on the part of the national government.[61]

Like anyone who has entered Brazil's public health care system, I have been overwhelmed by the scarcity of resources that it has, given the demands on it. I visited one hospital in Recife in 1990 that had holes in the floor, a shortage of janitorial staff, and antiquated equipment. I also received appropriate medical care for my asthma. Relative to many developing countries Brazil has a sophisticated network for public health, which the government reorganized in the 1980s.

> In an effort to improve access and equity, the 1988 Constitution extended a universal right to health care, fused the social security health services with those of the Ministry of Health (to form the

Sistema Unico de Saúde, sus), and decentralized financing to the states. It also introduced mechanisms for social participation by establishing "Councils" at municipal, state and federal levels of government to provide oversight of service provision and participation in the definition of priorities. A second set of reforms in the early 1990s transferred most of the responsibility for health care delivery to municipalities and implemented accompanying financial mechanisms for the financial allocation of federal funds to states and municipalities.[62]

While these reforms presented great challenges to the health care system, which now needed to cover the entire population, they represented not only a new commitment to public health but also an effort to give local communities say over how funds would be spent in their areas. Despite the significant challenges facing Brazil's public health system, this network and the universal care promised by the 1988 constitution represented an enormous achievement, which later permitted a broad response to the AIDS epidemic. By the end of the 1980s and early 1990s, people living with HIV had new access to support and new awareness of their legal rights. It was at this time that the public perception of AIDS began to change.

■ The Popular Awareness of AIDS

Agenor Miranda de Araújo Neto was a sweet, jovial, passionate man. He adored the work of Brazilian novelist Clarice Lispector and claimed to have read one of her books (*Água Viva*) 128 times. He was also a rock musician in Brazil, where he was known to his fans as Cazuza and was famous for his pranks and wild lifestyle. He tested HIV-positive in the late 1980s, a time when people living with the virus in Brazil faced intense discrimination. One homosexual was forced to leave a town in the northeast after people said they saw him "touching several fruits at the open-air market."[63] Such stories were not unique: another "domestic servant of a homosexual was 'accused' of having AIDS and then of spreading her virus by mixing her blood in the children's ketchup in supermarkets."[64]

People with AIDS were not only ill; they were frightened. Like their counterparts in the United States and Europe, they often sought to conceal their disease. Even celebrities tried to hide their condition. Lauro Carona, for example, was a famous Brazilian soap opera star who kept acting until he literally could no longer walk onto the set, but he kept his HIV status a secret from even his closest friends. Stunned fans learned that he had the disease when he died on July 21, 1989, an event that sparked a national debate about the treatment of people with AIDS.

In keeping with his fearless character, Cazuza announced publicly that he was HIV-positive. When he died of AIDS on July 7, 1990, at age thirty-two, a rock concert was taking place at the Jockey Club with the popular Brazilian rock band Legião Urbana. The event became an impromptu celebration of Cazuza's life, with the lead singer dedicating the first song to him and entwining verses from Cazuza's work into the group's own material. Cazuza's records continue to sell well, and the public remains fascinated by his life. His mother, Lúcia Araújo, founded an organization to care for children with AIDS and wrote a biography—*Só as Mães São Felizes* (*Only the Mothers Are Happy*)—which became a best seller and inspired a film. After 1989 the Brazilian perception of HIV/AIDS began to change. The disease had a public face.[65]

It would, however, be wrong to emphasize only the courage of individuals in creating a sea change in popular attitudes. An immense amount of effort also went into this task, as anyone realizes who has perused the AIDS education materials from this period. These were often in the form of extensive cartoon books that used the language of the street to inform sex workers and drug users about how to protect themselves. What is striking is how, with their combined efforts, NGOs seem to have reached out to every conceivable community affected by the disease in Brazil. A famous artist produced a poem about AIDS education in the format of a *literatura de cordel*. These are small pamphlets often sold on clotheslines in open-air markets and that cater to the poor.[66] One NGO in Bahia even produced a pamphlet on safe sex in six languages aimed at tourists: "AIDS has taught us to be more caring and respectful with our body. But it does not prevent us from using our erotic creativity. Explore the sources of safer sex that your body offers. In addition to using a condom, make sure no semen, pre-semen, or blood get into your partner's mouth or sores. Take care and do everything that gives you pleasure."[67] But these campaigns moved beyond safe-sex education. Many pamphlets sought to teach people living with HIV of their legal rights and carefully outlined how the provisions of the 1988 constitution could be used to protect people with HIV. They also spread information about how groups affected by HIV/AIDS were organizing to confront the disease.[68] These efforts helped to create dramatic shifts in popular attitudes and strengthened public health leaders as they sought to confront cultural and religious beliefs that ostracized AIDS patients.

■ Religion

While African religions claim many followers in Brazil, and there is a rapidly rising tide of Protestantism, the majority of Brazilians are at least nominal Catholics. The Catholic Church in Latin America is profoundly divided, with a senior hierarchy that has grown increasingly conservative over the last two decades and a grassroots clergy that is often concerned with issues of social justice. In most nations in Latin America, health workers attempting to implement effective anti-AIDS policies have found that this entails challenging the Catholic Church. In the Brazilian case, health authorities and government officials ultimately were able to reach an understanding with the Church, despite what seemed to be most inauspicious circumstances. In the early years of the epidemic some prominent figures within the Church condemned AIDS as God's punishment upon sinners.[69] These statements did not represent the views of the entire Church hierarchy, and similar statements could be found in other religious communities from the period. Nonetheless, the initial response of the Catholic Church to the AIDS epidemic often reflected the institution's concern for sexual morality (including opposition to both condom usage and sex education) rather than a desire to fight HIV/AIDS.

What is striking, then, is the evolution of the Church's stance on this issue in Brazil. Trends at the Vatican affected this process. In 1989 the pope asked that Catholics "treat people with AIDS as if they were Christ himself."[70] At the same time, leading figures in the fight against AIDS in Brazil were wise enough to realize that to succeed they needed the support of the Catholic Church. They therefore began an effort to reach out to leading Church figures not only to inform them about their efforts but also to incorporate them into their campaigns, as the comments of Pedro Chequer, the past president of the national AIDS program, made clear: "In the beginning, the Church wanted to control information, but this met with strong resistance from the Ministry of Health and from the AIDS Program. Abstinence, fidelity and marriage were just not for everyone; condoms were the most sensible option for many. Since 1997, we have been dealing with

Chairman of the Bishops Conference and the Church is now our great ally."[71] By the early 1990s the Catholic Church had established a number of projects to address the needs of people with HIV. Of course, it is possible to overemphasize the extent of the Catholic Church's cooperation, and the Church as an institution remains divided.[72] Yet despite these difficulties the Church has remained heavily engaged in the provision of services to people with AIDS, and the government has been able to implement its AIDS policies without starting a political war with the Church. Paulo Roberto Teixeira, the head of São Paulo's effort to fight sexually transmitted infections, including HIV, stressed this fact in my interview with him in July 2005. While some bishops had opposed government efforts, the majority of the Church understood why they were important. And health officials had worked to gain the Church's support. Teixeira told me that he knew of one condom distribution program in the schools. The health workers had interviewed local priests first and gained the support of the majority.[73] There have been similar experiences among other Brazilian AIDS workers. Rosemaire Munhoz, who worked in the Brazilian Health Ministry, emphasized this point: "The Church is divided, but there are some sectors within it that cooperate with the government. We know of priests and nuns who advise people to use condoms. And there's a church in Fortaleza where they have distributed condoms in the church itself."[74]

When discussing religion in Brazil, one must also remember the religious diversity within the country. In more than a decade of studying and traveling in Brazil, I have been struck by the omnipresence of African religions. In 1992 and 1993 I lived in Rio de Janeiro and rode the bus to visit friends in various neighborhoods on weekend nights. As I traveled through the different neighborhoods of the city, I might pass candles and food offerings left on a corner in Flamengo, or I might be struck by the simple beauty of a rock wall in Copacabana that was covered with candles that flickered against the night. Despite the ubiquity of practitioners of macumba, umbanda, and candomblé, it is difficult to determine their exact numbers.[75] Social scientists have found this a difficult issue to address, as religion in Brazil is syncretic, so that many people practice more than one faith. Given Brazil's history of state and Church repression, African religions are decentralized and often wear masks within masks.

In 1996 some Brazilian friends wanted me to hear jongo, a Brazilian musical form that they believed to be one of the roots of samba.[76] They took me to a house/bar in Santa Theresa (a neighborhood once home to nineteenth-century elites on a hillside overlooking Glória, which is now home to a sizable colony of artists) where there was to be a performance. The open-air courtyard of this residence was a bar on weeknights, but during the days it was also a site for worship of the *orixás*. The evening began with an invocation to the gods, to whom the owner spoke at length before carefully making a ritual pouring of alcohol on the bare soil of the courtyard. I was struck by the seriousness with which not only this man but also everyone present took this offering. This was not a show for tourists, nor was it affected. The same site could be both a bar and a site for worship, something that would be a sacrilege in a Christian context.

Both scholars and Brazilians were struck by the rapid growth of Protestant churches in the country during the 1990s. Wherever I have traveled in Brazil, there seems to be no poor neighborhood that lacks an evangelical church on every corner. Yet I suspect that the number of terreiros might be nearly as great, but they are generally invisible, much like the one I visited in Santa Theresa. Brazilians are also sometimes reluctant to admit to practicing African-based faiths, given their association with the era of slavery and the sense that they were somehow less "modern" than movements with roots in Europe and North America. But these practices are not confined to the poor or to Afro-Brazilians. In 1990 I did an immersion program in Recife and lived for part of the time in a house in Olinda. The owner was a man who headed a local terreiro that practiced umbanda. His girlfriend, who was the North American director of the program, and other members of his group were educated, middle class, and often white. African religions in Brazil cut across lines of class and race and have been significant in the response to AIDS.

By the late 1980s the Afro-Brazilian religious community had begun to rally to fight AIDS, in part because of the fear that members might be at particular risk. José Marmo da Silva, who headed the AIDS NGO, Odô Yá, explained the community's fears: "All epidemics are aggressive to the people of candomblé. Why? Because candomblé is in areas that lack health care, nature space, transportation, and education. Without information or education you cannot combat these epidemics."[77] His center, Odô Yá, had been started with help from the Institute for the Study of Religion, which sought to involve many religious groups, including followers of candomblé, in addressing the AIDS crisis.[78] His organization worked to bring religious leaders from within the community together to address the issue of AIDS: "We had discussion groups in which high priests and priestesses worked as consultants, where we tried to figure out what would be better for can-domblé, as well as what language to use."[79] The group produced pamphlets on AIDS using the imagery of candomblé to provide information and altered some rituals, such as the high priest's use of a shared razor to shave initi-ates. Da Silva argued that his community had the advantage of being able to discuss sex openly: "Other religions see sex as bad. But not candomblé. Sex is life. A source of *axé* (life force). Because all bodily fluids—sweat, sa-liva, semen, vaginal secretions—all of those have axé. The power of life. So this is a good thing. Sex is a beautiful thing. We don't keep anybody from having sex just as we don't keep anyone from sweating."[80] His organization weakened and changed both its name and its focus in the mid-1990s.[81] But it was only one of many such centers that intimately linked the prac-tice of African-based religions with the struggle against HIV/AIDS. One of the best examples of this association could be seen in a poster produced in 2001 by the Centro Baiano Anti-AIDS. The poster had beautiful colored pictures of the six leading orixás and the slogan Candomblé—Saúde—Axé (Candomblé=Health=Axé), together with contact information for the cen-ter.[82] The presence of this community in AIDS work has been enduring.

The Protestant community has perhaps come later to work against HIV/ AIDS. Given the rising concern within the evangelical movement about AIDS, this may change early in the new millennium.[83] But even with this com-munity, there was not large-scale, organized opposition to the Brazilian gov-ernment's sex education and condom provision drives in the 1990s. In-stead, Brazil has been fortunate in its ability to carry out education and anti-HIV/AIDS programs with support from numerous religious traditions, which facilitated significant changes in government policy in the mid-1990s.

■ The World Bank

Brazilian AIDS policy changed in the 1990s for many reasons, one of which was a lending decision by the World Bank. In 1944 the United States had sponsored a conference held at Bretton Woods, New Hampshire, that was attended by forty-five countries. Together, these nations founded three or-ganizations that would be the pillars of the modern world financial system: the World Bank, the International Monetary Fund, and the General Agree-ment on Trades and Tariffs (which later became the WTO). The main pur-pose of these bodies was to prevent another economic disaster like the one the world had suffered in the 1930s, which many nations blamed for the conflict that followed. The World Bank in particular was created to assist countries devastated by World War II, hence its name, the International Bank for Reconstruction and Development. Once its original reason for existence had ended, with the recovery of major European economies by the 1950s, the World Bank shifted its focus to development efforts in the Third World. It made loans at low interest rates to these countries, which then used the funds for key development projects. But the World Bank became a lightning rod for international criticism. According to one critique, the bank loaned developing economies funds that they were not realistically able to repay, for projects that they often did not need, thus increasing the problem of Third World indebtedness. Second, the World Bank often imposed conditions as part of its loans; known as "structural adjustment" packages, these conditions decreased government spending in key areas that benefited the population. Third, many environmentalists argued that the World Bank often financed grandiose development plans without adequate environmental oversight, which caused environmental destruction in areas as diverse as the Amazon and China.[84]

Some scholars believe that the intensifying criticism of the World Bank and the widespread perception of the structural adjustment programs it supported encouraged the World Bank to give renewed attention to HIV/ AIDS in the early 1990s.[85] At the same time, the widening epidemic in the poorest areas of the world was beginning to drain the economies of poor countries, which made HIV a legitimate development issue for the World Bank, as UNAIDS noted:

HIV/AIDS results in a large loss of human life and economic resources and is a major threat to the economic and social development of many countries in the developing world. HIV/AIDS calls for expensive and prolonged care in the health area; it is focused on adults at the most productive stage of their lives; it gives rise to complex legal and ethical questions; it affects all levels of society, but it has become the scourge of the most socio-economically underprivileged members of society, and it is spreading rapidly. Between 1986–1999 the WB spent over $750 million on 75 projects in an effort to control the epidemic in a number of different countries.[86]

These factors combined to encourage the World Bank to provide a major loan, AIDS I, to Brazil in 1993.

AIDS I entailed a loan of $165 million, which was matched by a $90 million disbursement by the Brazilian government for HIV/AIDS programs. This loan was made as part of a larger context in which another loan from the World Bank was being used to reshape the Brazilian health care system to make it more decentralized and responsive.[87] The official goal of these funds was never to provide free medications to AIDS patients. Instead, the Brazilian government wished to focus on AIDS prevention. From the start, it was dedicated to drawing NGOs into this effort, perhaps partly to blunt criticism of the World Bank from this community, but also because the World Bank believed "NGOs are often more effective and efficient in delivering HIV/STD services."[88] Rather than adopting a top-down approach, the loan entailed the inclusion of a variety of local and grassroots actors. The project required that significant resources devolve to Brazilian states (60 percent), and it also mandated the inclusion of NGOs. Indeed, NGOs, universities, and other organizations had participated in the negotiation of the accord.[89] This fact would have a dramatic impact on the AIDS NGO community in Brazil, given the sheer scale of the loan: "About 175 NGOs participated in the first AIDS/STD Control Project and there were about 400 projects financed."[90]

As Jane Galvão has argued, this money changed the calculus of what Brazil could do to fight the epidemic.[91] These resources helped the country make the dramatic decision to provide free medications to all people with AIDS. Paulo Roberto Teixeira, who had also helped Brazil negotiate its loan with the World Bank, stressed the fact that when Brazil negotiated its first loan, both the WHO and the World Bank were against the free provision of medications. Thus the 1994 accord had prohibited the use of these funds for this purpose. But, he said, the funds could be used to create the laboratories, testing equipment, surveillance systems, and institutional structure to make distribution of free medications possible.[92] It is ironic that the World Bank did not provide any funds for distribution of medications, which became the hallmark of Brazilian policy and the key to the effort's success. In the end, free distribution was a purely Brazilian decision that was implemented with both political will and organizational ability. Still, Teixeira stressed that the loans from the World Bank had been a key component in the creation of Brazil's HIV/AIDS program, even though the total amount of funds received had always been much smaller than the total resources invested by the Brazilian government. In his view, the first loan had been particularly important to the establishment of this program.[93] The result has been a program that UNAIDS now holds up as a model to other nations throughout the developing world.

■ Free Medication

Beginning in 1991 the government began to distribute AZT through the public health system. This represented a major advance, given that in the past, health authorities would "say in the press that AZT should not be purchased for patients in public hospitals because 'they're going to die anyway.'"[94] In 1993 Brazil began to produce AZT in its own laboratories.[95] But it was in 1996 that something truly remarkable happened. In July 1996 scientists at the Eleventh International AIDS Conference in Vancouver announced that HAART had proven to be extremely successful in limiting the replication of HIV. The so-called drug cocktail appeared to reduce the level of the virus to an undetectable level in a patient's blood. While the initial claims for this therapy would later prove exaggerated, the introduction of this treatment option represented a huge advance in AIDS therapy. The question was how available these medications would be in Brazil. In 2005 I spoke to two men who were members of GIV, an HIV support group founded by an HIV-positive man in 1990 in São Paulo. They told me that one of GIV's members in 1996 was an HIV-positive woman who attended the Eleventh International AIDS Conference in Vancouver. At the time she was very sick. She returned and told people about the cocktail. Her friends chipped in to buy her the medications, as she did not have the money, but she soon realized that this would not be sustainable. In desperation, she sued the state of São Paulo, with the argument that the state government had the responsibility to provide this medication to all those who needed it. She won.[96] This pressure from NGOs and the threat of similar lawsuits may have pushed the federal government to move with startling speed. On November 13, 1996, only five months after the Vancouver conference, law number 9313 came into force and gave HIV-positive people the right to free medications through the public health system. By 1997 this therapy had became widely available to those who needed it.

It is difficult to overstate the extent of the Brazilian achievement in creating the necessary infrastructure to provide care to people living with HIV. This entailed building a system of laboratories, health clinics, dispensaries, and drug factories normally only seen in the developed world. Yet the costs of providing this health care proved manageable because patients with HIV were not entering public hospitals for treatment for opportunistic infections. Moreover, people on regular treatment are less contagious, which also helped to contain the virus. Together with the aggressive education efforts of both the Brazilian government and NGOs, Brazil has proven to be enormously successful in controlling the spread of HIV.[97] The support of the World Bank had changed the funding climate in a manner that made this dramatic effort feasible.

The Brazilian government's successful program, however, occurred both in spite of and because of international pressures. In this sense, the story is almost a cautionary tale about the two faces of globalization. Brazil's policy led the country to enter a debate that drew in international pharmaceutical companies, the United States, the WTO, and international NGOs. In order to be able to provide medications to HIV-positive people, Brazil decided to produce generic versions of medications that were not covered by that nation's patent law.[98] On one hand, this decision was critical for Brazil to be able to afford to carry out its policy, as the decision sharply cut the cost of the drugs it provided, as the World Bank described: "The program has also achieved important savings through the local production of 7 of the 13 ARV drugs currently utilized. Moreover, price negotiations with international manufacturers for the other 6 medications have also helped to lower prices. Thus, from 1997 to 2001, the cost of ARV drugs was reduced by 54%, from an average per ART patient of US$4860 per year to US$2223."[99] But on the other hand, this decision angered pharmaceutical companies, which pressured the U.S. government both to file a complaint with the WTO and to invoke "the 'Special 301' provision of the country's Trade Act, which allows the United States to impose tariffs unilaterally on a country's exports to the United States if adequate IP standards are not met."[100]

■ Intellectual Property and TRIPS

The issues at stake were immense. Most commentators had long believed that developing countries would not be able to provide free medications to their people because, when antiretroviral therapy was introduced, it could easily cost US$10,000 a year for a single patient. From the Brazilian perspective, however, it made no sense to withhold medications that could save hundreds of thousands of lives in order to defend the interests of multinational pharmaceutical corporations that made only a fraction of their profits in the developing world. In this argument Brazil had the support of many international relations scholars, who were concerned about disparities in global health expenditures, based on statistics such as the following: "For example, 66 per cent of US government expenditure on research and development is devoted to military research, and 90 per cent of the global expenditure on medical research is on diseases causing 10 per cent of the global burden of disease. Moreover, of 1,223 new drugs developed between 1975 and 1997, only 13 were for the treatment of tropical diseases."[101] From this perspective, health is an international human rights issue, and this was most clear with AIDS: "A consortium of international organizations has estimated that fewer than 10 per cent of the people living with HIV/AIDS in developing countries have access to antiretroviral therapy. This proportion goes down to about 0.1 per cent in Africa."[102] International NGOs also argue that many drugs to which pharmaceutical companies own patents were discovered through public-sector funding, such as proved to the be the case with Briston-Myers Squibb's drug Taxol.[103] The pharmaceutical companies, however, argued that they were making immense investments to treat AIDS, and that if they could not recoup these, they would lose their incentive to continue their work. People in the United States would be unlikely to continue to pay high prices for these medications if they could import them from Mexico through Internet pharmacies. And these corporations pointed to the TRIPS agreement, the Trade-Related Aspects of Intellectual Property Rights clause within the WTO.

The TRIPS agreement was negotiated in 1994 and was intended to cover all aspects of intellectual property and patents. While it originated as part of the Uruguay round of the General Agreement on Tariffs and Trade, it is now a key provision of the WTO. The latter organization was created in 1995 and is far more powerful than the former, its parent. The signatories originally intended the TRIPS agreement to address the problem of intellectual piracy in which software, movies, medications, and other goods were being produced illegally in many developing nations without royalties being paid to intellectual property owners. By signing this treaty, countries agreed to recognize the rights of patent holders for twenty years. To the pharmaceutical companies, TRIPS provided a welcome tool to fight the production of generic drugs to treat AIDS. But TRIPS also contained an opt-out measure in cases of "national emergency." This appeared to create an open door for countries, particularly in Africa, that wanted to produce drugs to treat the AIDS epidemic, through rules on compulsory licensing and parallel importation.[104] These rules permitted countries to produce generic medications on their own where necessary, provided they paid the copyright owner a reasonable amount. But the legal standards governing these activities were unclear, and many nations feared the clause in TRIPS that allowed countries, such as the United State, to impose sanctions such as tariffs on countries that violated the act.[105] The drug companies also promised to use legal action to defend their interests. Brazil, however, was not intimidated by this threat and argued that it was in compliance with international law as it implemented its AIDS policy. For the pharmaceutical companies, Brazil represented a major threat. Its economy was too large to ignore, it had the capacity to produce the drugs on its own, and as the largest economy in Latin America, it could withstand great pressure.[106] India and South Africa also posed major problems. But if the drug companies were to keep the generic genie in the bottle, Brazil in particular had to be stopped. The power of Brazil's example was clear, as Tina Rosenburg described in 2001:

> But one major reason that only Brazil offers free triple therapy is that, until now, there was no Brazil to show it is possible. A year and a half ago, practically nobody was talking about using triple therapy in poor countries. Today it is rare to find a meeting of international leaders where this idea is not discussed. International organizations like the United Nations AIDS agency, UNAIDS, and nongovernment groups like Médecins Sans Frontières are starting to help countries try to replicate Brazil's program. Brazil has offered to transfer all its technology and provide training in the practicalities of treating patients to other countries that want to make drugs and will supply them to patients free.[107]

From the perspective of the pharmaceutical companies, Brazil represented a major threat.

As a result of this standoff, a lengthy battle ensued between the United States and the pharmaceutical companies, on one hand, and Brazil and international NGOs, on the other. For Brazil this was a critical issue. The threat that it might break companies' patents proved to be a powerful incentive for corporations to drop the price of their medications.[108] Without reducing these costs, the Brazilian government did not have sufficient resources to maintain its program. With the support of international NGOs,

Brazil brought intense political pressure to bear upon the U.S. government: "Importantly, the NGO network mobilized support from key international organizations: the World Bank, the United Nations Development Program (UNDP) and the WHO. The World Bank's support was crucial because the Bank has impeccable credentials in supporting and promoting the neo-liberal economic agenda of which IPR protection was a critical item."[109] In the summer of 2001 the U.S. government "retracted a complaint filed with the World Trade Organization over a law that enabled Brazil to produce cheap generic versions of antiretroviral drugs manufactured by multinational drug companies."[110] Major protests in Brazil shortly before this date reflected popular sentiments in Brazil.[111] These protests were probably less influential than the actions of the international NGOs, but the U.S. decision was viewed as a clear victory for countries like Thailand, South Africa, and Brazil. This success was followed by another at the Doha conference in Qatar, where developing countries such as Brazil managed to have the WTO adopt the wording they desired on compulsory licensing.[112]

The contest was not over, however. Pharmaceutical companies remained concerned, particularly after Brazil announced in July 2002 that it would "share its generic AIDS drugs and the technology used to produce them with some of the world's poorest countries."[113] But Brazil continued to enjoy international support. For example, this bilateral problem became a multi-lateral issue in October 2002 when Latin American nations refused to accept any provisions of the Free Trade Area of the Americas proposal that might limit countries' abilities to produce generic AIDS drugs.[114] This support, and the consistent efforts of NGOs (as well as intergovernmental organizations such as the United Nations Human Rights Commission), has allowed Brazil to continue to follow this policy without paying a significant economic penalty.[115] The Brazilian government has been able to use the issue of compulsory licensing as a powerful negotiating tactic with multinational pharmaceutical companies.[116] Indeed, Brazilians believe that their success will alter the implementation of TRIPS and that they have blazed a path for other developing countries to follow. Certainly, the general trend internationally tends to be toward a generous interpretation of TRIPS so as not to limit developing countries' access to HIV/AIDS medications, although this battle may not be over.[117] Still, after the anthrax attacks in the United States that followed September 11, the U.S. government itself adopted the threat of compulsory licensing in order to bring down the cost of the antibiotic Ciproflaxin.[118] Thus it would be difficult for the United States to then critique other nations providing medications for HIV. In 2002, Argentina, Barbados, Brazil, Costa Rica, and Uruguay provided free medication for all AIDS patients.[119] The cost of AIDS medications had fallen to $140 per year per patient in 2004.

One result of this history has been an atmosphere in Brazil marked by bitterness toward the United States. I interviewed twelve drug users and people living with HIV in São Paulo in July 2005. One theme that emerged among HIV-positive individuals was the belief that U.S. pharmaceutical companies had discovered a cure for HIV but were not releasing it because it would threaten their enormous profits.[120] I spoke about this urban legend with a member of GIV, an HIV NGO in São Paulo. "Jean" was an articulate, mature, fifty-something gay man. He told me that he, too, had heard these stories. He did not believe them because he thought that these companies could make an immense amount of money if they could find a cure, such as a vaccine.[121] These popular beliefs do not seem to have any credence among health professionals or AIDS educators. But the fact that these stories continued to circulate marks how the perception of the United States in Brazil has been shaped by this experience, even though Brazil emerged victorious.

■ AIDS II and AIDS III

Brazil's policy did not cost the country continued funding from the World Bank, even though this organization remains opposed to the free provision of medications. Indeed, as late as 1998 the World Bank was still concerned that the Brazilian policy of providing free medication was an economic mistake created by the political power of the HIV/AIDS community: "The government currently subsidizes AIDS/HIV patients to a greater extent than it does patients with other diseases. . . . The effective social mobilization of AIDS/HIV patients also has probably helped them to access public resources. The government has a policy of furnishing medications, including triple drug therapies, free of charge to patients. In 1997 the government spent roughly $400 million to supply these drugs."[122] The World Bank believed that this policy was economically unsustainable, even though it kept making loans to Brazil to fight HIV/AIDS. In October 1998 the World Bank loaned US$165 million to the Brazilian government, which was to be matched by a US$135 million contribution from the government itself. This program ran through 2002. The World Bank noted that the Brazilian effort was widely perceived as a success and that the Brazilian government had "contributed more than had been estimated at the time of negotiations."[123] AIDS II financed a wide range of projects. The official proposal mentioned mass media campaigns, condom distribution, a National Human Rights network, NGO projects, a counseling line, "about 80 group homes," support for the laboratory system, the "strengthening of STD diagnosis and treatment services," the "implementation of a centralized logistical control system for drugs and condoms," epidemiological surveillance, "National Reference Laboratories," training, and research.[124]

On June 26, 2003, the World Bank approved a third loan of $100 million to Brazil for AIDS III, which the Brazilian government matched with another $100 million. By this time, the Brazilian government's own funding to treat AIDS had increased dramatically. But the bank believed that its funding was still critical: "While in recent years Bank financing has made up only between 8 to 15 percent of federal financing for AIDS, it has financed key aspects of the program."[125] The World Bank realized that the Brazilian government's policy had reduced the prevalence of HIV.[126] This loan, however, still did not provide money to provide antiretroviral drugs. Instead the World Bank described itself as providing the infrastructure to make this possible, as was clarified by the bank's description of AIDS II: "While ARV drugs were not directly supported by this project, the project facilitated their use by financing the preparation of necessary protocols, mechanisms for patient adherence follow-up, studies to measure possible resistance to treatment, training for all staff involved in the provision of ART, and laboratory supplies."[127] Yet the World Bank continued to harbor doubts about the rising costs of treating all AIDS patients for free: "In 2000, treatment represented 80 percent of program costs. ARVs alone represented 69 percent of program costs. . . . Brazil has been successful in negotiating lower costs for many medications that are currently under patent protection, and has promoted the use of generic ARVs to reduce costs. However, given that it is unlikely that new cases of HIV will be stemmed in the near future, costs will continue to increase and new cost-cutting measures will have to be identified."[128] The irony is that the key international institution that supported Brazil as it changed thinking about HIV still has reservations about this policy. Of course, Brazil will have to continue solving serious problems, which will continue to include issues around generic medications and intellectual property, for the program to continue to succeed.

■ Challenges and National Pride

By early in the millennium Brazil had created an effective system to treat HIV-positive people, implemented a wide-ranging education campaign, and perceived itself as an international model for how to fight the disease. Yet significant challenges remained. The World Bank's AIDS III report noted that perhaps 600,000 Brazilians were HIV-positive, and among teenagers more women were infected with the disease than men.[129] In São Paulo half of all women infected "were women with a single partner."[130] The ratio of men to women has continued to decline, while the poor are increasingly affected. The disease is making progress into the most remote areas of Brazil, including the Amazon.[131] Poor garimpeiros have been moving into this region and bringing sexually transmitted diseases and HIV with them. The sheer cultural diversity of the region remains a major obstacle to HIV education efforts, as one study suggests. Brazilian and North American scholars evaluated a program in the Upper Rio Negro region, "a vast rain forest area (larger than the combined territory of Kentucky and Tennessee) which is inhabited by approximately 25,000 indigenous people from diverse tribes who can be categorized in four main linguistic groups (Tukano, Arawak, Maku and Yanomami). Population in this area is distributed in about 700 villages which are located along streams and rivers."[132] One can imagine the challenges of outreach among these native groups, especially given the number involved: "Due to cultural obstacles, ie. different language, sexual mores, and world view, Indians do not respond to AIDS prevention education programs developed in Portuguese by the Brazilian government. To effectively change their risky sexual behavior, culturally appropriate and gender-specific education materials were developed (ie. posters, pamphlets, 'flyers') and indigenous people from their villages trained to be peer educators and condom distributors."[133] This particular program was successful, but the diversity of languages and cultures makes this work difficult.

The Brazilian government is aware of this challenge, and AIDS III contains a specific component dedicated to Brazil's indigenous peoples, "215 different societies and cultures speaking 180 languages."[134] But all of these efforts are based on the assumption that AIDS education programs can change behavior. As Richard Parker has argued, it is not always clear that this is the case, despite some successes.[135] Brazil still has a very high rate of notified AIDS cases.[136] On a national level, there are also other concerns. "Jean," a member of GIV in São Paulo, worries about the future. Generally, in the past people had been given a two-month supply of medication at a time. Now they were at times only given a two-week supply, which meant that they would have to return to a hospital or clinic to receive more. He knew that Brazil looked good from abroad, but he said the country still had a long way to go.[137] It is true that despite its immense efforts, Brazil has not been able to control the epidemic in the same manner that Cuba has.

Despite all these caveats, the Brazilian achievements nonetheless are impressive: "Over the last 5 years, [Brazil] has achieved much in the fight against HIV/AIDS, including halving the mortality rate, cutting the HIV/AIDS hospitalization rate by 80%, and sharply reducing mother-to-child transmission."[138] While the epidemic has not stopped in Brazil, as the work of Célia Landmann Szwarcwald and other Brazilian epidemiologists has shown, it is decelerating. This has generated national pride in the program, which Brazil hopes to use as a model for other developing countries. When Brazil's AIDS program entered a crisis in 1999 and 2000 because of a lack of funds, widespread popular protests persuaded the government to solve the problem.[139]

Brazil is positioning itself as an international model for how developing countries can effectively fight AIDS. In August 2002 it announced that it signed an agreement with other Lusophone countries to share its technology to produce generic medications. This followed an announcement at the international AIDS conference in Barcelona that summer, where Brazil had pledged a small amount of money for ten pilot projects ($100,000 each) to promote the Brazilian model in other countries.[140] NGOs had been pressing Brazil to sell generic anti-HIV medications to other Latin American nations.[141] Given the scale of the funding, these projects might have a limited impact. They may have been equally significant as a measure of Brazilians' pride in their national AIDS program and their wish to draw international attention to their success. According to Paulo Roberto Teixeira more than forty countries now have exchanges to learn more about Brazil's program.[142] One HIV-positive man told me that Brazil is part of the First World in only three areas: soccer, banking systems, and medicines against HIV.[143] Brazil is now also sufficiently strong in this area that it can decide whether the conditions for accepting international AIDS assistance are compatible with Brazilian values. For example, in May 2005 Brazil announced that it would not accept approximately $40 million from USAID "because of a clause in the agreement condemning prostitution."[144] The Brazilian government's AIDS program had worked closely with sex workers' associations in the effort to control AIDS. While the U.S. funds would have supported AIDS work, they would also have undermined the local alliance. This infuriated public leaders.

"We can't control (the disease) with principles that are Manichean, theological, fundamentalist and Shiite," said Pedro Chequer, director of Brazil's AIDS program and chairman of the national commission that made the decision to turn down further U.S. money as long as the antiprostitution pledge requirement remains in place. He said the commission members, including cabinet ministers, scientists, church representatives, and outside activists, viewed U.S. demands as "interference that harms the Brazilian policy regarding diversity, ethical principles and human rights."[145]

Brazil's AIDS program has become a symbol of national pride and independence.

■ The Continuing Importance of NGOs

Another factor in the continuing success of Brazil's HIV program has been the enduring vitality of NGOs. I witnessed this myself in July 2005 when I conducted interviews regarding HIV in São Paulo. One group that I visited was Projeto Samaritano de São Francisco de Assis, which had its center far from São Paulo's core. This organization works to stop HIV as well as doing harm reduction with drug users. Like most NGOs that do work involving drugs in poor communities, this organization experienced difficulty with traffickers and had to ask their permission to work in the community. But the traffickers considered them to be "partners" and accepted their work. Projeto Samaritano had six volunteers, of whom at least one is HIV-positive and all of whom were clearly dedicated to their work. For example, when I arrived, the organization was having financial difficulties. Jacques (not his real name), who was giving me a tour, showed me their storeroom, which contained rice and diapers, so that people who were most at risk could have basic supplies. The diapers, he said, were especially important as the organization worked with approximately twenty HIV-positive children. Jacques said that they did not know what they would do when the diapers ran out. I offered to make a small donation, but Jacques did not want to take my money, saying that he felt awkward as I was a guest.

Projeto Samaritano has a partner institution, a brief walk away, that houses people who need residential treatment for drug addiction. People usually would stay for about ninety days while they detoxed. The staff was professional and passionate. One counselor, a well-dressed, fortyish, Afro-Brazilian woman, told me that sometimes the police brought people to the shelter in handcuffs. The staff would immediately insist that these be removed. I spoke with another counselor, whom I will call Edvida, who had used drugs for several years; she then quit using for two years before returning to drug use. She had been clean for four years when I saw her, and she ran the group counseling sessions at the center. I had lunch and talked to people interned in the facility; all were male, and most were in their early twenties. I had said that I did not want to interview them, as they were in recovery, and I did not want to invade a safe space. But they asked that I attend a brief support group meeting, led by Edvida, and it became clear that I would be rude to refuse. The meeting began with a holding of hands and a prayer. After a brief introduction, each person spoke about his experience. Claudia Carlini, my research assistant, and I later discussed the commonalities in their stories. Most of the men came from dysfunctional families, but in every case their families remained important to them. Their experience of drugs began with drinking and marijuana use. Then they "experimented" with drugs. It reminded me of an earlier interview I had done with a crack user in São Paulo who said, "I would tell someone don't experiment. Because you're going to like it."[146] In the end, though, what impressed me was the ability of these young men to speak articulately about their lives and the self-reflection they displayed about their addiction. In this favela, in which the traffickers had immense authority and the state seemed so weak, this organization was able to provide a key service. Indeed, its employees possessed a moral authority because of the respect that the community had for them, which enabled them to go places that government workers never could have entered.

This authority became clear to me when Claudia and I went into the community with two employees of Projeto Samaritano who were distributing clean syringes and condoms. We took two boxes of condoms, one with white wrappers and one with yellow. The yellow proved to be much more popular. We also brought what looked like a calendar but was in fact a photo board about different sexually transmitted diseases. This contained graphic photographs of genitalia with various forms of illness. Jacques, a fortyish man, carried a clear, plastic replica of the female reproductive system, which he would use to teach prostitutes about the female condom. Our first stop was a hotel used by prostitutes with their clients. The women greeted Jacques and his partner cheerfully at the door, and we descended the stairs into the building. The women were in their twenties, not particularly attractive, and dressed in skintight, tacky clothing. In Brazil it is common to call well-paid call girls "sex professionals," which indicates a measure of respect, while many other women in the sex trade are called "sex workers." In Portuguese, however, these women were prostitutes.

This hotel was run by a woman I will call Dona Marina. She was in her mid-seventies and no more than five feet tall. But she was a forceful personality. At one point some of the women at the top of the stairs were talking loudly. Dona Marina called out, "What's all that confusion up there!" Instantly, there was silence. Dona Marina gave me a tour of the hotel. Some rooms were for couples, while others were for prostitutes. Both sets of rooms were surprisingly clean. Towels and a bar of soap were carefully arranged on the beds. The rooms had tiles on the floors and walls, color televisions, and showers. The prostitutes had separate rooms where they lived, which were very different from the rooms where they worked. Dona Marina showed me one poorly lit, dirty room that looked like a cell and had a door of metal bars. For the women to go into their work rooms must have seemed a form of escape. At one point when we were walking back through the halls, Dona Marina walked up to a door and banged on it with her arm very loudly. She yelled, "Who's in there?" Then she turned and shrugged, "Fazenda programa." A prostitute servicing her client. She kept going.

Jacques and his partner, whom I will call Emilia, then set themselves up at a table in the lobby, where Jacques placed his model of the female reproductive system. This quickly attracted a small group of curious prostitutes who came over to try to figure out what this was. Jacques immediately began to show them how to use a female condom. One prostitute stepped in and took charge of the demonstration and tried to show her friends how to implant it on the model. She failed. Jacques ultimately took over and showed her how it was done. There was a great deal of laughter in this process. Jacques and Emilia bantered happily with the women. Jacques made the point to the women that they could insert the female condom up to eight hours before intercourse. The women seemed unconvinced that this was an attractive option.

Jacques then began to show the women the photos of genitalia affected by different sexually transmitted diseases. He stressed the need for early treatment and emphasized that the women should not believe that they were cured when the symptoms disappeared. The women seemed excited and interested and kept pointing at different pictures and discussing their own history of infection. I was concerned that the graphic photographs might frighten or even traumatize the women, but they did not show any signs of fear. What struck me were a couple of the questions that the women asked about HIV transmission. Despite their work, they still were not certain about how the disease could and could not be spread. When we left shortly afterward, all of the women had taken a string of condoms. They also had taken a few female condoms, although I doubted they would use them.

We then walked away from the commercial district, and in a few short blocks we entered another world. Open sewage flowed down a rivulet in the center of the unpaved street, which was covered in plastic garbage bags, soiled fabric, and a blizzard of paper. A concrete wall lined one side of the street, and there, hidden in the high grass, seven people were using crack. Emilia called out to them, and as we approached, she asked one young man to show me his crack pipe. He was embarrassed but took it out so that I could see what looked like a broken car antenna driven into a short length of pvc pipe. I had heard that sharing a crack pipe could be an HIV risk, as users' mouths were often cut and burned by the homemade pipes. The metal on the car antenna looked rough. As we walked away from this group, Emilia commented on the presence of a teenage girl with the group. Young and attractive, she had not been there the last time Emilia had passed through.

A small river of drainage flooded the street before us, so we detoured down another street, which Jacques said Emilia disliked. But he always insisted on walking it during their rounds. I could understand her reticence. Even the wild dogs looked miserable in this place. One cringing mutt had so little hair that its pink and wrinkled body looked as though it had been shaved. But people called out to Jacques and Emilia with a laugh and a smile as we passed, and they came running to get their condoms. There did not seem to be much demand for the drug kits, but men and women both wanted condoms. One crack addict began to follow us, barefoot, through the street. She was young and tall. The skin on her face and arm was marked by some kind of infection, and her teeth were blackened or missing. I was frightened of her, but Claudia was nonchalant. Jacques and Emilia stopped and began to talk with her, holding her by the arm and chatting quietly. Claudia and I shook her hand, very politely. It was late in the day, and I was tired. I found her Portuguese almost impossible to understand. I caught something about a baby, which I think had not been registered with the government. She wanted help. Emilia filled out a form and told her how to take this paperwork to the hospital. Jacques later explained to me that people were often reluctant to approach the bureaucracy and were more comfortable if they had these forms to explain what they needed. As we walked away, I looked down the squalid street and wondered how any infant could survive in this space.

Before we finished, we passed a small shop that was open to the street. The owner sat behind the counter; he seemed to sell only milk and liquor. An Afro-Brazilian man, his lone customer, sat in front of him on one of the few stools in the space. He looked stunned and weak. Although he was tall, I doubted that he weighed 100 pounds, and he reminded me of images I had seen of survivors liberated from concentration camps at the end of World War II. Although Emilia knew him, he did not recognize her when she tried to start a conversation. Jacques told me that two years ago he had been an exceptionally strong man who was quite intelligent and had managed to attend college for some time. But he had contracted HIV three or four years ago and then refused to accept that he had the disease. He had never taken medicine and must have sickened quickly. I thought that now it was too late. Emilia tried to persuade him to go to the hospital, but he seemed too confused to understand what was happening. She offered to wait with him while someone from the project arranged a car to take him to the hospital. He refused, again and again. In the end, the best that she could do was to leave a sheet of paper with the project's phone number with the bar's owner, who promised to call if the man changed his mind. Then we left.

What struck me from my visit to Projeto Samaritano, and to other NGOs focused on HIV and drug use, was that it would be difficult for the government to do this work. There were, in fact, support groups and similar organizations run by the municipal health authorities. I attended one support group for HIV-positive people who were having trouble keeping to their regimen, which was organized by São Paulo's CRT (Centro de Referência e Treinamento, Secretario de Estado de Saúde, SP). I listened to their stories and marveled at the honesty of these people: an HIV-positive man who had refused to leave his house for a year after the diagnosis, a young man who hated taking the medicine because he believed that the side effects (especially the shaking) had cost him successive jobs, the mother who married as a virgin and then was infected by her late husband, the man who arrived at the group for the first time, having tried to commit suicide the day before, because his CD-4 count was falling despite his religious adherence to the regimen.[147] This was a boot camp in which people confronted one another with brutal openness tempered by affection. They sought to help each other not only to keep using the correct regimen but also to accept the reality of being HIV-positive. The health professionals who facilitated the group were exceptional.

Still, the moral authority that Jacques and Emilia had allowed them to visit places that state employees could never enter. The fact that people at NGOs had often experienced the same problems as the people they served bonded them to their clients. NGOs were also able to tackle politically difficult issues. I visited Projeto Esperança in Guaianães, in eastern São Paulo. Their space had a series of connected buildings that played multiple roles. Some rooms were dedicated to a store to sell handicrafts produced by people in their support groups and a cafeteria that generated much-needed funds. The center also had a support group for people with HIV as well as drug users. They did not separate these populations because, in practice, they overlapped. Their clients could also take classes in this building on topics such as how to start a small business. Their organization was seventeen years old and had initially been founded to do work focused on HIV. With time, however, the importance of drugs had become clear, and drug use became a target of the group's efforts. The group had faced great difficulties, not least of which were the encounters with drug traffickers during their household visits. When I arrived, there had been a change in the leadership of the drug gangs in one of the favelas where they worked. These gangs were very organized and controlled access to the community. Although the workers continued to try, they were having great difficulty entering one particular favela.

The workers told me that when the project began, they had been naive and had worked hard to persuade people to stop using drugs. But with time they had to rethink their efforts, because this approach did not work; they decided that harm reduction was a more realistic goal. They also came to believe that there was not necessarily a hard line between users and ex-users. Indeed, some of the employees at the center were users or part-time users of drugs. I spoke with these people, and they told me that they sometimes felt that they knew more about drugs than health professionals, because they were the ones who went into the community to talk to people. And they had firsthand experience. One employee I met was an Afro-Brazilian male in his mid-thirties, whom I will call Alberto, who was an HIV-positive drug user. I also met with a quiet and professional woman, whom I will call Gabriela, who was a crack user. She showed me her crack pipe, of which she was quite proud. It was hand carved of wood, with a large colored stone set on top. When she smoked crack, she would wrap the rock in aluminum foil before putting it in the pipe bowl.

This led to a discussion of crack pipes, one aspect of harm reduction. Because crack users frequently make crack pipes out of whatever is available, as I had seen, they often have cuts and burns on their mouths. This creates a possible route for HIV transmission pipes are shared. Some people argued that this risk could be reduced by making quality crack pipes available. I later chatted with an acquaintance over a meal at Rascal's, a pizzeria. She had worked in the health services years before, as the organization wrestled with the issue of harm reduction. She had ended the experience badly frustrated: "This is it? After all this work on harm reduction this is the best we can come up with? Crack pipes?"[148] I was not quite sure what to say to Gabriela, who stressed that her pipe was not typical: "This one is nicer, obviously, because it is mine."[149]

At this point I had already interviewed several drug users, most of whom were addicted to crack. In no way did these calm, self-possessed people at the NGO match my image of drug users. Claudia, my work partner, said that she also had to rethink many of her own beliefs about drugs when she began working with Centro Brasileiro de Informações Sobre Drogas Psicotrópicas, a center within the Federal University of São Paulo. For example, she had believed that crack users would usually die in a short period and that they were always violent. I had also heard horrific stories of suffering from the drug users I had interviewed. It was difficult to reconcile the memory of these accounts with the dedicated workers who were planning to deliver condoms and supplies to the community that afternoon.

■ Drugs

I had decided to interview drug users because of the key role that they had played in Brazil's epidemic, particularly in São Paulo. Claudia Carlini had extensive experience administering large-scale studies regarding drugs, and she put me in touch with a wide range of drug users. Some of the interviews were amusing. One cocaine user and former drug trafficker kept warning me about the dangers of marijuana: "I use it myself, but only to sleep. Cocaine is better."[150] Another HIV-positive drug user came to the interview dressed exactly like me. I had interviewed Paulo Teixeira earlier that day, so I was dressed unusually well, in a button-down shirt, khakis, and a blue blazer. My interviewee was too, only he looked more natty because he had a shiny aluminum briefcase. It began to ring during the course of our interview. He answered his cell phone: "I can't talk right now. I'm doing an interview at the hospital."[151] But there were more moments of pathos and pain, such as the HIV-positive man in his mid-forties, a former injecting drug user, who was ashamed to talk because he lacked teeth. He had lost his wife five years earlier. She had been an IDU as well, and they had shared syringes in an era when needles had been illegal to purchase. He had outlived most of his friends. Now he was unemployed and had no financial resources. His mother and daughter were taking care of him. The municipal health service, CRT, was paying for him to receive dental implants, one at a time, to reconstruct his mouth.[152] But what I most remember was the end of an interview with a man who had spent years in Carandiru, the main prison complex in São Paulo. During our conversation he described the immense hardships of prison. Afterward we walked out into the hospital lobby, where a television was playing. We watched the screen as one of the immense buildings at Carandiru disappeared in a massive explosion. The government was converting the site into a park, which would also hold a major university building. I looked at his face as he watched the building disappear into the dust cloud, but I lacked the courage to ask him what he was feeling at that moment.[153]

Certain key themes recurred in my conversations with both drug users and professionals who worked with them. First, the appearance of HIV had discouraged injecting drug use and likely facilitated the rise of crack, which had arrived in Brazil around 1985. Most IDUs were age thirty-five or older. There was considerable discrimination against IDUs, so younger users were more likely to favor crack.[154] Heroin was too expensive for average people. Injecting cocaine was also no longer common. But cocaine use continued, and in Brazil it had never been an upper-class habit. Second, users never began their drug habits with crack or cocaine. Their experience of drugs always began with marijuana and alcohol. Another factor that became clear during my interviews was that despite the work of the NGOs, much work remained to be done in the field of education. For example, one former drug user said he had heard that if you were really healthy you could not catch HIV, even if you had unprotected sex with an HIV-positive person.[155] Another Afro-Brazilian man that I interviewed, whom I will call Oswaldo, did not know the difference between HIV and AIDS.

In all these narratives, job loss was always a key experience of addiction. Many drug users were still lamenting the loss of a job early in their addiction, and they viewed this as the end of their hope of a normal life. Eduardo was a forty-five-year-old man, an injecting drug user who was HIV-positive. He had five children, of whom one had died. He had used injecting drugs for nearly twenty years, and his arms were a mass of scars. He described the hold that drugs have by saying that people "trade family for drugs."[156] He recounted one period when he used drugs all day for twenty days straight with a friend; at the end of that time he began to spit blood. He entered the hospital, and by the time he left, his friend was dead. He recounted a sad story of suffering, but he was most wistful when he discussed the loss of his job.

I interviewed another man, "Oswaldo," who used crack, cocaine, marijuana, LSD, and "delerium tea." He stressed that people tend to be labeled according to the drug they use, but most people could use any drug in the moment. Of all my interviewees, I think he best captured the hold that drugs acquired over an addict's life. Oswaldo described how someone might experiment with crack by purchasing three rocks. They would try one and then think, "That was good. I think I'll have one more." Then they would have the next rock. They would try that and think, "That was good. I think I'll have one more." Then they think, "MORE! MORE! MORE!"[157] He suddenly screamed these words so loudly that I jumped in my chair. I found his experience, which was echoed by many other interviewees, difficult to reconcile with that of Alberto at Projeto Esperança. An employee of the center, he still used drugs on the weekend, usually when he had a little money left over at the end of the month.[158] I think that this variety of experience accounts for the ambivalence surrounding many conversations on harm reduction and drugs in Brazil today.

All of my interviewees stressed the importance of crack. On one hand, there was considerable discrimination against crack users. Even many traffickers did not like to sell it, because people often consume the drug where they purchase it, which attracts unwanted attention.[159] There was a hierarchy among drug users. Crack users were discriminated against even within this world, although they were not such outcasts as the IDUs. "Juscelino," an older man who had spent time in Carandiru for an assault he committed to feed his cocaine habit, told me of a man that he knew who tried to keep his use of crack hidden from his girlfriend. He waited until she had left for the day to use the drug. Once he had used crack, however, he would become obsessed with the idea that she would find him or that she was watching him from a hidden location within the apartment. One day he tore up the wooden floor underneath his front door because he was convinced that she hiding there and peering at him. Juscelino, who had spent 1991–95 and 2002–4 in prison, told me that the prisoners themselves banned crack, even though other drugs were freely available, because it made people too unpredictable and violent: "Rock, it's a sickness," he told me. "I'm afraid of it."[160]

Crack is also clearly associated with behaviors that increase the risk of HIV. Juscelino said that woman crack users sell everything to obtain the drug. He knew of a twelve-year-old child sold by his parents. Women usually ended up as prostitutes. He believed that it was easier to buy sex with crack than with money. Crack addicts were unlikely to use condoms when selling their bodies for drugs, in his opinion: "Condoms, they don't exist."[161] Paulo echoed these comments, saying that the popular phrase was "cocaine in the hand, pants on the floor."[162] He agreed with Juscelino's comments that women in this circumstance could not negotiate condom use. In Juscelino's opinion men were more likely to rob, rather than to sell themselves, to raise funds. Obviously, this could lead to prison, as in Juscelino's case, and a high risk of HIV infection while incarcerated. Paulo had spent time in pavilion nine at Carandiru. He told me that when you arrived there, you had to have sex every day. "If there are twenty-five men in the room, you will have to have sex with all of them."[163] Injecting drug use may be less common now than it was in the 1980s. But the continued epidemic of crack use in São Paulo and other major cities requires a comprehensive program to deal with drugs, if Brazil is to continue to contain the HIV epidemic.

■ Factors to Explain Brazil's Success

After speaking with drug users from different regions of São Paulo and witnessing the work of NGOs with this community, I believe that these organizations are critical to Brazil's success. I was also struck by the extent to which they received resources from abroad. When I visited GIV's well-run facility, they had just received a grant from an international organization called Red Hot that would let them offer computer classes.[164] Projeto Esperança had received support (including, for a time, interns, although this aspect of the program proved a failure) from Europe.[165] At the same time, the Brazilian state has also provided resources to NGOs, even in areas that have been politically challenging in other regions of the world. For example, according to Paulo Roberto Teixeira, there are more than 200 projects in Brazil that focus on harm reduction.[166] This mix of international resources and state support helps to explain the Brazilian model's achievements.

This model continues to face a number of challenges. When I spoke with Teixeira, he pragmatically described the weaknesses of the program. There is still a problem of late diagnosis, as I had seen myself with the members of Projeto Samaritano. In particular, this was a concern with people in poor social situations. The prisons remained a problem, and he said that there was a 12 to 13 percent rate of HIV within the prison system. He also remained concerned about vertical transmission, given the fragility of the perinatal health system. Only 60 percent of mothers had access to prenatal care, and access was particularly problematic in the northeast. Nevertheless, Brazil's program has clearly proved an immense success, which Teixeira said you could measure by the falling rates of HIV among those younger than twenty. This record, in a country with Brazil's immensity and social problems, has global implications.[167]

Teixeira pointed to three factors, which in his view were critical to Brazil's success. The first was the fact that Brazil had moved relatively quickly. He said that work to create such a program had begun in São Paulo in 1983, when there were four cases of HIV in the city. Second, the mobilization of society had proved critical. Groups that had been affected, the press, and civil society had united to face this threat. This process had involved sectors of the population that had been marginalized. The activism of health professionals, he believed, had been important to this process. Society had also accepted projects dedicated to harm reduction, and the legal system had supported universal access to care. Third, he believed that international forces were critical to Brazil's success. There had been a great interchange between civil society in Brazil, the United States, and Europe. Brazil had also received support from PAHO, in particular during the period from 1988 to 1995. The total amount of funding had been relatively small, but it had been used strategically. This had strengthened Brazil when it had taken an increasingly independent path after 1992. Finally, the loans from the World Bank had been key, even though, he argued, in real terms they had never exceeded 10 percent of Brazil's total expenditures on HIV. But they had great political and practical significance. They had organized the infra-structure, led to the consolidation of the program, and guaranteed the technical development and assessment that the program entailed. In his mind, the first loan had been the most important and had helped to establish a program that Brazil could maintain for the long term. There will not be an AIDS IV, according to Teixeira. It is not needed.[168]

■ Brazil as an Example

Perhaps the most important challenge that the global community faces to-day is whether it will be able to give access to antiretroviral medications to the tens of millions of people living with HIV. Given the scale of the challenge, it is not at all clear that states, NGOs, UNAIDS, and other international actors will succeed in this effort.[169] But as recently as the late 1990s, it appeared impossible to even consider such a commitment by developing countries, given that it would have entailed an annual expenditure per patient of US$10,000 to US$15,000 per year. Despite this overwhelming obstacle, a coalition of international actors rallied to overcome the barriers to the provision of these medications. In so doing, they changed what was in the realm of the possible. In 2004 the cost of antiretroviral treatment dropped to $140 a year because of an agreement with pharmaceutical companies negotiated by the Clinton Foundation.[170] As Tina Rosenburg argued in a widely read article in the *New York Times Sunday Magazine* in 2001, the question is no longer if nations and the international community can provide these medicines to the people who need them.[171] Rather, the question is whether there exists the political will to make this happen. While a broad coalition of international actors combined in this effort, Brazil was the key state participating in this complex undertaking, although Thailand and South Africa were also important. Brazil is not unique in Latin America in offering universal drug care to its HIV-positive citizens. But it is by far the largest of the countries to do so, it has the greatest cultural diversity, and it had the largest number of people living with HIV. Given the scale of the challenges, the success of the Brazilian achievement is immense. The same year that antiretroviral therapy was developed, the Brazilian government made a commitment to provide care to all citizens within reach of its federal clinics. It created the complex infrastructure necessary to make this possible and maintained it despite pressure from the United States and pharmaceutical companies. Now key figures such as Paul Farmer are undertaking similar initiatives in countries such as Haiti. The Brazilian model shows that providing these medications is not only possible, but it also makes good economic sense. Brazil has not only provided hope to its own people; it has also validated a new paradigm for AIDS care before the entire world community.

MEXICO AND CENTRAL AMERICA

I was nervous as I waited for Eva, a transgendered ex-prostitute, in a café in Oaxaca City, Mexico. All the other patrons in the café were young men. Perhaps arranging the meeting and interview for a public space would prove a mistake, but it had been her suggestion. When she arrived, I saw an attractive twenty-eight-year-old woman with long brunette hair, stylish black glasses, and simple but chic clothes. Despite her obvious care for her appearance, she also needed a shave. She greeted us, and the owner immediately stepped out from behind the bar. He came over, kissed her on both cheeks, then said, "When you are done, I have some pictures that I would like to show you." He left, and we began our interview. What struck me most during our conversation was her openness and dignity. Eva had become a sex worker like many young gay men and transvestites whose families could not accept their sexuality. When Eva's father had realized that his son perceived himself as a woman, he had rejected him, and Eva's relationship with his mother had also been difficult. Oaxaca City had a sizable, if disorganized, gay community and a small transvestite subculture. Anguished and in despair, Eva had begun to drink heavily and experiment with drugs. She had quickly fallen into sex work to survive, and into a world shared by transvestites.[1]

The gay sex workers in Oaxaca divided into two main groups. One group worked the bars and streets, especially near the zócolo *(city square). A slightly better-off group worked private clubs, especially the famous club 502, where there was protection from police harassment and violence and the clientele was upscale. Many patrons were foreign tourists who had come to Oaxaca City looking for sex.*

Prostitution in Mexico exists in a limbo where it is often neither strictly legal nor clearly illegal, although pimping is outlawed everywhere (although brothels are common, and enforcement is another issue). In many municipalities, including Oaxaca City, prostitution is regulated by the local government, which requires that sex workers undergo regular health checkups and carry a book (librito) that shows their compliance with this monthly testing program. The program was flawed, though. Eva said that she knew several people who would bribe authorities to have their book updated. Some of them were HIV-positive, Eva said, but continued their work because they "lacked a conscience or they were desperate." With time, Eva herself had left sex work. She realized that she wanted surgery to change her body, although she did not want to lose her male genitals. Such operations were now available in Oaxaca City, which is where she had her own procedure done. Other people went to Mexico City, although it was much more expensive there. Many gays, transvestites, and transgendered people also went to Mexico City because they believed that it would be a more open space. In Eva's experience, life in the capital proved to be very hard, and most of them returned to Oaxaca City. Many were HIV-positive when they returned. As for Eva, she had left sex work and remade her life. She still went out with her friends, but none of them drank. Her mother was now ill, and Eva took care of her. She had brought her mother to live with her. And Eva was HIV-negative.

The HIV/AIDS epidemic in Mexico and Central America is characterized by a contrast between the relatively low rate of HIV in Mexico and much higher rates in its southern neighbors. Within Central America the epidemic quickly became dominated by heterosexual transmission and a low female-to-male ratio. In the early 1990s, many observers were struck by the fact that Honduras, with only 17 percent of the population of Central America, had nearly 57 percent of the reported AIDS cases.[2] The reasons for this remain mysterious, as we will see. Since the 1990s the virus has spread within Central America. Within Mexico, however, the rate of HIV/AIDS has remained quite low, 0.3 percent of the population in 2004, according to UNAIDS. The director of CENSIDA, the Mexican federal government agency responsible for fighting AIDS, has estimated that in Mexico in 2004 there were between 116,000 and 177,000 people who were HIV-positive. This translates into a rate for Mexico that is much lower than not only most of its Central American neighbors to the south (with the exception of Nicaragua) but also the United States to the north. The HIV/AIDS rate in the United States in 2004 was 0.6 percent of the population, according to UNAIDS, roughly double that of its southern neighbor.[3] If these numbers are accurate, then something about Mexico has acted to control the spread of the virus. The question is whether Mexico will continue to contain the epidemic or whether its own rate of HIV will begin to climb rapidly. The history of the HIV/AIDS epidemic is littered with examples of countries that were complacent about the epidemic because of low rates of infection, only to see the virus spread with staggering speed. In this sense, Central America's past could be a foreshadowing of Mexico's future.

The history of the epidemic in Central America and Mexico can help us to understand the factors that have shaped its character and which may define Mexico's future. In Central America there is a bitter controversy over whether the contra wars of the 1980s helped to introduce the virus to the region. It is clear, however, that this conflict had one important result: it shielded Nicaragua from infection. This country still has the lowest HIV rate in the mainland of Latin America, although there are fears that this may change quickly. That Nicaragua's rate is so low is rather shocking, as elsewhere in the world armed conflict has generally been described as a driving factor behind the spread of AIDS. In the case of Mexico, enlightened policy decisions, strong NGOs, and cultural factors seem to have limited the virus's spread so far. But the country now faces a major challenge in that labor migration (both of Mexicans to the United States and of Central Americans through Mexico) seems to be changing the face of the epidemic. The disease is spreading in the poorest areas of the countryside. It is clear that a confluence of factors has worked to shield Mexico so far. But unless the connection between international migration and HIV/AIDS is addressed, the virus will continue its movement into remote areas, where middle-aged married women are being infected in surprising numbers. The experience of both war and migration are thus integral to the virus's movement through the region.

■ Mexico

Modern Mexico is an immense nation, more than three times the size of France, with approximately 100 million people. It is the second largest, most populous, and most powerful nation in Latin America, only after Brazil. The nation is fractured by climate, which varies from the high desert of the north to the moderate climate of the Valley of Mexico; by mountains, which can make even short trips in southern states take hours; and by ethnicity. One state, Oaxaca, has sixteen different ethnic groups, each of which has preserved its language, culture, and identity.[4] This diversity means that you can travel an hour's flight from Mexico City, the largest city on earth, and be in a remote area where many people do not speak Spanish as their first language, if at all. Despite recent investments in new highways and bridges, the importance of tourism, and a powerful central state, regional identities remain strong. At the same time, Mexico exports more migrants than any other nation on earth, and a significant percentage of the population now lives in the United States.

Modern Mexico's history has been shaped by a social revolution that began in 1910 and took between 1.5 and 2 million lives before it finished in the early 1920s. Out of this conflict came a new constitution in 1917 that recognized the social diversity of Mexico (for example, it defended the *ejidos*, the communal landholdings that were key to indigenous villages), and a new political party, the Partido Revolucionario Institucional (PRI). This party dominated Mexican politics, through co-option and corruption, until the end of the century. Elections were held every six years, but the PRI would always win, not only because the elections would be rigged, but also because most groups in Mexican society feared social unrest if the PRI lost.

In 1994 Mexico signed the North American Free Trade Agreement with Canada and the United States, which ushered in a period of rapid economic change at the same time that the PRI found it increasingly difficult to manage new political demands, and the party was racked by scandals. Under the leadership of President Ernesto Zedillo, who was committed to a meaningful democratization of the Mexican political system, truly fair elections were held in 2000. Vicente Fox, a former Coca-Cola executive, won the presidency at the head of the right-wing National Action Party (PAN). Under his leadership Mexico continued to undergo a period of rapid economic and social change. Although Mexico is often described as a conservative society in which the Church retains immense power, this image fails to capture the complexity and dynamism of this country.

■ AIDS in Mexico: The Early Hysteria

AIDS first appeared in Mexico in 1983. The earliest case was a homosexual man who had a history of multiple trips to San Francisco. This was a forerunner of many early cases, which were concentrated in the gay community among middle- to upper-class men who lived in major urban centers. Tim Frasca later interviewed leaders in the HIV/AIDS community in Mexico City, many of whom said that the initial reaction to the appearance of AIDS was one of skepticism: "I remember it perfectly well: (*the gay groups*) said AIDS doesn't exist. It's just an invention by Ronald Reagan to control our sexuality."[5] It soon became clear, however, that this disease was horribly real. Although some academics, such as Carlos del Rio and Jaime Sepúlveda, have correctly lauded the rapid response of the Mexican state to the epidemic, it is also true that Mexico was not exempt from the same hysteria and panic surrounding the disease that marked its emergence in other countries.[6] Many people at first downplayed the risk that HIV posed to most Mexicans because it was viewed as being a foreign disease that mostly affected homosexuals. Some of the statements made by experts now appear ridiculous, such as the comment of doctor Manuel Cervantes Reyes, who was the head of the Mexican Medical Association, who said that "Acquired Immune Deficiency Syndrome will not ravish Mexico as much as developed countries such as the United States, given that our population has a wide range of natural defenses from being in contact from an early age with a broad spectrum of germs."[7]

If people were complacent about the risk that the disease could spread through unprotected heterosexual sex, they were terrified about the possibility of catching it from homosexuals through the most casual of contact. Max Mejía has collected a series of horrifying stories of the discrimination that gays faced. They were rounded up by health authorities and compelled to take an HIV test. In May 1987 there was a witch hunt against homosexuals in the Yucatan, which fortunately the secretary of health took an active part in denouncing.[8] These sentiments were fueled by an irresponsible press and often were justified using religious rhetoric.[9] Mejía argues that by 1986 the hysteria had begun to decline. But as my student Paula Anderson noted in her M.A. thesis, in "1991, when gay and lesbian groups in Guadalajara, Mexico were planning to host the International Gay and Lesbian Association in the city, clashes between political, governmental and conservative religious groups erupted. Graffiti campaigns with messages like '*Haz Patria. Mata a un Homosexual*' (Be patriotic. Kill a homosexual) and '*Muerte a los Homosexuales*' (Death to homosexuals) materialized around the city."[10]

Sadly, this hysteria influenced the state's response to the epidemic, as Carter Wilson's work makes clear. Wilson spent time at an AIDS clinic in a social security (Instituto de Servicios Sociales a los Trabajadores del Estado [ISSTE]) hospital in Mérida, Yucatán, in 1992 and 1994. His book, *Hidden in the Blood*, captures the dedication of the clinic doctors at a time when the medical treatments for AIDS were of limited use, despite the existence of AZT and treatments for opportunistic infections. But other doctors still succumbed to the general hysteria, as one letter from an AIDS patient's sister written in February 1992 made clear.

> Señor director, by means of the present I want to register my complaint against Dr. ——, a doctor in your clinic, since he has consistently dealt badly with my brother, Professor ——, who it seems now carries the illness known as SIDA, according to the doctor my brother can no longer travel by bus or airplane to the city of Chetumal, because he would infect the other passengers, the doctor even told me my brother ought not be admitted to the ISSTE (clinic) because of the possibility that *he* or the nurses or the other patients hospitalized there could become infected by being in contact with my brother, he also told me that my brother *and my sister in law* would be confined in Mérida and not allowed to leave, he also told me that even my mother and I would have to take an examination since surely we are also infected, and even if we ran off to Chetumal they would track us down there in order to make us take this examination, moreover he stated that my brother had had sex with a homosexual, and that *he* was the chief source of the infection. Dr. Ramirez, I beg your consideration because my family does not know what to do.[11]

Such attitudes were also not unknown in the higher levels of the administration. The head of the AIDS clinic described one encounter he had, when "the top administrator for the D.F. who was at the conference button-holed him and said *his* current biggest problem was that at the IMSS [Instituto

Mexicano del Seguro Social] hospitals in the capital there were a lot of doctors who were clearly *putos*, and who also clearly had the disease. How, he asked Alejandro, was he going to get them out?"[12]

■ The Government Response

Despite such examples, Carlos del Rio and Jaime Sepúlveda are correct that overall the Mexican state has mounted an effective response to the epidemic. In 1986 the government created CONASIDA, a national AIDS council, dedicated to coordinating the state's response to the epidemic. State governments also began creating their agencies to fight AIDS, which were called COESIDA. That year there were 226 reported cases of AIDS in Mexico.[13] Also in 1986 the national government created a surveillance system. In May of the following year the government banned private blood clinics, which paid donors for their donations. This step, combined with mandatory testing of blood donations, almost eliminated blood-borne transmission of HIV. As del Rio and Sepúlveda noted, this step was especially important because transmission by blood had helped to fuel the "heterosexualization" of the epidemic.[14] These authors also stressed the fact that Mexico regulates rather than bans commercial sex work, with the exception of "the Federal District where Mexico City is located, and the states of Mexico, Puebla, and Guanajuato."[15] In most areas commercial sex workers are confined to certain areas of the city, are required to undergo regular health checkups, and must carry a book documenting their compliance with these requirements. What is striking is that infection rates for commercial sex workers in most parts of Mexico have remained low, both in areas where sex work is regulated and in areas where it is banned (such as Mexico City), perhaps because of the infrequency of IV drug use among this population or perhaps because prostitutes have used condoms.[16] It may be, however, that sex workers have been easier to approach and to regulate because in many municipalities they are already compelled to have regular meetings with health care providers. In this sense, the government's approach to this social ill may have already laid the framework for an effective response to the epidemic.

As early 1987 and 1988 the government also launched a significant education effort.[17] The initial campaign faced a conservative backlash because the key point of the effort was to make condoms acceptable to the general public. This effort united many different groups from rural areas to the capital, where "a conservative group named ProVida—'Prolife,' mocked as 'PROSIDA' ('PROAIDS') by the more progressive AIDS activists— . . . became a boisterous opponent of CONASIDA's efforts. In 1989, the group filed a lawsuit against CONASIDA and the Secretariat of Health, charging that the governmental AIDS program promoted promiscuity. . . . It also organized a political march on the Secretariat of Health during which participants burned condoms."[18] Interestingly, part of the opposition to the initial campaign in 1987 came from within the Ministry of government itself. The state was as divided as civil society.[19] The Ministry of Health responded to such pressures by revising the campaign, as Castro and Leyva have described, and developing strategies to target specific groups in society. Since 1996 the government has worked very hard to target adolescents in this effort.[20]

Overall, the general populace seems to have acquired considerable information on AIDS, although areas of weakness remain and conservative groups are still leading a vigorous effort against education efforts.[21] Carrillo relates one anecdote that captures the pressures that some groups face. In Guadalajara, when one AIDS education session "was offered by Ser Humano in mid-1995, the police were contacted anonymously and told that the organization was going to be holding 'a homosexual orgy' in its locale. A squad team showed up ready to close down the place. Fortunately, the educators were quick to contact the state AIDS council, and the police were convinced that what was being offered was AIDS prevention training."[22] Still, the rapid growth of NGOs dedicated to fighting for gay issues and fighting AIDS during the late 1980s and early 1990s helped to keep the pressure on the government to continue its efforts and reinforced the government's AIDS education measures.[23] A wide range of outreach efforts, from local radio advertising to a national phone line to answer questions about AIDS, continue to make information on AIDS available.

The government has also taken steps to provide antiretroviral drugs to the general population and to fight HIV among pregnant women. At first these medications were only available to people covered by social security or other state health plans. Various NGOs lobbied the government very hard from the late 1990s to the early part of the new millennium. The introduction of these medications led to a dramatic drop in mortality from AIDS in Mexico.[24] On August 5, 2003, President Vicente Fox pledged to make these medications available to all Mexicans who were HIV-positive. Mexico had participated in a multinational agreement in the spring of 2003 that would reduce the prices paid by Latin American countries for antiretroviral medications and help to make this pledge feasible.[25] Serious questions remain about the effectiveness of this effort on a national level, because there are wide differences in how well different Mexican states have responded. Still, this will hopefully put an end to the black market in AIDS medications in which "mercy smugglers" illegally bring the medications into Mexico from the United States. For many people with HIV, these smugglers had been the key to survival:

> Patricia, a 33-year old mother of two living in a tiny Michoacan village, said she contracted HIV from her husband after he returned from work in the United States. He died, leaving her to raise her children by harvesting corn and lentils. Patricia, who asked that her last name not be used, spent the family's entire savings—$2,500—purchasing AIDS medications for herself. When the money ran out, a friend's son who lived in California offered to bring her unused medication from clinics near his home. Patricia believes that she would be gravely ill—if not dead—without his help. "It's only because of the goodwill of others that I can make it," she said.[26]

The provision of free medications has ended much of this need, but many desperate people with HIV sell their medications in order to survive.[27] Overall, the governmental response to the epidemic in Mexico has been relatively successful. In 2002 Mexico was ranked ninety-seventh in the world in terms of its HIV rate.[28] But it is also true that Mexico could have devoted more resources to the epidemic. For example, in 2002 President Fox's administration dedicated "less than 1 percent of the national health budget to people with AIDS."[29] There has thus been substantial room for the Mexican state to augment the resources it spends in this area.

There are two questions about Mexico's response to the epidemic. Are the government's actions, as successful as they have been, the main reason that the epidemic has so far been contained? Will Mexico's epidemic remain relatively contained, or is the face of the epidemic about to change abruptly? The disease remains concentrated in the three major Mexican cities and along the northern border, where injecting drug use may be one of the factors driving the epidemic. In most of the country IV drug use is not common, and sex remains the main means of transmission. Men who have sex with men continue to account for roughly half of all HIV infections, and the percentage of gay men in the nation's capital who are HIV-positive remains disturbingly high. But heterosexual transmission is becoming more important to the virus's spread, and the epidemic is making inroads in the countryside.[30] Early in the epidemic most women who were infected with the virus were exposed to it through a blood transfusion.[31] Now they are most likely to receive it from a sexual partner, usually their husband. Finally, HIV/AIDS has moved from the upper and middle class to workers and the poor.[32] In June 2004 there were 72,864 cases of AIDS reported in Mexico, of which 69.1 percent had died.[33] It is true that this is not a large number relative to the size of Mexico's population. But it will take a sustained and thoughtful effort to maintain Mexico's success with HIV/AIDS.

■ Mexican Sexual Culture

It is not immediately clear why Mexico's experience with HIV should be markedly different from that of some of its Central American neighbors, when Mexico's sexual culture appears to be quite similar. There is an extensive literature on AIDS and sexuality in Mexico.[34] Scholars working in the field have found a similar complex of sexual beliefs as in most other Latin countries. Mexican men are expected to exhibit machismo, a behavior that is characterized by their confidence and dominance of women. Extramarital affairs are tolerated by men and viewed as a sign of virility. Men are inducted into sexual activity at a young age, often with friends or family who take them to prostitutes.[35] Women, in contrast, are expected to remain virgin until marriage and not to exhibit strong sexual desire after the wedding. This sense that "good" women do not enjoy sex further pushes men to visit sex workers for sex acts that they could not ask for within their homes. The valuing of virginity also decreases the number of sex partners available to young men, which leads them to sex workers and, in particular, a subculture of transvestites. In this respect Mexico is similar to many other sexually conservative societies that tolerate sex between men and transvestites as a form of exploration. This is the case, for example, in sexually conservative Java in Indonesia.[36]

The contradiction within the belief system between a critique of homosexuality (equated with effeminacy) and sexual relations with transvestites entails that these relations be veiled with secrecy outside a close circle of male friends. But it also reflects the same duality about intermale sexual relations that is prevalent throughout Latin America. Men who penetrate other men, and are thus seen as dominant and macho, are not viewed as homosexual. On the other hand, someone who is penetrated is believed to lose all qualities of maleness by participating in this act. It is this subgroup of men who have sex only with men that is defined as being homosexual. These sexual patterns do not vary greatly from those of other Latin nations, as the beautifully written work of Silvana Paternostro has shown.

There are regional variations within Mexican sexual identity that are important. In Oaxaca, for example, there is a region in the south called the isthmus where there is a long-standing indigenous tradition of a third gender, in which men are transvestites. There is, of course, nothing uniquely Mexican in this tradition, which is found in many other cultures. Chris Beyrer discusses similar sexual identities in Asia in an area stretching from India to Thailand and from Cambodia to Malaysia.[37] In the isthmus of Oaxaca these people are called *muxe*, a Zapotec term. They play an important role in local sexual culture, as the reporter Julie Pecheur found: "'Because a woman's virginity before marriage is still very important in our society, many young boys are initiated by muxe,' says Yudith López Saynes, the director of Gunaxhii Guendanabani, an association dedicated to AIDS prevention. 'It is widely accepted, but with AIDS now people are more cautious.'"[38]

Although they wear women's clothing and have relationships with young men in the village, muxe are an accepted feature of local society. Indeed, when conducting interviews on AIDS and gay culture in Oaxaca, I heard repeatedly the phrase "Every mother wants a muxe." Unlike other children, a muxe was expected to remain home and care for parents in their old age.[39] This rather passive construction of this gender, however, denies the active role of muxe in local gay culture. Gays have helped to organize *velas*, or saint's days festivals, in Oaxaca in order to raise awareness of the issue of AIDS. These celebrations subvert the traditionally religious orientation of these festivals and create an unusually safe place for gays to congregate and celebrate in public in small-town Mexico. The impetus for these velas comes out of the isthmus, where muxe leaders have long organized these affairs. One such vela, Las Auténticas Intrepidas Buscadoras del Peligro, evolved into a traveling drag act to raise awareness of AIDS. It received grant funds to take the show on the road throughout Oaxaca.[40] The existence of the muxe perhaps creates a social space that has permitted political organization and thus facilitates gay awareness elsewhere in Mexico.

Yet these variations do not change the fact that Mexico's sexual culture is a conservative Latin morality that does not seem dissimilar from that of its southern neighbors. Michael Higgins and Tanya Coen have a telling anecdote about prostitutes in Oaxaca who knitted as they waited for their clientele in Oaxaca City. The place where this group of women waited was not particularly distinctive as being involved in the sex industry, and the women's dress did not mark them as prostitutes: "The block they work has few inexpensive hotels (where they take their clients), a few residential units, and a variety of small shops and stores. Unlike the *chicas*, the knitters do not openly solicit clients or even call much attention to themselves beyond their knitting. The fact that they are standing around at midday on the street is enough to communicate that they are prostitutes."[41] The fact that the women are marked as sex workers because they are standing around knitting reflects the rigid gender roles that still shape Mexican society and are accompanied by macho sexual roles for males. It appears difficult, therefore, to explain Mexico's low HIV rate with reference to particular sexual mores.

■ Oaxaca

The challenges facing Mexico and the reasons for its success to date can be seen by considering the experience of Oaxaca, a relatively poor rural state in southern Mexico. As recently as the 1930s the state was very difficult to access from Mexico City, which is now perhaps an eight-hour drive to the north. An ethnically diverse state, it has very high rates of out-migration from indigenous villages, which send migrants to Texas and Southern California. The influence of indigenous cultures is one of the defining characteristics of Oaxaca, as survey results find that at least 40 percent of the state's population is indigenous (using language as the main criterion); if other measures to define ethnicity are used, the figure may reach 70 percent.[42] The migration of young men from these communities is critical to the survival of rural indigenous villages, in which the basis of the economy is subsistence agriculture and handicraft production for the tourist market.[43] These tasks are gendered, so that the men often spend lengthy periods of time abroad, while the women sell their products directly in Oaxaca.

My graduate student, Paula Jean Anderson, had written her M.A. thesis on AIDS in women in Oaxaca to examine the factors that made many housewives particularly vulnerable to the virus from a conflict resolution perspective. Her thoughtful study had examined the cultural factors that influenced the disease's epidemiology, but I wanted to look more at the state and NGO response to the epidemic, particularly in a state characterized by poverty. As Anderson said in her thesis, while AIDS is a significant problem, many Mexican states also lack basic health services. This can be seen in mortality statistics, for "the principal causes of death reported in Oaxaca in 2002 (were), in order of occurrence: infectious intestinal illnesses, malignant tumors, pneumonia, homicides, accidents, cirrhosis and other liver diseases, and measles. According to a 1992 report, 23.9 percent of Oaxaca's households lacked electricity, 41.9 percent lacked running water, and 61.1 percent had no sewers. The infant mortality rate in Oaxaca is the highest in Mexico: 33 deaths for every 1000 live births. By comparison, the rest of Mexico is 27 for every 1000 live births."[44]

Given this social context, Oaxaca seemed a useful example of a state with scarce resources in which AIDS was only one of several pressing problems. As of June 2004 there had been 2,298 reported cases of AIDS in Oaxaca, of whom 60 percent (1,379) had died. Of these cases, 1,866 were men and 432 were women. According to Servicios de Salud de Oaxaca, 39 percent of AIDS cases had been reported in the central valleys that house Oaxaca City, while the isthmus had another 23 percent.[45] The majority of people had become infected through unprotected heterosexual sex. In the summer of 2004 I traveled to Oaxaca to interview people in the gay community, doctors, and employees at COESIDA and AIDS prevention organizations to better understand the epidemic.

In the course of this research trip I was very impressed by the response of Oaxacan society and state government to the epidemic and to a confluence of factors that may have helped the state to contain this virus so far. COESIDA in Oaxaca is a strong organization. Well-organized NGOs, such as Frente Común Contra el SIDA, help to keep this organization responsive to the needs of people with AIDS. MEXFAM, a private organization devoted to family planning, helps to ensure condom availability and sex education. Both MEXFAM and COESIDA have outreach programs in the countryside, critical in such an ethnically diverse state. The federal government makes free medication available to people with AIDS. HIV tests are readily available. It is true that the rate of infection is increasing and that the reported numbers are likely too low. But it is also true that by regional standards Mexico has a relatively low rate of HIV. This rate might be low because the government has provided health testing to sex workers and because

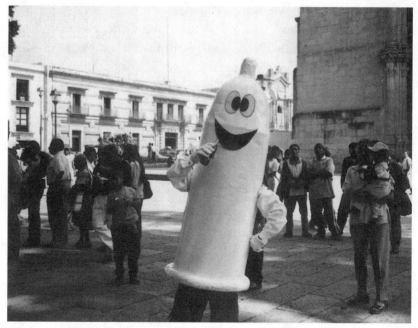

This image of "Señor Condón" was taken in downtown Oaxaca City. Photo by
Paula Anderson.

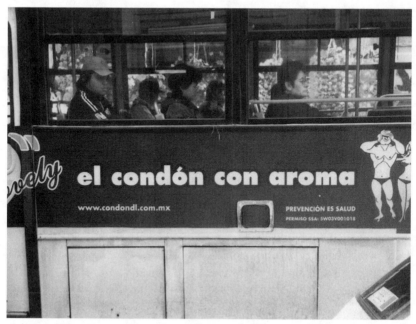

This Mexican bus carries an ad for condoms. Photo by Paula Anderson.

MEXICO AND CENTRAL AMERICA

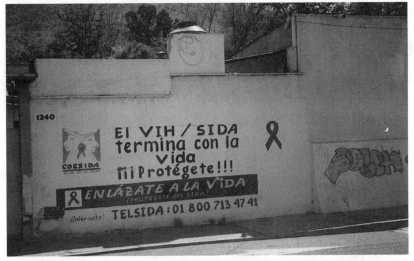

This billboard in Oaxaca, Mexico, calls for safe sex. Photo by Paula Anderson.

IV drug use is uncommon in the culture. But the reasons for Mexico's low HIV rate may lie in cultural and social responses that are partly outside the central government's control but, rather, may come from the local or state level. Oaxaca is unusually successful in fighting the AIDS epidemic. Indeed, Bill Wolf of Frente Común Contra el SIDA referred to what he thought of as a "Oaxacan Model" for fighting AIDS. The basis of this model is a strong state response partnered with cooperation with civil society. This model is significant because if it can work in Oaxaca, a poor, largely rural, and ethnically diverse state, then it can probably work in many other locations.

■ MEXFAM

The size of the average family in Mexico has plummeted sharply over the last three decades, from 4.5 children per mother in 1970 to 2.5 per mother in 1988 alone.[46] The rate still continues to decline, although now more slowly. A large part of the credit must go to MEXFAM, an organization that makes all forms of birth control available at low prices and carries out extensive family planning campaigns. I toured a clinic in Oaxaca City that was small but clean and well maintained. The surgery room was well equipped; the waiting room had a large television set and comfortable furniture. The director who gave me a tour clearly took pride in her center. The organiza-

MEXICO AND CENTRAL AMERICA

tion is completely private, and much of the funding comes from international donors, such as the Bill and Melinda Gates Foundation.

While this was the only MEXFAM clinic in the city, the clinic also had a rural coordinator who traveled to remote parts of the state. The employees went into schools to talk to children about sexuality, birth control, and AIDS. The clinic sold condoms for a peso each. It also had agreements with three pharmacies to provide condoms cheaply. As part of this arrangement, MEX-FAM sells condoms to the pharmacies at a low price, with the condition that the stores also keep their prices down when they, in turn, sell the condoms. Another part of this understanding is that the pharmacies will readily provide condoms to all who ask for them. The person behind the counter will not be shocked if a fifteen-year-old asks for a condom. This organization clearly did a great deal both to make family planning available to average Mexicans and to ensure that information on AIDS and sexual issues was widely available. Given the rapid decline in family size, MEXFAM's work has clearly been effective.

■ The Catholic Church

One point that struck me was that the MEXFAM employee said that the organization had never had any trouble with the Catholic Church. Personally, he had the sense that the Church knew that this work had to happen and that family size had to be brought down.[47] I heard similar statements repeated over and over again during my interviews. At COESIDA I met with an employee who was responsible for managing a half-hour radio program that played weekly on Saturdays at 11:00 A.M. and was also available on the World Wide Web. The show had a "chat" format, rather than being structured as an interview. Some parts were prerecorded to include interviews with people in the street or small dramas with COESIDA employees drafted as actors. The show covered AIDS but also touched on many other issues concerning human sexuality. Given the limited resources of COESIDA, this was doubtless a useful means to ensure that AIDS information was made available in the countryside. I asked this employee, "Maria," if her organization had ever had difficulty with the Church. She said that they had only received a single, very long letter of complaint based on religious grounds.[48]

It is true that the Catholic Church on numerous occasions has spoken out against AIDS education efforts in Mexico. It argues that condoms are not a sure means to prevent AIDS and that sex education can promote promiscuity. But the Church's teachings in this area, much like those on family planning, are widely ignored by the populace.[49] Indeed, one almost has the sense that in some areas, the Church's resistance is largely pro forma. I met with Bill Wolf, the head of Frente Común Contra el SIDA, an important organization in Oaxaca. An enormously energetic and committed man, Wolf had helped to found the organization and still managed its activities in 2004. He told me that when he and his allies were discussing founding this organization, he decided to go to the local bishop and ask his support. Other people thought he was crazy. But he and a female friend went to the bishop and outlined their plans for the organization. The bishop listened very carefully and at the end of the meeting said, "I must reiterate the Church of Rome's position on the use of condoms. That said, in all other ways, you have my support."[50] Wolf left the meeting feeling rather disappointed, but his friends said, "That's great! What did you expect?" Indeed, Wolf said that the only people who ever asked about the Church were from outside the country. He had the Church's silence, which was all that he needed. "I don't need them to hand out condoms. We can do that ourselves."

The Mexican state may have an advantage in this dichotomy between the letter of the Church's teachings and the real experience of most Mexicans. Unlike some other Latin American nations, where battles with the Church have been bitter, in Mexico the Church for the most part has not successfully blocked education efforts. This does not mean that there are not conservative voices within the Church, and there are examples of the Church trying to block the government's AIDS programs. This may be particularly true in northern Mexico, which historically has had a more conservative Church. But in much of Mexico, it seems that the Church tolerates the efforts of the state and NGOs to conduct AIDS education and provide condoms. In instances where the Church is uncooperative, the Mexican people seem to largely ignore the Church's teachings on these issues.[51]

■ COESIDA

In the state of Oaxaca, the fight against AIDS has been helped by an unusually strong COESIDA, the state AIDS organization. At the national level, Mexico's anti-AIDS effort is led by CENSIDA (formerly CONASIDA), which sets guidelines and oversees policy decisions. But each state is responsible for creating its own agency, which is responsible for the practical implementation of anti-AIDS efforts. This highly federal system means that some states (such as Guadalajara, Michoacán, and Oaxaca) have extremely effective organizations, while in other states COESIDA appears to be little more than a phone line.[52] Frente Común did a phone survey of COESIDAS in southern states about 2002. It found two functioning COESIDAS, but in the other six states the organization seemed to lack even a telephone.[53] This means that it is difficult to discuss a coherent response to AIDS at the state level in Mexico. In Oaxaca, COESIDA has historically been a strong organization since its foundation in 1994, which in part reflects the close ties between the head of COESIDA and the outgoing governor.

COESIDA in Oaxaca City is housed in a three-story building.[54] A clinic on the first floor attends to the needs of HIV-positive people, the second floor has an outreach center, on the third floor there are the administrative offices, and on the roof there is a small area that serves as a laboratory. The technician in the laboratory said that they do HIV tests in this space but the work for CD-4 and viral load counts has to be done in Mexico City. From this center a comprehensive AIDS education effort is managed. COESIDA outreach workers make trips out into the countryside to small villages that have high rates of migration to the United States. Because it is very difficult to have access to the migrants, who spend much of the year out of the country, COESIDA's philosophy is that the state needs to educate the entire village, in particular the young who will be migrants themselves someday. COESIDA also manages a half-hour radio program every week, sends out news bulletins to the local press, and runs a phone help line. The work is difficult because the employees never know when the phone rings if it will be someone in crisis or even suicidal. People often call during the "window period" after they have been exposed but before they can take the test to tell if they have been infected. The employees keep track of the calls that they receive and use them to shape the topics covered in the radio show. Sometimes people even call from other states because directory assistance refers them to COESIDA, Oaxaca. The organization also does outreach into the prison system.[55] The clinic on the ground floor does not have the facilities or beds to hospitalize patients. Patients who enter the system undergo an evaluation that includes CD-4 and viral load counts. Based on test results, patients are classified as being stage one, two, or three, with the last being the most serious. If patients are at stage three, they are referred to state hospitals in the city.[56]

The local offices of COESIDA also had a lawyer who was responsible for dealing with the legal and human rights issues that people with HIV faced. According to the lawyer, the single key problem was confidentiality. Despite the law, nurses and others would sometimes share information on an individual's HIV status. This led to one of the most common complaints: maltreatment at work when an employer learned of an employee's HIV status. The employer would then often try to make the employee's job so unpleasant that he or she would decide to leave. The lawyer found her work frustrating at times because people often made complaints but rarely followed up. It was often also hard to contact people because, in their fear, they often provided false addresses and phone numbers. Family violence was also a major problem. Men would blame their wives for infecting them, even though the opposite was often true, and would beat their spouses. She said that when men were ill, their spouses always cared for them. But when the women were ill, the men washed their hands of the problem and left.[57] I was impressed both by the difficulty of her job and by her dedication. One particular anecdote captured for me the scale of the challenge that she faced and why it was essential for COESIDA to have such a person. A woman died in a small town perhaps a two-hour drive outside Oaxaca City. This community, called Miahuatlán, is renowned both for its machismo and for its high rates of violence. When the town fathers learned that the woman had passed away from AIDS, they refused to allow her to be buried. Upon hearing the lawyer tell this story, Liliana, my research assistant, said, "What, did they think that she was going to infect the dead?" A complaint arrived at COESIDA, and the lawyer prepared to travel to the town. But when the local authorities heard she was coming, their resistance collapsed and the woman was quickly buried.

One factor that impressed me about COESIDA was its openness to the community. When I met with the heads of local gay organizations in Oaxaca, they told me that they knew the senior officials by name at COESIDA and had met with them. The organization does face challenges. One senior official, Dr. Q, told me that she was worried that a new governor was taking power who might have different priorities for state expenditures. Doctors at COESIDA were already paid much less than doctors at IMSS. In some states COESIDA almost did not exist. It is true that state and federal governments together paid for antiretroviral medications. But in some states people had to gain access to these medications from agencies other than COESIDA, because of these weakness of this organization. Dr. Q also recognized the cultural challenges COESIDA faced. She said that in some parts of the state a band still plays on the wedding night while the couple consummated the relationship. Then the bloody sheet would be hung out the window. In this context, in which such a high price was put on female virginity, many men's first sexual experience was with other men. Wives found it extremely difficult to negotiate condom use with their partners. Dr. Q. believed that the disease in Mexico would follow the path taken in other countries, where it would increasingly affect women. Nonetheless, this official continued to take great pride in COESIDA's accomplishments in Oaxaca and the dedication of its employees.[58]

■ Nongovernmental Organizations

The government's work has also been aided by the proliferation of NGOS that have appeared to fight AIDS. Mexico witnessed the same proliferation of HIV/AIDS organizations during the late 1980s that Brazil experienced.[59] These organizations have a broad presence: "there are more than 300 NGOS throughout the country distributed among most of the 32 states of the republic, but with a high concentration in Mexico City."[60] There are perhaps more than 200 organizations dedicated to fighting AIDS in Mexico City. In Oaxaca there are 8 NGOS dedicated to fighting AIDS, of which the most influential is probably Frente Común Contra el SIDA. This particular organization came out of the arts community and from the start had powerful people on its board. The organization carries out a wide range of AIDS education activities. It has an office, Condón-Manía, near the zócolo in the heart of Oaxaca City, which sells condoms and hands out AIDS information. Perhaps forty people a day will drop by the center, for a total of over a thousand people a month. Of the people who asked for condoms, 87 percent were male and 13 percent were female. The organization also has information packets that include audiocassettes in different regional languages, from Mazatec to Zapotec. Frente has handed out more than 2,300 of these packets so that anyone can give the Frente's AIDS education talk using their materials. Some packets have even wound up in migrant communities in the United States. The organization has also worked with the media in Oaxaca City, which agreed to sign a five-point accord. This agreement said that the media would respect the confidentiality of AIDS patients, report on positive developments, use correct terminology, and let NGOS check figures

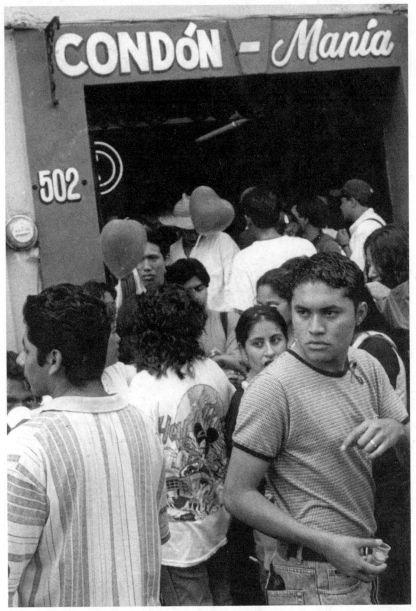

This image was taken in 1997 at the opening of Condón-Manía, a condom store and informational center run by Frente Común Contra el SIDA in Oaxaca, Mexico. The Peruvian singer Tania Libertad sang in the street and cut the ribbon. The street (J. P. García) was closed for two hours as hundreds of Oaxaqueños partied to the popular rock band Los Sonidos. Cantera magazine called it "a pioneering event in Mexico." Photo by Russell Ellison.

before they were published. Bill Wolf of Frente Común is now trying to take this accord to the national level.[61]

Wolf believes that the number of AIDS cases reported in a region depends on the number of AIDS NGOs active in the area and the strength of the state COESIDA. This may explain why nearly a quarter of AIDS cases in Oaxaca are reported from the isthmus, a largely rural area. This area has an active and organized gay community, which may facilitate AIDS reporting. On the other hand, states that have low numbers of reported AIDS cases may in fact only have a poor organization to collect this data.[62] Some organizers in the NGO community also have concerns that politics may affect AIDS reporting. One person showed me a chart with the number of AIDS cases reported per year. These figures showed a marked drop in the number of reported cases every time there was a change in the government. The activist interpreted this to mean that the outgoing secretary of health wanted to show good numbers when he or she was leaving the position. Dr. Q at COESIDA offered a very different perspective. She acknowledged that their numbers were not perfect, but their calculations indicated that they were accurate to within 30 percent.[63]

The relationships between the NGOs and COESIDA are inherently strained.[64] Frente Común, for example, pressured COESIDA to provide figures on the number of patients receiving antiretroviral therapy. COESIDA did not want to do this, but at the NGO's request the secretary of health asked that COESIDA provide this information. It turned out that the numbers were not as high as Frente's organizers believed they should have been. In 2004 there were perhaps 919 people living with AIDS (these were not people who had only been infected) in the state of Oaxaca, of whom 369 were seen by COESIDA, and 272 were receiving antiretroviral medicine from that organization. As Miguel Ángel Ramírez Almanza argued in a press bulletin, the others may have been receiving their medications from other state organizations: IMSS, ISSTE, or Pemex. But the question remained: Why were all patients seen by COESIDA not receiving medication?[65] In theory there is universal access to medication, and in Mexico City and the Federal District the coverage is quite good. But in the countryside it is a different matter, and whether patients receive access to the medications may depend on their individual savvy and knowledge. For this reason, after Frente obtained its numbers from COESIDA, the NGO pushed COESIDA for permission to undertake a survey to gain further information on patients and what they were taking. This survey found that of the 153 people surveyed, only 69 said that they were

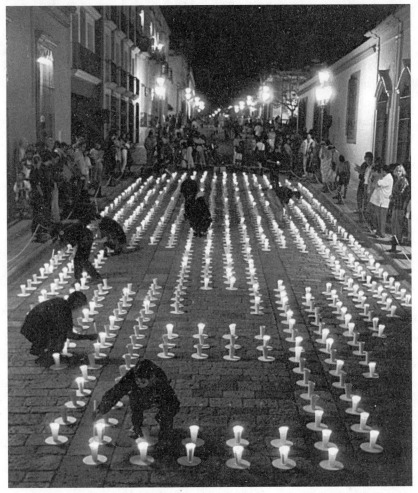

An AIDS memorial in Oaxaca City, Mexico. Each candle represented one person lost to HIV/AIDS. Photo by Russell Ellison.

receiving a complete cocktail of three medications. Thirty-one patients did not receive any medicine, 2 patients were receiving one medicine, and 20 patients received two medicines. Thirty-one patients did not respond.[66] Frente also has a number of other concerns about the care that HIV-positive people receive. For example, the state does not pay for CD-4 and viral load counts. The tests are too expensive for many rural people living with HIV, as "a CD4 count test cost 350 pesos (US $35) in 2002, and a viral load test 1,250 pesos (US $100)."[67] Thus some people whose condition is not verified by testing might not be given drugs that are in short supply.

MEXICO AND CENTRAL AMERICA

COESIDA in Oaxaca City is an unusually strong organization. But the surveillance and pressure of NGOs will be necessary to ensure that everyone who needs treatment receives it. According to figures provided by the head of CENSIDA, the national AIDS organization, a large percentage of people with AIDS in Mexico may not be receiving any medical attention. The figures show that of the 72,864 reported cases of AIDS in Mexico, 50,349 have died, and 16,712 receive attention from a variety of sources (IMSS, ISSTE, Secretariat of Health, Pemex). This leaves thousands of people who are not receiving any care at all.[68] Oaxaca may have challenges, but the situation in some other Mexican states must be far worse, given that in some states COESIDA is more a name than a reality.

■ The Gay Community

The gay community in Mexico began to organize in the mid- to late 1980s. The movement began in Mexico City and was very much influenced by the example of similar movements in the United States. But gay organizations tend to be new and relatively weak outside the three major cities in the nation. One scholar in Oaxaca City questioned whether there was truly a gay community in the state. In my interviews, however, I sensed that this may be changing. I met with three members of Vinni Gaxhea, a gay organization that was founded around 1999.[69] The name of the organization comes from a Zapotec word meaning "different people." Members stressed the importance in Oaxaca of the sexual culture of the isthmus, where many parents welcomed children who were muxe. This created a space in which gays could be visible. Nonetheless, in Oaxaca City the gay community was plagued by many problems, not the least of which was lack of self-esteem. The problem of men having sex with men but not defining themselves as being gay also made organization difficult. To counter this, one man I spoke with had organized three major velas, all of which proved to by huge successes. Still, the work of Vinni Gaxhea would take a great deal of time, which is why members focused much of their effort on the young. AIDS education was not their main purpose. They had too many other challenges to face. Still, information on AIDS did seem to be available to the gay community. One young gay man, "Julio," who worked at a local language school, told me that the gay community was not doing a lot of work around HIV education in Oaxaca City.[70] On the other hand, even though the gov-

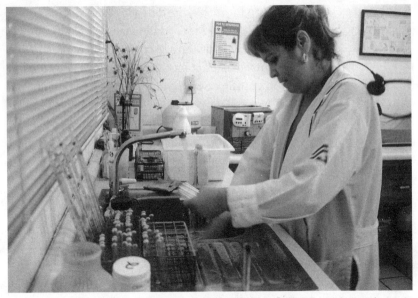

A blood laboratory in Melaque, Mexico. This particular laboratory is to the north, outside the main district of storefronts and businesses, but is close to a local pharmacy. The laboratory is run by one licensed doctor and a technician. The laboratory does HIV tests, but testing for diabetes is a larger part of its work. Photo by Jana Kopp.

ernment could do more, there was sufficient AIDS education information available through organizations such as Frente. The gay community is now organizing and is playing an important role in efforts to contain HIV/AIDS in major urban centers that, until now, have been most affected by the virus. Much more work, however, remains to be done in smaller state capitals and in the countryside. The state has, perhaps, been more thorough in its efforts to reach sex workers.

■ Regulating Sex Workers

In Mexico, sex work is regulated in the majority of states and municipalities. Prostitutes are required to have a small book that demonstrates that they have regular health checkups and that they do not have a venereal disease. Even states and cities that do not mandate this program often ask the prostitutes to volunteer. This is the case, for example, in Mexico City, where many men expect this from sex workers:

When they come looking to buy sex in the dim alleys and side streets of this sprawling city, many Mexican men look for something else first: a small white identity card. Bearing a photograph, pseudonym, and the stamped dates of blood tests, the card grants no formal rights to the women who carry it. But it identifies its holder as one of thousands of Mexico City prostitutes who have volunteered for training and regular blood tests in an all out effort to combat the spread of the AIDS virus. "It's a question of life or death, and the men are beginning to realize that," said a 32-year old prostitute who works near Mexico City's historic Zócolo, or main square. "Now they want to see the card before they decide whom to go with."[71]

As the experience of Eva suggests, these men are foolish if they believe that these test results alone can protect them from AIDS. Prostitutes may bribe state officials to stamp their books without the test results. Historically, however, the regulation of sex workers has caused a decrease in the spread of sexually transmitted diseases.[72]

As early as 1992 it was clear that far more housewives than sex workers were being infected in Mexico, by a factor of at least ten.[73] This ratio has not wavered greatly with time and holds true throughout the country. In Oaxaca, one senior official made the point that the epidemic is not being driven by sex workers by showing me the state health department's statistics that indicated the professions of people who had been diagnosed with AIDS (not who were only HIV-positive). Twenty-four sex workers had been diagnosed, which represented a total of 1.04 percent of this population. Among housewives, 286 had been diagnosed, which represented 12.45 percent of the total number of AIDS cases in the state.[74] In interpreting these figures it is important to remember that sex workers in Oaxaca and most Mexican states must undergo regular health checks, so they would be far more likely to be diagnosed with HIV/AIDS.

David Bellis, in particular, has done considerable work on AIDS and prostitution in the United States and Mexico. He interviewed sex workers in multiple Mexican cities during 1996 and 1998, as well as in Southern California in 1988. One key question he examined was why sex workers in the United States were more at risk for HIV than their Mexican counterparts. While there are many possible reasons, one crucial difference he uncovered was that Mexican sex workers were far less likely than their northern counterparts to inject drugs. As he described it, the "differences between the Mexican and American FSWs (female street sex workers) were startling. The

Mexicans were *choir girls* compared to their beaten up, sick, toothless, heroin-addicted Southern California sisters. Many more of the Americans had been through the drug/jail/john wringer compared with the Mexicans."[75] Mexican statistics support the argument that IV drug use is not a major risk factor for HIV transmission to date in Mexico, as a "negligible .07 percent of female AIDS cases—less than one in a thousand—are attributed to IDU."[76] Bellis's work also found that Mexican sex workers were more likely to "have monthly medical checkups," to have customers who wanted to use condoms, to require "condom use, including for fellatio," and to have "sex with fewer clients per day."[77] Also, according to Bellis, these women were less likely to use IV drugs, to keep working if they became HIV-positive, and to "report that customers do not like to use condoms."[78] Bellis summarized his findings that "Mexican FSWs have contained the spread of HIV infection and STDs by (1) avoiding IDU; (2) careful precautions with clients; and (3) legal prostitution with mandatory medical examinations and testing for STDS and HIV. Mexico presents a clear-headed view of prostitution. It is tolerated and controlled, not by arrests and marginalizing, but by zoning, licensing, and periodic examination of FSWS for STDS."[79] In this area, Mexico seems to have an advantage not only over many developing countries but also over the United States, where in the early 1990s the HIV rates among sex workers in some cities were truly appalling.

■ Migration and Women

Mexico's low rate of AIDS may be explained by a number of advantages its society and government possess. Intravenous drug use is rare except along the northern border, although it has emerged as a problem in some areas such as Tijuana.[80] Organizations such as MEXFAM have made sure that family planning information and AIDS education are widely available. The state response in the national capital and major urban centers has been strong. The fact that sex work is regulated but not prohibited in much of the country has meant that prostitutes have regular health checkups and the state has the chance to provide them with AIDS education materials. At the same time, one has to be struck by the fractured nature of the response to AIDS, given the federalization of the government's AIDS organizations. Outside the largest states with the major urban centers, there were many small and rural states in which COESIDA exists more in name than reality. Given epidemiological trends, this is worrying. One major challenge the Mexican government faces is addressing the problem of AIDS in the migrant community. This will entail working in the most remote areas of Mexico and across the lines of class and ethnicity. The state of Oaxaca has clearly shown that this is possible. But this work will have to be done throughout the nation if Mexico is to retain its unusually low rate of HIV.

It is a commonplace in American political discourse that the border between Mexico and the United States is the only location in the world where a wealthy First World nation abuts a developing country. Mexico has a long tradition of sending migrant labor to the United States, and this has sharply accelerated since the 1980s.[81] As particular regions have sent workers to the United States, historical ties have drawn migrants from specific Mexican states to particular regions in the United States. For example, in my home state of Oregon many Mexican laborers come from Jalisco and Michoacán. Most migrants from Oaxaca probably travel to Southern California and Texas.[82] While for decades these migrants were stigmatized in their own country, since the inauguration of President Vicente Fox the Mexican state has sought to welcome these people home and remove any sense of shame they might face. In part, this was a recognition of economic reality. As an article in the Oaxacan daily *La Jornada* noted in 2004, remissions from migrants were the most reliable influx of foreign funds in the balance of payment and enable Mexico to pay the interest on the national debt.[83] The migrants, often poor and uneducated men from rural areas or urban slums, had become essential to Mexico's national economy. Moreover, the sheer numbers of migrants made a force to be reckoned with. In the late 1990s, the percentage of the U.S. population from Mexico was "equal to 8 percent of total Mexican population."[84]

Migrants are also a significant group in the changing face of Mexico's AIDS epidemic. The work of Shiraz Miraz and others has shown that the majority of migrants are young men whose life expectancy is two-thirds the national average. They are poorly educated and are often drawn from small communities in rural Mexico. They travel to the United States on a difficult journey during which they may face demands for sex either for money or for help crossing the border. Although 70 percent of migrant workers are married, they spend months away from their families, spouses, and partners in a new environment.[85] Extensive research has shown that men often experiment with new sexual experiences while abroad and are more likely to use the services of sex workers, and a portion experiment with drugs, including injecting drug use.[86] Migrants sometimes pool their funds and share a sex worker on payday, a practice that makes them "milk brothers."[87] Some migrants also claimed that sex with another man was a way for them "to stay faithful to his wife."[88] Hispanics in the U.S. have an incidence of AIDS "three times that of non-Hispanic whites."[89] The cultural factors that place Latin Americans living in the United States at risk for HIV are complex. One study of Puerto Rican women found that only one variable seemed to indicate who was most at danger. The statistics suggested that "AIDS risk increases as preference for English increases."[90] Still, the marginality, new opportunities, and isolation that migrants face create social spaces for the transmission of HIV. Many migrants also report that they are afraid to use the health care system because they may face deportation.[91] This means that not only are they likely to take risks while in the north; they may also be less likely to seek treatment if they acquire a sexually transmitted disease. When these migrants return to their small towns, often for a saint's day, a portion of them may be HIV-positive. Once home, they often demand sexual practices learned in the United States. As one migrant said, "I have changed. Other things are known over there and when I come back, well, I feel free to do it with my wife."[92] These cultural factors create opportunities for the transmission of HIV.

Mexico's status as a transit point on the route to the United States also encouraged the spread of HIV. Central Americans traveling through the country were vulnerable to sexual exploitation and violence. In Oaxaca, for example, there was a population of female migrants from Honduras, Guatemala, and El Salvador, many of whom ended up in the sex trade industry. The police had frequent contact with them when they went to the brothels.[93] Some women who came to Mexico had no intention of working in the sex industry but became trapped along the way. This was particularly the case in Chiapas.[94] Elmer García Mesa, who worked for the government AIDS program in Chiapas, gave an interview in which he said that the disease in the region was being driven by undocumented Central American women. He told a reporter that "this illness has been 'ruralized' because Central Americans enter the country with the hope of reaching the United States, and remained in the region in the area temporarily or permanently, and basically they have infected the inhabitants of rural zones."[95]

One point that everyone stressed during my interviews in Oaxaca was that it was important not to stigmatize the migrants, who are already among the most marginalized groups in Mexican society: poor, rural, uneducated, and often indigenous. The media has given considerable attention to the issue of AIDS and migrants, which is perhaps dangerous. The tone of one article from the journal *Noticias* in 2003 was perhaps typical. It quoted authorities in the Mixteca region of Oaxaca who said that the growing number of AIDS cases in the area was largely due to the phenomenon of migration and that there was a major problem with people returning from abroad and infecting their partners. The article went on to speak about other dangers these migrants posed, because with their return there were "automobile accidents, since they drive in a state of drunkenness and they run a great risk of hitting other vehicles, causing countless damage to property and placing at risk the lives of third parties, according to police sources. They remark that this increase (of automobile accidents) is provoked by the excess of alcohol that the migrants consume in the city, above all the youth given that when they return to their places of origin they take part in countless parties, consuming alcoholic drinks in excess, this being the dark side of migration."[96] The headline of this article was "Undocumented Migrants the Main Carriers of AIDS." Another headline that same year in *El Tiempo* was "50% of the People Who Emigrate to the United States Prostitute Themselves." The reported claimed that "50% of the people that emigrate to the United States prostitute themselves in their first year of residence, and upon their return they bring with them a high probability of having been infected with some type of sexually transmitted disease, such as AIDS."[97] The article failed to provide much detail or evidence for this assertion.

It is difficult for the government and for NGOs to reach migrants. According to one person I interviewed at COESIDA, there are some villages in Oaxaca from which so many travel that the only people who remain are the young, the elderly, and the mothers.[98] Migrants are often on the road and are generally paid under the table. They are difficult to reach to give AIDS brochures. Another employee I spoke with at COESIDA worked in particular with women, and she found it very difficult to prepare women to negotiate condom use with returning husbands and boyfriends. She said that you could imagine the situation of a housewife whose husband has spent months in the north. When he returns, "if she suddenly hands him a condom and asks him to use it, she's going to get punched."[99] Studies have found that migrants' wives generally did not take any action to protect themselves from being infected by their partner even when they believed the partner was unfaithful.[100] This is easy to understand, given the women's poverty and marginalization, the cost of condoms, and the difficulty of negotiating safe sex with their partners. But another study also found that the majority of farm-working migrant women in the United States agreed with the statement, "I can't catch AIDS because of I'm faithful to my husband."[101] The lack of education and the lack of power place migrants' wives in danger.

Paula Anderson's work provides a rich description of the social factors that make women vulnerable to HIV in Oaxaca. In rural areas, communities exist in states of crushing poverty that places women's health at risk. This deprivation is reflected in the fact that "many women in Oaxaca suffer from chronic malnutrition. In many regions of the state women suffer from a 20 percent lack of calories and in regions of extreme poverty, up to 40 percent. As a result this population is at extreme risk of suffering a multitude of illnesses."[102] Female mortality rates are high, and in rural areas there are few social services provided by the government. It is not unusual for women in rural areas to be married at age fifteen, to have children very shortly after marriage, and to spend lengthy periods alone with the children because their husbands are abroad.[103] Anderson's research also revealed that as recently as the 1980s, birth control was uncommon, abortion remained a leading cause of maternal death, and the homicide rate was strikingly high, as "homicides rank fourth as a cause of death in Oaxaca."[104] Finally, traditional gender roles stress the self-sacrificing and sexless nature of mothers, an ideal described as "marianismo."[105] While women are placed in socially vulnerable positions, culturally and religiously they are also expected to submit to their husbands, to accept suffering as their position in life, and to avoid reflecting on their sexuality. Given this social reality, Anderson argued that it would be impossible to address the problem of AIDS in rural Mexico without confronting the social issues that disempower women and make them vulnerable to the disease.

This work is critical because these rural, indigenous women are now strikingly vulnerable to AIDS. An all-too-typical pattern has been for a woman to learn that she is infected with HIV in Oaxaca when her husband travels to the hospital to die from AIDS: "In Mexico, the first woman infected by HIV was a housewife of 52 years of age, whose unique risk factor was to have had sexual relations without any kind of protection with her husband."[106] It remains a staggering fact that in much of Mexico, more housewives than sex workers are becoming HIV-positive. At the start of 2003, 11 sex workers, 208 housewives, and 263 migrants, "of whom only seven were women," had tested positive for the virus in Oaxaca.[107] The sex workers are aware that they are at risk and they protect themselves. Migrants and their spouses do not. One Oaxacan woman described her experience of being told she was HIV-positive: "But I couldn't understand it. It's much more than ignorance. I had heard of that illness, but for me, it was an illness for those people. For example, the women who dedicate themselves to (pause) . . . how do you say it? . . . those women right? The ones who sell sex. Or gay men. For me this illness is for them, among them. For me . . . I hadn't thought about it. I had heard about it but I thought that it wasn't for me because I am a woman of the house, dedicated to my children, to my husband."[108] When these women realize that they are infected, they have to immediately address multiple issues, of which the threat to their life may only be one.

Victoria May Eaton carried out extensive interviews with women who attended COESIDA for her undergraduate thesis, a remarkable document that captures the voices of many women dealing with HIV infection. The story of one migrant's wife echoed the experience of many of her peers and conveys a sense of the particular challenges these women face:

> She was infected by her husband. María, twenty-eight years old, sat before me in a white room at COESIDA (Consejo estatal para la prevención y control del SIDA—State Council for the Prevention of Control of AIDS) and began to tell her story. Her frail frame barely filled the chair that she sat in across the table from me. She smiled nervously. Her husband had left to work in the United States for two years. Three months after he returned, he became very sick, and María needed to take care of him along with her two children: a girl aged three years and another girl aged ten months. María tested positive in July, as did their youngest daughter. The three year old will need to be watched carefully during the next year or so. María told me of the day she received her results. She felt depressed, resentful, and worst of all, she felt a strong hatred towards her husband. Her husband was sick, but he had not told her right away. Now they have a baby who is also sick with "this illness." They have told his family, and received support. María will not tell her family. She says it will be bad for her father; but she thinks that they suspect something.[109]

Perhaps the most difficult part of her experience was not the disease with which María lived but, rather, the discrimination that she feared, as became clear when Eaton asked her about her plans: "I ask María when she will go back home so that maybe I can speak with her after she comes back from the trip to Mexico City. Her head pulls up (she has been looking at the table), and her eyes widen. 'I can't go home,' she says. 'Where I come from, they kill people with AIDS.'"[110] This story captures the sense of isolation that many women feel. Yet their experience is intimately linked to migration, although the majority of these women have never traveled to the United States.[111]

The realization that Mexico's relationship with the United States has shaped the epidemic of HIV/AIDS is nothing new. As early as 1988, Jaime Sepúlveda pointed out that in Mexico, with the exception of the nation's two major urban centers, "the highest rates of AIDS are found in those states that border our giant neighbor."[112] The association has continued through time, and now migration is the main factor driving the spread of the virus in rural Mexico. According to Mario Bronfman, who has done considerable work on the subject, in 1998 10 percent of AIDS cases had "a history of residence in the United States."[113] In 2000 some other health officials estimated that 30 percent of those infected with HIV in rural areas of the country had been infected in the United States.[114] In some states, such as Hidalgo, it may be that most new infections are among migrants.[115] The movement of the virus into rural areas has thus reflected a larger process of human migration: "In the beginning of the epidemic there were no cases of rural AIDS. At present, however, rural cases make up 5 per cent of the total. This phenomenon is inevitably associated with migration, being an indicator of the growing impact of migration on epidemiological trends. . . . This percentage is unequally distributed in the country, with states such as Hidalgo and Zacatecas reporting that rural cases exceed 20 per cent of total cases."[116]

People at COESIDA in Oaxaca are well aware of this. Dr. Q told me that she believed migration was becoming a critical factor in the spread of the virus in Oaxaca. Most likely, she believed, the disease in Mexico would follow the path of other countries and increasingly affect women.[117] If this trend is to be stopped, a nonjudgmental, international effort will need to reach out to the migrants and their partners on both sides of the border. It is also important to recognize that the threat of HIV moves in more than one direction. Many Mexican border cities see heavy usage of sex workers by young men, many of whom "are long-haul truck drivers from regions throughout the U.S., primarily the Midwest."[118] Any effort to deal with the challenge will have to be an integrated response involving the state and national governments of both nations. There are some positive examples, but not enough.[119] There may also be a limited amount of time to meet this challenge, although in 2000 rural areas were "estimated to account for about 10% of the total. But a recent government study suggested that the disease is spreading much faster in rural areas than in the cities—with a more than 80% rise in cases in some outlying provinces since 1994."[120] In the mid-1990s the rate of increase of HIV infections was "sharpest in Aguascalientes, Durango and Guanajuato states, which have large numbers of migrants working in the United States."[121] Mexico may be unusual in its success to date controlling HIV, but many other nations have had lower rates than their neighbors, only to see the epidemic flare to frightening levels because of apathy. Mexico needs to act to address AIDS in the countryside with a comprehensive program that will mandate the creation of effective COESIDAS in all states. But migration cannot be addressed without considering the women who are being infected in Mexico.[122] Any effort that focuses solely on their partners will fail. Mexico will therefore need to undertake a long-term project to improve rural health services and to address the inequalities and violence that women face if it is to prevent the feminization of this epidemic, as has happened in so many other countries.

■ Central America

Central America consists of seven nations: Guatemala, Belize, Honduras, El Salvador, Nicaragua, Costa Rica, and Panama. The latter country historically formed part of Colombia until 1903, when President Theodore Roosevelt supported a local rebellion in favor of independence so that the United States could build a canal across the isthmus. The fact that the United States created this country indicates the extent of U.S. influence in the region. U.S. filibusters also invaded Nicaragua during the 1850s and managed to briefly dominate the country under their leader William Walker. He reestablished slavery and made English the official language before a combined army of the Central American nations expelled him. He was executed in 1860 after trying to invade the region yet again. The United States also invaded Nicaragua in 1912. The last marines did not leave until 1933. After a lengthy guerrilla war the head of the U.S.-created National Guard, Anastasio Somoza García, made himself dictator with the backing of the United States. He ruled the country until his assassination in 1956. His sons, each in turn, inherited the presidency. President Dwight Eisenhower also ordered Alan Dulles and the CIA to overthrow President Arbenz of Guatemala in 1954 out of the conviction that he was a Communist. Throughout the Cold War the United States, believing that all reform movements were associated with Communism, supported the social status quo in the region as part of an alliance with local elites. With the large and dissatisfied indigenous population in Guatemala, the extreme social inequality of El Salvador, and the unpopular dictatorship of Nicaragua, this policy contributed to the revolutionary movements and civil wars that wracked the region beginning in the 1970s.[123]

By 1979 guerrilla groups were fighting throughout the Guatemalan countryside, while the military had begun a brutal counterinsurgency campaign that with time evolved into something approaching a race war. In El Salvador the military had long had a key role in the political system. As early as 1970 guerrilla activity had broken out in rural areas, and by the end of the decade the country was in the midst of a true civil war. The government responded with brutal repression that only fueled the insurgency. In Nicaragua a guerrilla movement, the National Sandinista Liberation Front, had been founded in 1967. In 1972 an earthquake devastated the country's capital, Managua. In the wake of this disaster, most Nicaraguans believed not only that the government had proved ineffectual but also that President Anastasio Somoza Debayle had stolen much of the funds and supplies donated from abroad for reconstruction. This anger impelled a national insurgency that toppled Somoza's government in 1979. The party that emerged in the nation's leadership was Marxist, though democratic and committed to a widespread program of social reforms. President Ronald Reagan of the United States responded by launching a campaign to overthrow the government through the CIA. As part of this program the United States funneled money to a guerrilla army of dissidents—many of whom at first were former Somocistas—organized by the CIA on Nicaragua's northern border in Honduras. At its peak in the mid-1980s this army may have had 15,000 men. In return for hosting the "contras" and U.S. troops, Honduras received military aid and training and Washington's economic support.[124]

Some Central American countries escaped the violence. Costa Rica had abolished its army in 1949 and gradually adopted social welfare policies that reduced social inequality, provided good quality health care, and reduced political conflict. During the civil wars of the 1980s Costa Rica defied Washington and supported the Nicaraguan government. Belize is an English-speaking state that received its independence from Britain in 1981. Even during the 1980s it remained relatively isolated from the political turmoil of its neighbors. Honduras allied with the United States during the 1980s and served as a base for the contra armies. Several guerrilla groups also existed in Honduras during the 1980s. But the contras fought in Nicaragua, and Nicaraguan troops did not follow them over the border, fearing an American reaction. The guerrilla groups were small and fairly ineffectual. Honduras was relatively peaceful compared with El Salvador, Nicaragua, or Guatemala. Panama's political history during this period was complex. Panama's strongman, General Manuel Antonio Noriega, would ultimately become engaged in a confrontation with the United States that would see President George H. W. Bush send the U.S. army to invade the country to capture him, after which U.S. soldiers brought him back to Florida to face drug charges. He was convicted. But the country did not experience a civil war during this period. Nonetheless, the entire region suffered in the warfare and unrest of the 1980s, which generated large numbers of refugees, devastated the economy, and absorbed all the political energies of Central America's leadership.

In the end the violence was brought to an end because of a peace plan generated within the region itself. Costa Rican president Oscar Arias proposed an agreement that all countries involved in the conflict accepted in August 1987. This pact entailed "a cease-fire, national reconciliation, amnesty, democratization, termination of external aid to insurgent movements, and free elections."[125] Nicaragua, El Salvador, and Guatemala each reached an agreement between the government and the rebels that brought the fighting to an end by 1996, when Guatemala's guerrilla groups laid down their arms. The Sandinistas in Nicaragua lost a free election in 1990 that brought a moderate conservative government into power, which dismantled many of the social programs the Sandinistas had implemented. In El Salvador the dominant right-wing party won an election in 1994, which nonetheless saw the party headed by the former guerrillas become a meaningful political party. The transformation within the region is striking, despite the organized crime and drug trafficking that continue to bring violence to Central America.

With its lack of natural resources, relative poverty, extreme inequality, overreliance on export crops such as coffee and bananas, weak democratic institutions, and frequent outside interventions, Central America has long faced serious challenges. The wars and political unrest of the 1980s left the region exhausted, with hundreds of thousands of refugees in Mexico and the United States, and with serious economic challenges. It was in this context that AIDS arrived in Central America. In 2004 the statistics showed that the incidence was "highest in Belize (2 percent adult prevalence), Panama (1.5 percent adult prevalence), Guatemala (1.0 percent adult prevalence), and El Salvador and Costa Rica (0.6 percent adult prevalence), and Nicaragua (0.2 percent adult prevalence)."[126] The history of this disease in this region cannot be understood apart from this history of war, which created migration outside the region, sealed borders, and exhausted governments.

■ War and AIDS

From the emergence of AIDS, the spread of the disease has been associated with military conflict, which has particularly affected the HIV rate among women.[127] Conflicts tend to spread HIV for a number of reasons.[128] Wars may so weaken national governments that they cannot implement AIDS prevention programs. Rural areas or entire sections of the country may be cut off from the government's health authority. For governments struggling to survive, HIV/AIDS may not be a priority, and warfare consumes resources that could otherwise be devoted to health education and programs. For people facing daily risks in a war zone, the long-term dangers of HIV/AIDS may also not be their immediate concern. During warfare the social order tends to collapse, and many women are put in a position where they have difficulty denying men sex for protection or resources.

Armies at war can also introduce or accelerate the transmission of HIV. In many developing countries the HIV rate among soldiers is higher than in the general population and may be over 50 percent in some armies in southern Africa.[129] One study that surveyed the region in 2005 suggests that the rates may be significantly higher than even this staggering figure:

Malawi, which has an adult infection rate of 15.96 percent, has an estimated 75 percent of its military personnel infected with HIV. Uganda, which is considered one of the world's success stories for its commitment to combating AIDS and its success in bringing its adult infection rate down to 8.3 percent, has a 66 percent infection rate in its military. This is nearly eight times the infection rate of the population as a whole. In Zimbabwe, estimates show that 80 percent of the military personnel are HIV-positive. Even more amazingly, the Zimbabwean government itself admitted in 1993 that up to 70 percent of its officer corps was HIV-positive. Estimates for the South African Defense Forces peg the infection rate around 40 percent, double that of the adult population as a whole. However, there exists a wide degree of variation within that estimate. Some units, such as those in KwaZulu-Natal, have an estimated rate of infection of 90 percent.[130]

By the mid-1990s some army units in Thailand had a 10 percent HIV rate, while in Cambodia the rate reached 30 percent.[131] Historically, most soldiers are more likely to visit prostitutes and to have multiple partners.[132] The movement of soldiers thus presents opportunities for the transmission of the virus. The first appearance of AIDS in Uganda (the African state most affected by AIDS early in the pandemic) was associated with the Tanzanian invasion that overthrew Idi Amin in 1978–79. The virus initially infected people in those subcounties through which the victorious troops traveled.[133] In civil wars from Colombia to Kosovo, combatants also have used rape as an instrument of terror, which can leave women not only traumatized by also HIV-positive.[134]

The displacement of large numbers of people also creates opportunities for HIV to spread to new groups. From Africa to Southeast Asia, guerrilla groups have turned to trafficking women to support their activities. Soldiers stationed abroad for peacekeeping may have financial resources denied to local communities and have often fueled the sex trade, as has been the case in Kosovo. In Cambodia in the early 1990s, United Nations peacekeepers seem to have contributed to the rapid spread of HIV, which particularly affected women.[135] High rates of HIV tend to weaken the state, which may lead to social unrest and exacerbate regional conflicts.[136]

One of the most important aspects of warfare is that it seals borders, which in most cases appears to have accelerated the spread of HIV/AIDS. Warfare impedes the ability of UNAIDS and other organizations to acquire accurate information about HIV rates and epidemiology. Danger and chaos also restrict the ability of NGOs to educate and pressure governments to act, which has been the case in Burma and the Democratic Republic of the Congo. For this reason, in many developing nations at war it is difficult to obtain good information about HIV rates, although it is clear that they are escalating. But in a few rare cases war seems to have had a paradoxical effect, in that it may have isolated some nations from the spread of HIV/

AIDS. This appears to have been the case in Nicaragua in the 1980s, during which the Nicaraguan contras conducted warfare along the nation's border without penetrating deep into the country or challenging the local authority of the state. Instead Honduras bore the brunt of the early AIDS epidemic in Central America, which raised the question of how the conflict influenced the epidemic in this country, when the disease took a different path in Honduras's neighbors.

■ Honduras and Nicaragua

The AIDS epidemic truly began in Honduras, which still has the highest rate for Central America. Honduras is also the poorest country in Central America, if not in all of mainland Latin America.[137] It very quickly became the epicenter for the disease. In the late 1990s the country had "only 20% of the population of Central America, but 60% of all the AIDS cases, according to UN officials."[138] Indeed, the sharply higher rates of HIV in Honduras early in the epidemic caused some researchers to worry that there might be something distinctive about the variant of HIV found in the country. Epidemiological research, however, failed to find an unusually aggressive subtype of HIV.[139] But the statistics remained too striking to ignore. In 1995 Honduras had 4,619 reported cases of AIDS, more than the total of all other Central American nations combined. El Salvador, in second place, had 1,248.[140] Terrifying predictions circulated in 1994 that by 2010 one Honduran in five might be infected with the virus.[141] In some communities, such as the Garífuna people of the northern coast, the rate of HIV was particularly elevated at perhaps one person in fifty.[142] This holds with a pattern that has found that in the Caribbean coast region of Honduras and Belize, "the epidemic is generalized and affects both urban and rural populations. The Garífuna Afrocentroamerican ethnic group that inhabits this area has been particularly affected."[143] Elsewhere, sex workers in San Pedro Sula were seropositive in 14 to 21 percent of cases.[144] Given that the country shared a common language, history, culture, and geography with its neighbors, what could account for these rates, if the figures were accurate?

One common argument was that the virus had been introduced either by U.S. troops or by the large numbers of contra fighters. Some local academic leaders pointed to the fact that the presence of U.S. troops had created a huge industry in the sex trade:

According to Juan Almendares, a US-trained Honduran doctor and former Rector of Honduras National Autonomous University, the presence of foreign troops in Honduras has created or exacerbated some serious health problems. To escape from poverty, thousands of Honduran girls have become prostitutes. In the city of Comayagua (near the US military base of Palmerola) there are an estimated 3000 prostitutes, about 60% of the total number of prostitutes in the whole country. This high level of prostitution has contributed to a pronounced increase in sexually transmitted diseases, including penicillin resistant gonorrhea. Teachers in Comayagua have noted venereal sores even in primary school children. Honduras also has the highest number of people with AIDS in Central America.[145]

This opinion was held by more than a single academic. One study identified "a special group of women that don't consider themselves sex workers, but who attended to the soldiers at the Palmerola base in the city of Comayagua. The majority of them are very young, many of them students that live in Comayagua or that come to this city on the weekends and meet with the North-Americans in discotecs and restaurants that have restricted access."[146] Another study suggested that the city of Comayagua had served as an entry point for HIV into Honduras "through the troops of the United States stationed at the military base of Palmerola." This study also surveyed sex workers in the city of Comayagua and found that of sixty-five prostitutes, ten proved to be HIV-positive in 1990.[147]

Based on this evidence, the rapid spread of the disease could have been caused by Honduras's unique position as a station for U.S. troops and CIA forces during the civil war. This might explain the rapid spread of the virus and the fact that the disease so quickly became dominated by heterosexual transmission. The first reported AIDS case in Honduras in 1985 was a man of "bisexual conduct who had lived in San Francisco, California."[148] Yet he was exceptional because from the very start the Honduran epidemic was dominated by heterosexuals. Indeed, the percentage of cases of gay men in Honduras has always been strikingly low. As early as 1993 gay men accounted for no more than 7.1 percent of all cases among men in the country, while heterosexual men accounted for 71.2 percent.[149] It was not that the infection rate among gay men was unusually low. One study reported in 2003 that 13 percent of all men having sex with men were HIV-positive in Honduras. For transvestites the figure was 23.5 percent.[150] But they were not the majority of people infected. Sex workers seem to have been more important in the spread of the virus. In 2003 more than 10 percent of all sex workers were infected with HIV.[151] Half of all men who were infected in the early 1990s reported having used the services of prostitutes.[152] If this were the case, was it possible that U.S. policy contributed to the AIDS epidemic not only in Honduras but also elsewhere in Central America? One author, D. Summerfield, presented this argument in the *Lancet* in 1991:

> There are striking variations in AIDS case detection rates between the countries of the Central American isthmus, and the politics of this troubled region seem to have been playing a part. By the end of August, 1990, Honduras had reported 626 cases to the World Health Organization (WHO), El Salvador had reported 192, Panama 180, Costa Rica 169, Guatemala 80, and Nicaragua only 8. Analysis of World Bank and other data suggests a correlation between the number of known cases in each country and the extent of military and economic aid delivered by the US during the 1980s, measured in terms of dollars and by the numbers of US military and other personnel stationed there.[153]

Many questions, however, remain with this argument, as the Honduran case makes clear.

The geography of the epidemic does not seem to match clearly with the hypothesis that the virus emerged around U.S. military bases and the contra staging points. From the start, the disease focused on the two main cities of San Pedro Sula and Tegucigalpa, which between them accounted for more than half of all reported AIDS cases. During the period from 1985 to 1993, San Pedro Sula reported 1,004 cases of AIDS, while Tegucigalpa reported 371 cases out of the 2,510 identified in the country. Comayagua, the fourth largest city in the country, reported 58 cases.[154] It hardly seemed an epicenter for the disease. Some specialists argued AIDS was introduced into San Pedro Sula "by Caribbean sailors long before there were military maneuvers on U.S. bases in the west of the country."[155]

The idea that the contra army might have spread the virus in Honduras has also been undercut by the Nicaraguan experience. With the end of the war the contras were repatriated and reincorporated into Nicaraguan society. But this failed to bring with it a sharp rise in the incidence of HIV/AIDS, in part because careful study proved that few contras were infected.

It has been feared that the return of large numbers of Nicaraguans from countries where HIV and AIDS are more prevalent than in Nicaragua could have a significant impact on the development of the AIDS epidemic. Sera collected from Nicaraguan refugee camps in San Salvador during 1984 revealed no cases of anti-HIV seropositivity in 182 samples. In Nicaragua, testing for antibody to HIV was performed during the process of demobilization and repatriation, but coverage was not complete because of the voluntary nature of testing and intermittent lack of testing kits. Of the 6,002 Contras screened, only one had confirmed HIV infection. Around 13,000 people have been officially repatriated from Honduras, half of whom are less than 15 years of age. Four adults, two men and two women, who reported themselves as heterosexual have been found to be seropositive.[156]

The locations of the contra camps also did not match the areas with high incidence of HIV. As Nicola Low and her colleagues noted, about "60% of the people with AIDS in Honduras are from the seven largest cities and towns in central and north western Honduras. Contras and their families lived in rural towns and military camps on the southern border with Nicaragua, where the impact of AIDS has been less."[157] The Honduran AIDS epidemic began in the north, while the contra camps lay in the south.[158] The return of the contras proved not to bring a major AIDS epidemic to Nicaragua.

Indeed, Nicaragua's HIV rate remains the lowest in Central America, despite the rapid privatization of the health care system after the Sandinistas lost an election in February 1990. In less than three years after the Sandinistas left power, the funds for public health "declined by 40 percent, in line with a Structural Adjustment Plan imposed by the International Monetary Fund."[159] In 1995 Nicaragua was "the poorest country in Central America and its economy was continuing to deteriorate."[160] The general level of AIDS education and awareness in Nicaragua in the early 1990s was not high, as "over 40 percent of adults in Managua think that HIV can be spread through public toilets, by sharing drinking vessels, or by mosquitos."[161] There have been concerns that the confidentiality of test results in Nicaragua was not maintained. The Ministry of Education opposed handing out condoms in schools because it might lead to promiscuity. The Catholic Church in Nicaragua also fought hard against condom use. Government officials criticized homosexuals, while the "Minister of Health himself recently claimed that AIDS was not an issue for Nicaraguans, only for foreigners."[162] For all these reasons, Nicaragua would have seemed to have been a country terribly vulnerable to HIV/AIDS.[163]

Despite these facts, the first case of AIDS did not appear in Nicaragua until 1987, and in 1994 "Nicaragua had the lowest number of cases of HIV/AIDS in Central America and the lowest prevalence and incidence of HIV/AIDS in Latin America."[164] In 1995 the nation had reported 117 cases of AIDS.[165] The disease largely remained confined to the capital of Managua, which had 57 percent of the total cases.[166] In 2003 UNAIDS reported that the HIV seroprevalence rate among adults was 0.2 percent.[167] One study in 2003 found that the HIV rate among commercial sex workers was only 0.3 percent, and in the capital the rate was 0 percent.[168] Given the similarities between Nicaragua and its northern neighbor Honduras, this continuing low level of HIV infection appears mysterious. One argument has been that isolation imposed by the war may explain Nicaragua's low rate of HIV/AIDS.

The relationship between rates of AIDS cases and U.S. involvement in the countries of Central America suggests that the ten years of low-intensity warfare raged by the United States against Nicaragua delayed the arrival of HIV. This effect is in direct contrast to observations of the spread of the virus in Central and Southern Africa. In Uganda, which has the highest number of AIDS cases in Africa, recruitment practices and subsequent troop movements explain much of the variation in AIDS case rates among districts. Social disruption and the growth of prostitution around military camps are proposed as factors that will propagate HIV infection in countries such as Mozambique and Angola which have had low intensity wars. Nevertheless, the incidence of AIDS in these two countries is currently much lower than in central Africa and it could therefore be argued that, as in Nicaragua, the entry of HIV has been delayed by the isolation experienced by these countries.[169]

The civil wars of Central America in the 1980s do seem to have shaped the epidemic, but not in the manner that might have been expected. The two countries in the region that currently have the highest incidence of HIV are Panama and Belize, neither of which experienced the years of warfare that their neighbors in El Salvador, Nicaragua, and Guatemala endured.[170]

The connection between warfare and AIDS in Central America remains complex. It is unclear if U.S. soldiers helped to introduce the virus to Honduras, although if that was the case, there should have been more infections in the areas where the troops were stationed. The U.S. military also monitors HIV rates among servicemen and -women, and no studies have indicated a high incidence of seropositivity among troops stationed in Central America. One of the most mysterious aspects of AIDS is its ability to devastate one country, such as Honduras, while a statistically and culturally similar neighbor escapes its wrath. There is no clear explanation for why the HIV/AIDS epidemic in Honduras emerged so early or cut such an aggressive path through the population of young heterosexuals.[171] It seems likely, however, that war not only isolated Nicaragua from the virus for a decade but also may have slowed the virus's spread elsewhere in the region. If so, that effect is now gone.

Honduras is making a successful effort to address its epidemic. In 1995 the Ministry of Health predicted that between "10% and 17% of sexually active adults" in San Pedro Sula would by HIV-positive in 2000. This did not happen.[172] Instead the government's efforts managed to slow, but not stop, the transmission of the virus despite multiple challenges.[173] By the late 1990s the government realized the urgency of the situation and responded vigorously to contain the epidemic: "In 1998, the HIV/AIDS department designed the first national strategic plan, incorporating extensive multisectoral participation by people living with HIV/AIDS, various sectors of government, civil society, chambers of commerce and the religious sector. In 1999, the Honduran government passed legislation to protect the rights of people with HIV/AIDS."[174] This energetic response, combined with the obvious scale of the problem, drew support from international aid organizations, such as USAID. The Honduran government began to provide antiretroviral treatment for pregnant women in 2000, then sought to expand this program to HIV-positive people attending public health services in 2001.[175]

In 2002 the Honduran government launched a major effort to fight AIDS with the help of the United Nations. Kofi Annan spoke at the inauguration of the national AIDS forum in Honduras and described its promise: "The launching of this forum is precisely the type of innovative response that we need to fight this epidemic."[176] Major problems remain, as one "study in three urban prisons in Honduras has revealed HIV prevalence of almost 7% among male prisoners in general, and almost 5% among those aged sixteen to twenty years."[177] In 2003 1.6 percent of all adults were HIV-positive, according to UNAIDS.[178] Such figures show the potential that the virus has to rapidly expand from a distinct group. As such, Honduras serves both as a sign of hope and a warning. It illustrates how quickly the disease can emerge and how it may still be possible for a government to address this crisis. No longer is Honduras the epicenter of the virus in the region. In 2003 the government spent 18.9 percent of its budget on health care, which represented a respectable commitment for such a poor country.[179] The focus of the disease has moved.

■ Elsewhere in Central America

HIV/AIDS is now making significant inroads in many Central American nations. In Belize the first AIDS case was not reported until 1986. But the virus has quickly spread into the most populated areas. The adult HIV prevalence rate was 2 percent in 2003. Most cases are transmitted through unprotected heterosexual sex.[180] This figure is disturbingly high and especially surprising given that Belize was the country in Central America that was most isolated from violence during the civil wars of the late 1970s and 1980s.

In contrast, Costa Rica has done relatively well, even though its strong social welfare system has not exempted the country from all the problems of its neighbors. Costa Rica has a significant problem with a transnational sex trade industry, patronized by pedophiles from the developed world.[181] The nation is also dealing with a major problem with street children, of whom perhaps 16 percent are from other countries. Of these children a large percentage (71 percent, according to one study) report that they are "sexually exploited."[182] Costa Rica responded very slowly to the emergence of the disease: "The Ministry of Health did not allocate funds to combat AIDS in 1986 and 1987 on the assumption that AIDS was a small problem compared to others."[183] Nor did the government make AIDS education a priority. As late as 1988, one study found that nothing "is being done to educate male and female sex workers on prevention of AIDS infection."[184] This may explain why that year the majority of Costa Rican women surveyed did not know that condoms were a good means to prevent AIDS.[185] The disease was also accompanied by discrimination by both the medical profession and the Ministry of Health, which caused great suffering within the gay community. Gays have tried to organized and fight back.[186]

Tim Frasca's work describes how one HIV/AIDS organization in Costa Rica drew admiration throughout the region. When it imploded, however, no organization stepped forward to replace it. The network of NGOS that work with HIV/AIDS remains weak in the country.[187] The Costa Rican government's priorities do not seem to have improved with time. In 2001 Frasca interviewed people working with HIV/AIDS in Costa Rica who conveyed the sense of apathy within the government: "On the official side, Carlos Valerio, who pushes the AIDS issue from within the government, calls the second half of the 1990s a 'black hole' for AIDS, a time in which prevention work essentially came to a halt. A very recent national AIDS plan was finally drawn up sometime in 2000, but the admirably complete document may not be taken very seriously by those who count: one government official lent me the office's only copy and asked me to be sure to bring it back later."[188] Much time and energy that could have been spent fighting the disease was instead wasted fighting against homophobia. Costa Rica was hardly the model of an enlightened response to the disease.

Despite these factors, HIV/AIDS continues to spread more slowly in Costa Rica than in its neighbors. The adult seroprevalence rate was only 0.6 percent in 2003.[189] It is difficult to explain this success, given clear weaknesses in Costa Rica's response to the virus, except to say that this may indicate the powerful effect that a strong public health system can have upon the spread of the virus, even in a relatively poor developing country. Costa Rica is unique in the region in having a universal social security system, while "free medical services are provided to the whole rural population. A network of modern hospitals and clinics serves the whole territory, but there is tolerance of private medicine. Current health indicators place Costa Rica closer to the industrial countries than to the less developed countries."[190] As part of this strong health response, Costa Rica provides HIV/AIDS medications to all people with HIV. This policy was adopted because a court ruling required the government to do so, not because the government made fighting HIV a priority.[191] It may be that the nation's social welfare net has limited the spread of HIV, even in the absence of a specific government commitment to fight the disease.

On the other hand, El Salvador has also maintained a relatively low rate of infection, with only 0.6 percent of all adults estimated to be living with HIV in 2003.[192] This physically small nation was home to 6.4 million people that year, who faced the lingering effects of the war, economic difficulties, and severe income inequality. Yet the virus had failed to spread as rapidly as in some neighboring countries. The official government reports illustrate that "between 1984 and June 2001, infection rates among high-risk groups ranged from 10 percent among commercial sex workers to 6 percent among sexually transmitted infection (STI) patients. A seroprevalence study conducted at the national maternity hospital in 2001 measured a 1 percent HIV infection rate among pregnant women. HIV infection among blood donors is thought to be low."[193] Another study reported in 2003 that the seropositivity rate for sex workers was 3.7 percent in port cities and 3.5 percent in the capital.[194] The virus clearly had the potential for rapid spread. But the government's response to the disease was neither energetic nor enlightened. Until 2002, when a Supreme Court ruling struck down the relevant statute, El Salvador's AIDS law required people applying for a job to provide the results of a mandatory AIDS test.[195] Yet, until now, the virus has not expanded in El Salvador as it has in Panama or Belize. Like Nicaragua, El Salvador seems to have somehow been protected from an acceleration of the virus during the civil war, which may have delayed the introduction of the disease.

In 2003 Panama reported an HIV seroprevalence rate of 1.5 percent, according to UNAIDS. That same year the country spent 18.5 percent of its government budget on health care.[196] Many of the early efforts at AIDS education were impeded by stereotypes and discrimination. One AIDS education book, reprinted five times by the Ministry of Education, contained poster-like images of a scheming prostitute (the mental tag-line read, "He doesn't imagine that I have AIDS") and threatened families.[197] Since the mid-1990s, the nation has made significant efforts to control the virus, but these measures have come too slowly. Sex workers are required to take regular tests for HIV, and their employers are responsible to make sure this happens.[198] According to PASCA (Proyeto Acción SIDA de Centroamérica), in 1999 Panama's Social Security board decided "to provide HAART to all beneficiaries infected with HIV/AIDS."[199] In 2001 the Ministry of Health budgeted $2.1 million to provide HAART to people living with HIV/AIDS. The private sector has also become involved with the creation of a National AIDS Business Council.[200] Even so, the Panamanian government has perhaps been less successful than Honduras in containing the virus.

The virus also seems to be making quicker headway in Guatemala, where in 2003, 1 percent of all adults were seropositive, according to UNAIDS. This nation of nearly 12 million people is also struggling to overcome the debilitating effects of its civil war. It has also faced a major challenge from the Catholic Church, which early in the epidemic fought AIDS education campaigns with particular vehemence. In 1997 the Church successfully halted the government's effort to launch a major AIDS campaign:

MEXICO AND CENTRAL AMERICA

The program's initial phase consisted of raising the general population's consciousness of the dangers and nature of the disease, achieving marked success. The campaign was set to begin giving instruction on preventative techniques, however certain religious elements are opposed to the campaign's promotion of condom use. Thus, continued funding was suspended pending further debate. According to AIDS educator Laura Asturias, "religious fundamentalism is taking hold in some government sectors and in educational centers in an overwhelming way."[201]

Still, Guatemala's Catholic Church is not a monolith, and progress has been made. In 2002 Frasca found one part of the Guatemalan Church that had "an active and enthusiastic program addressing the issue (HIV), a program that consciously attempts to break out of the church's traditional care-provision role in the health sphere to include discussions of prevention and at least some of sexuality."[202] Such action is clearly needed. In 2003 one report found that in the port of San José 8.7 percent of commercial sex workers were HIV-positive, while in the capital the rate was 4.2 percent. The same report stated 11.5 percent of gay men were seropositive.[203]

Guatemala has made some progress to fight the disease. A recent law "requires the Ministry of Education to integrate HIV/AIDS/STI information into school curricula, beginning in the fifth grade."[204] The Ministry of Public Health has also launched a number of significant initiatives to control the disease. In 2002, "President Portillo passed an executive order approving emergency funds (Q 500,000) to purchase ARV's for PLWHA [people living with HIV/AIDS] attending public health services."[205] But so far the scale of funds and effort has proved far too small. The government has dragged its feet on providing these medications.[206] Guatemala has the largest number of AIDS orphans in Central America.[207] It is significant that Guatemala spent only 14 percent of its annual government budget on health care in 2003, while Belize spent 10.4 percent. El Salvador spent 22 percent, and Nicaragua spent 22.3 percent, which was more even than Costa Rica at 20.7 percent.[208] These differences may be a major factor in explaining discrepancies in the region's epidemic. Since Guatemala has the largest population in Central America, there are real reasons for concern about the future of the HIV/AIDS epidemic in that country.[209]

The reasons why the epidemic may have become unusually severe in Central America are manifold. In part, there are high levels of mobility in the region, with the exception of those countries isolated by the civil wars of the 1980s: "Increased mobility along the region's highways and industrial corridors has exacerbated the spread of the epidemic. Central America has a history of interregional and extra-regional migration due to civil unrest, demand for seasonal labor, more open border policies, improved regional transportation routes, and proximity to the United States."[210] Many migrants have been pushed into sex work. One study, which examined Mexico's southern border, found that "93 per cent of sex workers were undocumented migrants from Central America, who stay in the country for about three months. Their clients included truck drivers, military men, customs and local security agents, all of whom are mobile populations."[211]

There is a series of transit points throughout Central America where young, poorly educated migrants spend time on their journey. One thorough study interviewed migrants in these areas from Chetumal, Mexico, to Mercado Central, Panama. One clear theme that emerged was the vulnerability of women:

> Violence, poverty, and corruption by border authorities and police are common to all the transit stations. Deportees reported mistreatment and violence more frequently, whereas those in (the) process of migrating were more likely to comment on their migration experience and expectations. Women are often forced to exchange sex in order to cross borders, and these same authorities demand cash from others attempting to cross. In this environment, transactional sex, survival and non-consensual sex are carried out in conditions that place individuals at risk of HIV infection; condom use is infrequent. These situations tend to affect migrant women who are already vulnerable for other reasons.[212]

Sadly, this same study reported not only that most women on the journey reported having nonconsensual sex while migrating, but also that in all of the transit areas the locals blamed the migrants for social problems such as drugs and sex work. Many female migrants become victims of human traffickers. One Guatemalan study found a large number of Salvadoran sex workers within the country.[213] Migrant women are attractive to human traffickers because they have left their social networks and no one will report them missing. The level of AIDS education among migrants is also painfully low, as some "agricultural workers reported that alcohol and perfume applied to the penis will prevent HIV transmission."[214] As in Mexico, migrants are heavily stigmatized at a same time when it is increasingly important to undertake AIDS prevention efforts in this population. If Central America is to address this problem, it must undertake a multilateral effort that extends beyond the region itself.

■ Reasons for Hope

Central American nations are collaborating around the effort to bring anti-retroviral drugs to the people who need them. Great progress has been made, as "in 2002, each country (with the exception of Nicaragua) covered in the Central American regional program (of USAID) expanded the numbers of people with access to antiretroviral treatment through both the social security institutes and the Ministry of Health. Costa Rica and Panama have the highest coverage as more than 90 percent of HIV-infected individuals qualify for assistance. The Global Fund to Fight AIDS, Tuberculosis, and Malaria will begin disbursements to Honduras and has approved proposals from Costa Rica, Nicaragua, and El Salvador."[215] For these efforts to succeed, however, the question of cost had to be addressed. For this reason the countries of the region came together to begin multilateral negotiations with major producers of medications. In 2003 Central America reached an agreement with five pharmaceutical companies to reduce the cost of antiretroviral drugs by 55 percent.[216] Some commentators have questioned whether the Free Trade Area of the Americas will privilege intellectual property over patients and threaten the ability of the poor to gain access to the medicines they need.[217] The drugs also remained very expensive for poor countries. The agreement "will lower the cost of treatment per patient in Central America—now between US$2500 and US$2800—to between US$1035 and US$1453, the health secretaries of the six Central American nations announced."[218] Yet the cost of providing antiretrovirals remains the largest component of the AIDS budget of most countries.[219] And these drugs still cost much more than they do in Brazil, which means that health care providers in nations such as Guatemala will perhaps continue to have to make terrible choices.

> Twenty-six children, age 2 months to 11 years, live in Mauricio's hospice, a modest home on a residential street on the outskirts of Antigua. A dozen adult patients are also at the facility. The hospice

receives private funding and donations, so every child with HIV can be given the so-called AIDS cocktail of medications, currently the most effective treatment. But since the drugs cost $800 to $1000 a month per person, hospice officials say they can rarely afford to give them to adults. Sofia Lopez, 26, a mother with AIDS lays dying without medicine. Doctors said her infection had progressed to her brain. She can no longer speak. She nods and holds up fingers to answer questions. When Lopez feels strong enough, she holds and kisses her 3 month old daughter, ANA. The baby smiles and kicks the air, her brown hair framed by a white bonnet, as doctors explain she is months away from being another AIDS orphan.[220]

It is true that the countries of this region are trying to create a unified effort to fight HIV/AIDS. At the current time only Costa Rica provides anti-retroviral medications to all HIV-positive people. El Salvador has a new law that provides "limited access," while Honduras, Panama, and Guatemala have limited coverage.[221] In Belize and Nicaragua "access through public health systems is negligible."[222]

The contrast between Mexico and Central America is striking. Mexico's epidemic remains at relatively low levels because of good government policy, cultural factors such as a low rate of injecting drug use, and the aggressive efforts of NGOs. The disease, however, seems to be making inroads into rural areas, driven in part by migration. The question remains what the future will be for this key Latin American nation. Central America perhaps provides us with some insights. In this region the epidemic fractured because of a variety of factors, one of which is that the civil wars of the 1980s may have isolated some countries, such as Nicaragua, and delayed the introduction of the virus. But the epidemic has spread much more widely in Central America than in most Latin American nations. One key factor may be migration, which is also critical in the Mexican experience. One implication from the epidemic's history is that no country in isolation can address the epidemic, given the importance of international factors, whether it be reaching migrants on their journey to the United States or presenting a common front to negotiate lower drug prices from the major pharmaceutical companies. The region will need to unite to fight to contain this disease.

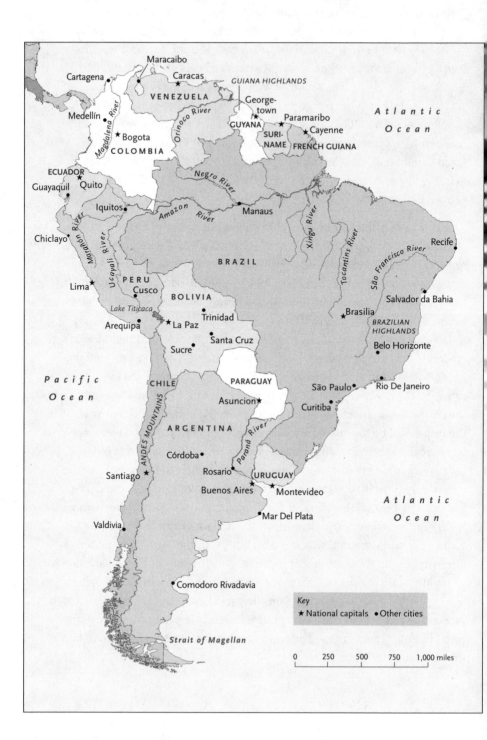

Cartagena

Maracaibo

Caracas

GUIANA HIGHLANDS

VENEZUELA

Medellín

Orinoco River

Georgetown

Paramaribo

Atlantic

Ocean

GUYANA

Bogota

Magdalena River

SURI-
NAME

Cayenne

COLOMBIA

FRENCH GUIANA

ECUADOR

Quito

Negro River

Guayaquil

Iquitos

Amazon River

Manaus

Chiclayo

Marañón River

Ucayali River

Xingu River

Tocantins River

São Francisco River

Recife

BRAZIL

Lima

PERU

Cusco

Salvador da Bahia

Lake Titicaca

BOLIVIA

Trinidad

Brasilia

Arequipa

La Paz

BRAZILIAN
HIGHLANDS

Sucre

Santa Cruz

Belo Horizonte

Pacific

Ocean

CHILE

PARAGUAY

São Paulo

Rio De Janeiro

ANDES MOUNTAINS

Asuncion

Curitiba

ARGENTINA

Paraná River

Córdoba

Santiago

Rosario

URUGUAY

Buenos Aires

Montevideo

Atlantic

Ocean

Valdivia

Mar Del Plata

Comodoro Rivadavia

Key

★ National capitals   ● Other cities

Strait of Magellan

0   250   500   750   1,000 miles

SPANISH SOUTH AMERICA

*Early in 1998 the Brazilian player Eduardo Esidio arrived in
Peru with the intention of playing for an important club such
as the Universitario de Deportes. He submitted to an HIV test,
among other medical exams, without knowing what was being
done, and was informed of the results at a meeting at which
there were present the doctors, the president of the club, and the
Argentine trainer. According to Esidio, they said to him that he
could not play in Peru. Stunned by the news, the player traveled
to Brazil. His absence was the excuse for the team authorities
of the sports club to try to rescind his contract. Afterwards, with
commendable courage, Esidio returned to Lima in order to make
them respect the contract, something to which the club finally
agreed. In little time, the athlete became one of the best Peruvian
soccer players and one of the symbols of the struggle against the
discrimination that people living with HIV suffer.*[1]

In Spanish South America the HIV/AIDS epidemic is characterized by a division between two regions. On one hand, there
are the Andean nations, which are defined by PAHO as Bolivia,
Colombia, Ecuador, Peru, and Venezuela. In most of these
countries the disease has not spread as rapidly to women as
elsewhere in Latin America, and the core of the epidemic remains men who have sex with men. This latter group counted
for 46.4 percent of all AIDS cases in the Andean nations in
2002.[2] On the other hand, in the countries of the Southern
Cone (defined by PAHO as Argentina, Chile, Paraguay, and
Uruguay) the epidemic was much more diverse.[3] On the sur-

face this disparity is rather surprising, in particular because relatively developed countries such as Argentina have a higher incidence of HIV than less-developed countries such as Bolivia. Part of the explanation for this disparity (which may now be changing) may lie in part in the global drug trade and how it has affected countries in the region.

The countries that supply cocaine to the world market (Peru, Bolivia, and Ecuador) are some of the poorest in Latin America. Colombia is relatively wealthier and serves not only as a producer but also as a distributor. These nations tend not to have high rates of IV drug use. Colombia has an emerging problem with basuco, a waste product from the production of cocaine, which is used to give a high. But this product is highly impure, is less attractive to the upscale market, and is not injected. According to PAHO, injecting drug use accounts for only 0.2 percent of all cases of AIDS in the Andean region—a fifth of 1 percent.[4] This figure is not likely to remain so low, particularly in Colombia. But the region's role in the drug trade has clearly been defined as a supplier for wealthier nations within the Americas and Europe, and consumption has not yet made a major impact on the region's drug epidemic. Instead, the poverty and drug violence of the region, which during the 1980s and 1990s helped to fuel not only the Shining Path in Peru but also the bitter drug wars of Colombia, has isolated Andean nations. Neither Peru nor Colombia has had tourism flows or investment commensurate with its offerings and opportunities, while Bolivia is not a major site for foreign investment. Much like the civil wars in Central America and southern Africa during the 1980s, this instability and violence in the Andes may have initially isolated these countries and delayed the initial spread of HIV, although the Colombian experience suggests that this pattern may not hold true for the future.

The countries of the Southern Cone have had a different experience both with the drug trade and with HIV. Some of these countries, such as Chile, Uruguay, and Paraguay, are not major drug producers, while the latter two nations are only moderate drug consumers. As such they have so far been largely untouched by the violence and challenges that the drug trade has brought to Andean nations. On the other hand, there is Argentina, which has an HIV epidemic that has been driven by IV drug use, much like its neighbor Brazil. The size of Argentina's population makes injecting drug use the single largest category for exposure among AIDS cases in the Southern Cone and skews the statistics for the entire region. According to PAHO, 34.3 percent of all AIDS cases in the Southern Cone are a result of IV drug use, the single largest category for exposure.[5] This is approximately 170 times the rate for this category in Andean nations, where the comparable figure is 0.2 percent. And this is true even though some Southern Cone nations (such as Chile) have a relatively minor problem with iv drug use. Overall, in the Southern Cone the hiv/aids epidemic has moved more quickly into the heterosexual population, and women tend to represent a larger percentage of infections. In this respect, the position of nations in the continent's drug trade may be one factor that helps to drive the regional epidemiology of hiv/aids.

■ Spanish South America: The Andean States

The Andes run down the western edge of South America, from Colombia in the north to Tierra del Fuego in the south. The Andes are the longest mountain range on earth, and their average height is staggering, as "thirty-two peaks exceed 20,000 feet."[6] Bordered by the great grasslands (llanos and pampas) in Colombia, Venezuela, and Argentina as well as by the Amazon River for most of their central range, the Andes have long divided South America into two cultural regions. The Andes have been home to a plethora of civilizations over thousands of years, of which the Inca are but the most well known. The dark images in the pottery of the Moche, the stunning goldwork of the Chibcha, and the vast ruins of Tihuanaco testify to the cultural wealth of this land. The fact that the Andes fractured the landscape into microclimates, so that geographically proximate regions could support production of everything from tropical fruits to herds of Alpine guanacos, created opportunities for rich networks of trade. The dense human populations, combined with the mineral wealth of the Andes, made this region attractive to Spanish conquistadors who did not yet know how to conquer the Amazon or to dominate the nomadic peoples of the pampas. The Andes would be the focus of Spanish administration and settlement in South America for three centuries.

The legacy of Spanish imperial rule would be Andean societies characterized by social conservatism, great disparities in wealth, a highly unequal system of land distribution, and a racial caste system in which politics was dominated by people of European decent, while the bottom of the social ladder was held by a rural and impoverished native class, which mostly was ignored by the state, except for regular demands for labor services.

This legacy has fueled political instability and social unrest throughout the twentieth century. Indeed, as Orin Starn has argued, while anthropologists continued to focus on the rich cultural heritage of the Andes throughout the 1980s, they largely ignored the social suffering and state neglect that was the most important aspect of the area's experience during this period.[7] This neglect was particularly true in the cases of Ecuador, Colombia, and Peru.

The heart of Spanish colonial rule in South America, Peru remained a quintessentially conservative society after independence. By the early twentieth century, key groups refused to continue to accept their marginal position in Peruvian society, and their resentments gave rise in the 1930s to clashes between a quasi-Marxist movement, the Apristas, and the Peruvian army. These struggles swelled, so that by the mid-1960s the government was fighting a brutal conflict with peasant guerrillas. In 1968 the military seized power, in large measure in order to carry out the social reforms that officers believed were necessary to prevent a revolution. The regime implemented land reform, enacted measures to win the support of the peasantry, and tried to organize the squatter settlements surrounding Lima. Yet these measures failed to end violent political dissent. In 1980 a guerrilla movement called Sendero Luminoso, the Shining Path, appeared in Ayacucho under the leadership of Abimail Guzmán, a charismatic philosophy professor. A violent group, heavily influenced by Maoism, its influence quickly spread so that by 1990 it seemed that it might succeed in overthrowing the state. It was soon joined by a second guerrilla group, the Movimento Revolucionario Túpac Amaru, which had stronger ties in urban areas. Simultaneously, the drug industry continued to organized and grow in rural Peru, where it forged alliances not only with Sendero Luminoso but also with corrupt factions within the state itself.

This guerrilla threat was ultimately smashed with state violence under President Alberto Fujimori, who was elected in 1990. His ruthless and successful campaign initially won him great popularity, even after he closed the congress in 1992. In the end, however, Fujimori's government proved so corrupt that he fled to Japan, which then refused to extradite him to face criminal charges in Peru. His neoliberal reforms also weakened the state as it faced threats such as a cholera epidemic in 1991 and a growing problem with multi-drug-resistant tuberculosis, which reflected the general level of social suffering.[8] This political context influenced the epidemic of HIV/AIDS in Peru. One might have expected that HIV/AIDS would not have been a high priority for the state. It is surprising, therefore, that in the midst of this chaos the government's public health service continued to work, and Peru has implemented what is widely seen as an effective anti-HIV/AIDS program.

Although Peru is a major producer of coca (the raw material for cocaine), Colombia controls the distribution networks for cocaine, which mean that the drug trade has profound implications for Colombian society. Colombia likely has the bloodiest history in twentieth-century South America. At the end of the War of a Thousand Days (1899–1903) the country had lost more than 100,000 lives and was too exhausted to withstand U.S. expansionism. President Theodore Roosevelt supported a political revolution in Panama in 1904 that created a new nation, so that the United States could build a canal across the isthmus. While the bitterness over this loss fed nationalist sentiments in Colombia, the nation remained polarized between the liberal and conservative parties. When the presidential candidate for the liberal party, Jorge Eliecer Gaitán, was murdered in Bogotá on April 9, 1948, there were massive riots, and widespread violence in the countryside killed perhaps 300,000 people before 1957. In some sense, the violence never truly ended. President Alvaro Uribe came to power in May 2002 and implemented an aggressive military policy to defeat the guerrilla insurgency, with support from international donors of which the United States is the most important. The government has had to fight not only powerful guerrilla organizations such as the FARC (Revolutionary Armed Forces of Colombia), which dates back to the 1960s, but also right-wing paramilitary organizations founded in the 1980s. The ensuing conflict has created a society that suffers from random violence, widespread kidnapings, internal refugees, and political terror.[9]

All of these problems have been exacerbated by the drug trade. Colombia has a tradition as a smuggling center that dates back to the colonial period, when it was a source for black market emeralds. With the rise of cocaine during the 1970s, Colombians moved to dominate the distribution of this product. According to the U.S. government Colombian "traffickers still provide 90 percent of the cocaine used in the United States and 50 percent of the heroin," although much of the raw product may be created in Peru or Bolivia.[10] During the early 1990s, the Colombian state first fought and won a war with drug lord Pablo Escobar, then managed to cripple the Cali cartel. This was a terrifying period in Colombian history, when Escobar exploded car bombs outside government buildings in Bogotá in order to break the will of the state. Ordinary Colombians seemed exhausted and confused by the violence when I was in Bogotá in June and July 1993. They appeared less frightened by the car bomb campaign than the constant stories of random violence, which ensnared ordinary people who offended the wrong group or took an unlucky turn on a rural road. Escobar's death in 1993 was a victory for the government, but it failed to end Colombia's civil war. New drug lords continued not only to smuggle increasing amounts of cocaine but also to corrupt senior government officials. In part because drug traffickers contributed to President Ernesto Samper's election campaign, the United States twice decertified Colombia under the Foreign Assistance Act during the 1990s.[11]

The Colombian government's struggle with its enemies has been made much more difficult by the complex ties between the drug lords and all political actors in Colombia; thus a military solution to the conflict is elusive.[12] The Colombian military claims that it needs U.S. aid to fight the guerrillas, whom it alleges are in alliance with the drug lords. In March 1998 General Harold Bedoya Pizzaro, former chief of the armed forces, stated that the armed forces were the only part of the state untouched by the drug trade.[13] Moreover, he argued that the guerrillas were in fact in the cocaine business. Reputedly, the guerrillas received $600 million a year for guarding drug crops in their territory. General Fernando Tapias, then commander of the Colombian armed forces, made a similar argument in July 1999, when he claimed that the rebels' drug wealth gave them an advantage over the military. For this reason, he argued that Colombia needed U.S. support to fight the drug wars.[14] The Colombian army has successfully employed this argument to justify requests for U.S. military aid into the new millennium, by equating the guerrillas they fight with the drug trade the United States opposes.

The challenge, however, is that factions of the armed forces are also involved in the cocaine trade, both directly and in alliance with paramilitary organizations. These paramilitary groups are generally led by large landholders, such as ranchers, who are particularly powerful in northwestern Colombia. Some of these organizations have turned to drugs to finance themselves, according even to U.S. officials. A series of scandals suggests that senior generals have links not only with the paramilitaries but also with the cocaine trade. President Samper survived an impeachment attempt following allegations that he accepted campaign funds from drug lords. Then, on a 1996 trip to New York, his presidential jet was found to hold four kilos of cocaine, which led to the arrest of three air force officers. In November 1998 a Colombian c-130 air force plane landed in Fort Lauderdale, Florida, with 600 kilos of cocaine.[15] The security chief for the air force base in Bogotá was arrested, along with several other members of the air force. General Jose Manuel Sandoval, the minister of the air force, resigned after denying the existence of a "blue cartel," a reference to air force involvement in drug smuggling. In March 1997 even the Colombian defense minister, Guillermo Alberto Gonzalez, had to resign after revelations concerning his ties to a drug trafficker.[16] Of course, some time has passed since these embarrassing revelations. President Alvaro Uribe has a reputation for honest administration and ruthless will that has served him well in the struggle with guerrillas and the drug lords. But the narcotics trade remains a national problem that forces every Colombian president to make compromises. Uribe's recent deal with the paramilitaries gives them amnesties for their crimes and allows them to keep funds raised through drug trafficking. And both the guerrillas and the paramilitaries remain powerful political actors.

Despite the more than $3 billion that the United States has spent on Plan Colombia (an effort to strengthen the Colombian state and attack the drug trade), cocaine production in Colombia has not declined. Massive aerial spraying of weed killer on coca plants has not put a dent in exports, which supporters of this policy term a "paradox" but Colombians explain in practical terms: "General Jorge Daniel Castro, director of the Colombian national police and one of Colombia's primary experts on the issue, described the Plan Colombia drug-enforcement paradox as a 'complex phenomenon' but added when pressed that he believed the traffickers were simply replanting the coca and opium plants almost as soon as the spray planes left."[17] The end to Colombia's conflict may still not be in sight, and the large numbers of internal refugees, the areas of the countryside outside government control, the climate of violence that devalues human life, and the spread of drug consumption among Colombians themselves may all facilitate the spread of HIV/AIDS.

Like Peru and Colombia, Bolivia is a nation characterized by social inequalities and political instability. Famous in the colonial period for the immense wealth of the silver mines discovered in 1545 at Potosi, little of the funds from the silver remained in Bolivia, which is now one of the most impoverished countries in Latin America. In 1879 Chile and Bolivia went to war, a conflict that ended in 1882 with Chile annexing Bolivia's maritime territories, thereby leaving the nation landlocked and isolated. These two key historical facts dominate much of Bolivia's political debate to the present, as the nation discusses how to develop its natural gas resources and how that development might engage it with its old nemesis, Chile.[18] The country's indigenous majority (which speaks Aymara, Quechua, and Guarani, as well as Spanish) has argued that the production of this resource in alliance with multinational corporations will leave few benefits in Bolivia. The fact that the government planned to export the natural gas by means of a pipeline through Chile (for export to Mexico and the United States) only exacerbated resentments, which grew so severe as to raise the question of the nation's territorial integrity.[19] In October 2003 widespread protests forced President Gonzalo Sánchez de Losada to resign. He was replaced by President Carlos Mesa, a conservative politician who has sought to reach out to the nation's indigenous population, which supported the popular protests.[20]

The debate over natural gas development grew so bitter because it overlay older divisions within Bolivian society. The indigenous majority has long perceived itself as being neglected by the government. Bolivia is likely the largest producer of coca in the Andes, and many poor, rural communities rely on this crop. In the past, the Bolivian government often lacked the will to fight the drug trade. Indeed, in 1980 the Bolivian military seized power in the "cocaine-coup," which was so named because of close ties between senior officers and drug traffickers, who exchanged protection for profits.[21] A democracy since 1982, Bolivia now participates in coca crop eradication and spraying campaigns, but these measures have angered rural communities. Coca growers have formed an organized political movement that now holds considerable influence. In December 2005 Bolivians elected a nationalist president, Evo Morales, who had close ties to the coca growers. Like other Andean nations, the drug trade has had a significant impact on the nation and has exacerbated Bolivia's existing political problems. Nonetheless, the nation has been only lightly touched by the HIV pandemic and has perhaps the lowest incidence of HIV in the Americas.

Ecuador also has a significant native population that has emerged on the political stage to challenge the state, in particular around the development of the country's petroleum resources. Successive presidents—Abdalá Bucarem in 1997, Jamil Mahuad in January 2000, and Lucio Gutierrez in April 2005—fled the presidency in the face of popular discontent. As Allen Gerlach has described, at the root of this anger has been resentment within the native community about the exploitation of petroleum in the Amazon and how this has failed to benefit local communities.[22] Ecuador, however, has been more fortunate than some of its Andean neighbors, in that the drug war has had less of an impact. Ecuador does produce coca, but it is probably more important as a transshipment point for both cocaine and heroin, which often depart from the port cities of Guayaquil and Manta. The nation as a whole, however, has not witnessed the political violence and social tension that drugs have fostered in neighboring countries.[23] Until recently the HIV/AIDS epidemic seemed to be controlled in the country, despite some concern about rising numbers in port cities on the coast, but there are now hints that the epidemic may be moving to a new level.[24]

Of all Andean societies, Venezuela has perhaps been affected least by the drug trade, even though it remains a significant shipment site for cocaine and heroin. The nation's political debates and social issues have been shaped not by narcotics but by petroleum. A nation of 25 million people on the north coast of South America, Venezuela has a wealth of petroleum resources, but a large percentage of the population lives in poverty. Among the working class and the poor there has been a widespread perception that the political system and the state were corrupt, and that the funds from the nation's oil wealth have been misspent and wasted. This dissatisfaction created an opportunity for nationalist officer Hugo Chavez, who organized a coup in 1992 that failed. But after the president was forced from power for corruption in 1993, popular disgust with the nation's existing political leadership returned Chavez to the political arena, and he was elected president in 1998. He was reelected in 2000 to a six-year term and soon began a wide-ranging series of reforms that drew him into conflict with both the nation's traditional political leadership and the middle class. A drawn-out political crisis then ensued that climaxed when Chavez was overthrown by a coup on April 11, 2002, only to return to power three days later. This led to a general strike against Chavez and popular protests calling for a referendum on his presidency. When this referendum was held on August 15, 2004, Chavez emerged victorious. To his critics Chavez is a dangerous demagogue who represents a return to the worst traditions of Latin American populism. To his supporters, Chavez is the advocate of the poor who is attacked because of his willingness to reform a corrupt political system that has failed to benefit the indigent. Venezuela's recent political history has been characterized by uncertainty and conflict. But this unrest has not been driven by the drug trade, which has not had the same political impact in Venezuela as in other Andean nations. Venezuela is, however, similar to other Andean countries in that its HIV/AIDS epidemic does not seem to be driven by drug injectors, unlike many countries of the Southern Cone.

■ HIV/AIDS in the Andes: Men Who Have Sex with Men

The HIV/AIDS epidemic in the Andes is evolving, but it has remained one largely driven by men having sex with men: "As of May 2000, MSM [men who have sex with men] accounted for 42% of the total cumulative AIDS cases reported in the Andean region (Peru, Colombia, Venezuela, Ecuador and Bolivia) and had the highest prevalence rates."[25] Intravenous drug use remains a negligible factor in the disease's progression in the region.[26] It is difficult to believe, however, that the epidemic will remain confined to men having sex with men, because of research on sexual practices in Andean nations. One study in Peru found that a high percentage of men having sex with men also had sex with women. Although the rate of condom use was low, one of the study's striking findings was that in this group of men (442 men participated in the study) heterosexual sex was particularly unlikely to be always associated with condom use: "Of those who reported having sex with at least one woman in the last year, only a minority reported always using condoms: 10.5% of heterosexuals, 20.0% of bisexuals, and 18.5% of homosexuals."[27]

This fact places Andean wives at particular risk, as they are not aware of the need to negotiate safe sex with their husbands. In Colombia, Silvana Paternostro learned that "eighty percent of the wives who had tested HIV-positive at Bogotá's Simón Bolivar Hospital had been infected because of the bisexual activity of their husbands. Most of these women had married as virgins."[28] Paternostro's remarkable book, a study of sexuality and gender in Latin America, took as its starting place her own experience growing up in Barranquilla, Colombia, and the realization that the man she dated as a teenager likely also had sexual relationships with prostitutes or transvestites he met at a nightclub called El Gusano.[29] She sought to understand how Latin men, whose identity was defined in opposition to homosexuality (which they equated with effeminacy), could have sex with transvestites without this calling into question their identity. Sometimes the answer she received was surprisingly succinct: "I asked an epidemiologist in Bogotá if he had an explanation. He answered by citing a popular phrase: 'Soy tan

macho que me cojo otro hombre.' I am so macho, I even fuck another man."[30]
As her research continued, Paternostro was struck by the pervasiveness of this behavior: "'I have a client who comes around on Sundays pushing a stroller,' a teenage male prostitute tells me in Bogotá, 'usually around lunchtime. He leaves the baby and his wife at the restaurant and comes to me while they eat.'"[31]

The key to the acceptance of men having sex with men is social invisibility. These connections are made only in certain carefully prescribed times and places, which are kept entirely separate from most public events. In the same city where Paternostro grew up, it "was stipulated in the official decree of Barranquilla's Carnival that homosexuals were not allowed to participate in the grand Batalla de Flores, the official parade that opens the three days of uninterrupted and uninhibited celebration."[32] As a result there is a rich web of networks and spaces that are defined as gay, but they are often only identified as such at particular times. I saw this at a small, upper-class shopping mall in Bogotá in 1993. This building had several floors, each of which could be viewed from the escalators and waist-high walls ringing the central courtyard. As the day ended, families and women flowed out from the mall, while men continued to enter the building, either singly or in small groups. These men circled the floors and rode the escalators, while other men stood against the pillars and watched them. The transformation in the space was striking, but what left the deepest impression was not the peregrinations of the men but, rather, the hesitancy of the women and parents who briefly entered the space. At this moment, the locale was clearly defined as gay, and outsiders were uncomfortable, even though this was a public location in a Latin culture that sometimes showed severe discrimination against homosexuals. These spaces only remain invisible with the collusion of society as a whole. They may not be discussed, but everyone is aware of them.

HIV has spread widely through the gay community in South America. One study examined 13,847 men in seven South American countries. The highest rate of infection among men who have sex with men was found in Bolivia, which was also the country with the lowest rate of HIV as a whole. Even in countries in which the gay community may be the most hidden, HIV infects more than 10 percent of the population of men who have sex with men.[33] The linkages between the gay and bisexual community and broader society are widespread. In this context, there is no wall dividing the AIDS/HIV epidemic in the gay community from that in the straight. The male-to-female sex ratio remains higher in the Andes than in any other part of Latin America.[34] But what is most surprising is that it has taken so long for the epidemic to evolve outside this group in the Andean region, although this does seem to be happening, as the example of Colombia suggests.

■ Colombia and Peru

It is strange that it is harder to obtain information on HIV/AIDS in the Andes, with its large nations and significant populations, than in Central America. As Geeta Rao Gupta wrote in 2002, there "is relatively little HIV/AIDS trend data for the Andean Area of South America. The best data have been collected for Colombia and Peru. Relatively less is known about Bolivia, Ecuador and Venezuela."[35] For this reason, I will focus my discussion of the Andean region on the former two nations. Still, it remains difficult to gain information on these countries, in particular for Colombia. As the U.S. Census Bureau notes, there "is little information pertaining to the HIV epidemic in Colombia."[36] The ongoing violence and uncertainty have limited foreign assistance and rural fieldwork, so it is difficult to create a clear statistical picture of the HIV/AIDS epidemic in the country. We do know, however, that the face of the Colombian epidemic has been changing, and that the percentage of people acquiring the disease through unprotected heterosexual sex has been climbing.[37] It is also clear that the nation is at the forefront of the HIV epidemic in the region: "National statistics show that Colombia ranks first in the Andean region with a cumulative total of 17,785 HIV/AIDS cases to January 2000."[38] Colombia is the fourth largest country in South America, with a population of 45 million people. For these reasons, an understanding of the epidemic's history and some factors particular to the Colombian experience of HIV/AIDS is significant.

According the Ministry of Health, the first case of AIDS in Colombia was reported in 1983. The patient was a twenty-three-year-old woman who lived in the port city of Cali, where she served a clientele that included sailors.[39] Some of the other early patients had a clear connection to Africa. In 1984 two men from Zaire, friends who both worked for "an airline that covered African routes," developed HIV.[40] Sonia Goméz Goméz has described the medical hysteria that surrounded the treatment of the initial cases, which makes it clear that Colombia was not immune to the same terror witnessed everywhere else when the disease first surfaced. One member of the medical staff remembered how they obsessively rinsed a public phone used by an AIDS patient with a disinfectant so harsh that after eight days the phone company "almost killed me because the apparatus was ruined."[41] Other employees washed their hands until they were raw and painful. Goméz Goméz includes a photo of health personnel from this period in their improvised AIDS clothing, with gloves, boots, cap, and eyeglasses.[42] At this time the disease was largely confined to the homosexual community: "In 1987, 82.4% of cases corresponded to homosexuals, 14.7% bisexuals and 2.9% to heterosexuals."[43] The total numbers remained low. As of June 1990, 1,492 Colombians had tested HIV-positive, of which 711 had developed AIDS and 357 had died. Of these cases, 92 percent were men. Although many cases had been diagnosed in the capital, many parts of the country had reported the illness.[44]

The health services quickly rallied, and in some areas, such as Antioquia, they created sophisticated integrated services for people living with HIV.[45] In 1991 Colombia also enacted relatively enlightened legislation regarding HIV/AIDS.[46] But health workers and educators soon encountered the same challenges faced by others confronting AIDS. One problem was that information did not necessarily change behavior, given the constraints that people faced, as the experience one doctor had with a Colombian sex worker makes clear:

One day a prostitute came to the State Health Service for Antioquia in order to do the AIDS test. The doctor, very satisfied because the test was negative, sat down to chat with her in order to give her the good news and in order to instruct her how to practice safe sex to avoid being a future victim of the illness. When the professional stopped talking about the use of the condom, she stood up and said "Until later, doctor, we will see each other again when I am infected." Looking at his shocked face, she explained to him: "My clients don't like condoms and if I tell them that they can't use it, at my side they will find someone who will attend them without it. So, if I fall out of work, are you going to give me money to buy food for my kids?"[47]

Most sex workers did not have even this level of knowledge. One study found that in the capital, "57.5% of child sex workers did not have information about the illness. And among those that had received information, 45% had not understood it."[48] Nor was the lack of information confined to sex workers. Government research "done in 1993, based on answers from 18,000 Colombians, found that 54.5% did not know that AIDS caused death, and only half had knowledge that it was transmitted sexually."[49]

By 1993 the face of the Colombian HIV epidemic was already changing. That year 46.7 percent of all HIV infections were reported to have come through heterosexual sex. Over 40 percent of the total cases were reported in the capital, but only the departments in the far eastern llanos had not yet had any cases.[50] The disease was no longer confined to gay men or to urban areas. The continuing challenge that Colombia has faced has been that the guerrilla insurgency has placed sections of the countryside beyond the control of the state. There are large numbers of displaced persons, many of whom have gravitated to urban slums where few services are available. Rape has been used as an instrument of political terror, which also forces some internal refugees into sex work.[51] The drug industry has also begun to turn to the Colombian market to supplement its sales. In particular, HIV cases are beginning to appear among heroin users for the first time. Colombian "officials blame the increase on traffickers trying to create a local market for heroin they cannot smuggle into the United States, and perhaps a 1994 court ruling legalizing the personal use of narcotics."[52] Many street children use basuco, a drug that mixes cocaine with impurities from the production process. It causes rapid physical damage and undermines judgment, so users undertake risky acts. The social upheaval caused by violence and the drug trade has created conditions that can facilitate the spread of the virus. Research has found that the HIV rate is significantly higher among people who have been forced to flee their home areas because of the fighting: "In Sucre and Cordoba it has been found that one out of every 100 displaced people is living with HIV. Research into these areas is in its infancy in this country. Ricardo Garcia, UNAIDS adviser in Colombia says that there is almost a direct relationship between the spread of the virus and the conflict."[53] For this reason, the Global Fund to Fight AIDS, Tuberculosis, and Malaria is focusing its funding in Colombia on displaced persons: "The overall goal of the project is to reduce the vulnerability of 600,000 adolescents and youths to STIs, HIV and AIDS, in 86 localities in 48 municipalities involved in situations of forced displacement."[54] This international initiative will bring much-needed resources to the problem, but the ongoing violence hampers HIV prevention activities in many respects.

The violence has discouraged foreign researchers from collaborating with their Colombian counterparts. There are few multinational researchers conducting studies in Colombia. Current information suggests that the HIV rates are not high, but they are rising. In 2003 the BBC News service published a report that 240,000 people had been infected by the virus, which "means that HIV is present in the blood of one of every 175 Colombians: 0.6 per cent of the population. It is the fifth leading cause of death in the working-age population, according to DANE Administrative Department of statistics. The most troubling issue is that the rate of infection is not slowing down but accelerating."[55] Despite gaps in the statistical analyses of the epidemic in Colombia, the latter fact seems to emerge as a consensus point. The HIV epidemic is also increasingly affecting women: "In the beginning there was one HIV-positive woman for every 20 men, but today the proportion is almost one out of two. In ten years there will be gender equity. The Atlantic Coast and Norte de Santander department have already anticipated this move."[56] Overall, the government response to this effort has not been adequate, despite some impressive activities in some departments, as UNAIDS has noted: "The National AIDS Council (NAC) was formed in 1997 as the main governing body to deal with HIV/AIDS, but it has not been functional and met only twice during 2003. In the second half of 2003, a review and evaluation of the National Strategic Plan was conducted. According to this evaluation, only 38% of planned activities were executed, and only 36% of the necessary financial resources were allocated."[57] To address this problem may require not only international resources but also pressure on the Colombian government to make HIV a priority.

The situation in Peru is perhaps somewhat brighter, given the end of large-scale guerrilla movements in the country and the relatively successful response by the government to the epidemic. Much of our information on this country comes from two key sources: a history of AIDS in Peru by Marcos Cueto and a multiregional study by a team led by Carlos Cáceres Palacios. Cueto's history describes how, after an initial period of apathy and hysteria, the Peruvian state and society responded well to HIV, even though the disease appeared "during the hard years of hyperinflation, misgovernment and political violence."[58] Cueto and others have argued that, ironically, social and political misery may have delayed the onset of the epidemic. Many well-to-do, urban gays—the first group affected by HIV elsewhere in Latin America—emigrated abroad, given harsh conditions within the country. Perhaps more important, Cueto and others have suggested that the fear of political violence probably also limited tourism, which may have delayed the initial spread of the epidemic.[59]

The study of Cáceres Palacios and his colleagues suggests that this argument should perhaps be qualified. Their careful work contained qualitative and quantitative research on the HIV epidemic during the period from 1991 to 1995, with a focus on three Peruvian cities: Chiclayo, on the desert coast; Cusco, in the high Andes; and Iquitos, in the Peruvian Amazon. Their thorough study was particularly significant and represents the most careful work to date on the epidemic throughout the country as a whole because most other studies to this date had focused on Lima and Callao. Their study pointed out limitations and weaknesses in the surveillance program by the government agency charged with fighting HIV/AIDS. Significant regional differences also existed in the spread of the virus. In Cusco, for example, heterosexual sex was more important to the spread of the virus, and the proportion of perinatal cases was surprisingly high. In all areas sexual transmission was central to the spread of the epidemic, while drugs were a relatively unimportant factor.[60] And their work found that sexual tourism was taking place on a significant scale, which had implications for Peru's HIV epidemic.[61]

Multiple groups engaged in sex with tourists in Iquitos and Cusco. One group of women in Iquitos, called *gringueras*, engaged in sexual relationships for the same reason as the *jineteras* of Cuba, in that sex was not directly exchanged for money:

> They are young women who look for the company of tourists in order to receive invitations, money, and in the best of all cases to leave the country. They also call themselves "the gringuerillas" and a type of youth—which frequents the bars that they inhabit—calls them "hamburgers" in the sense that they are "fast food for gringos." They indicate that this practice dates back approximately ten years and that the first "gringueras" belonged to the middle class. They go out with foreigners that provide them the ability to purchase things and there always exists the possibility for them to marry one and to realize their dream of traveling abroad.[62]

Even with sexual tourism, the drug trade seems to be shaping the social practices that affect the HIV epidemic, because this study found that their "main market currently consists of the personnel that work for the DEA (the narcotics office of the United States), followed by tourists and foreign workers in the city."[63] Similar groups exist in Cusco, where they are called *bricheros* and *bricheras*. The gay equivalents in Iquitos and Cusco are called *maperos,* who have attained a measure of international fame. In this case, however, money tends to play a more dominant role in the relationship.[64] Iquitos also has a reputation as a site that attracts European and North American pedophiles. It is clear, therefore, that if Peru's dangerous reputation limited tourism in the 1980s, and hence the spread of the virus, the situation has changed.

Indeed, in may respects Peru's early epidemic looked much like that in most Andean countries. Many of the early cases were among gay men, often returning from abroad, who lived in the capital. An overwhelming majority of cases were spread by sexual transmission. With time, the number of bisexuals and women infected increased, so that by 2000 18 percent of all cases were among women.[65] Cáceres Palacios's study found the same mix of knowledge, attitudes, and practices familiar to HIV researchers working in other Latin American countries. Infidelity was a cultural expectation for men. In "monogamous" relationships, women perceived that they had to accept that their husbands would sometimes cheat. Some poor but straight men had gay sex for money. Most homosexual men did not use condoms with stable partners. Sex workers did not consistently use condoms. A fear of offending the Church limited the emphasis on condoms in early education campaigns. In general, the rate of condom use remained low, despite women's expectations that their partners were being unfaithful to them.[66] In this circumstance, it is surprising that Peru's epidemic of HIV/AIDS has not spread more quickly. It is perhaps even more surprising that much of the credit for this must go to the Peruvian government, for—despite flaws in the surveillance system and other challenges—it has expended considerable effort since the 1990s to address the epidemic.

The Peruvian state truly began to respond to the epidemic in 1985, but as Cueto has made clear, it was not viewed initially as a high priority, given the multiple challenges that the Peruvian health system faced. Indeed, Peru's HIV incidence appeared relatively low in a Latin American context.[67] Political reasons may also explain the state's slow response to the disease: "The lack of political and economic support in the official efforts against AIDS during these years also resulted from the practical nonexistence of gay organizations and of NGOs dedicated to the themes of sexual and reproductive health."[68] During the 1980s Peru suffered a brutal civil war, which was followed by a period of authoritarian rule under Alberto Fujimori, who closed the congress in 1992. In most of Latin America, HIV/AIDS emerged during a period of democratization. Peru was the exception, and the experience of war and authoritarian rule shaped Peru's reaction to HIV.[69] Indeed, in Lima there were mass roundups of gays, who were compelled to undergo testing for HIV. It was not that Peruvian leaders did not address HIV. Tim Frasca recounts how Fujimori once "inaugurated a continent-wide AIDS and sexually transmitted disease conference by promoting condom use from the pulpit of the city's main cathedral."[70] But in Peru the response to HIV would initially come from the top down, not from the grass roots, and it would be greatly influenced by international support.

Cueto's work emphasized the critical role played by the U.S. Navy Medical Research Institute Detachment (NAMRID) in Peru. NAMRID became the center that facilitated the voluntary testing of groups at risk, and impressive numbers of people participated in these efforts. NAMRID also taught Peruvians basic skills, such as using rubber gloves, and the center's support helped the Peruvian state to clean up the blood banks. By 1989 and 1990 NAMRID began to transfer its work to the Peruvian state, which by then had the capability to undertake essential tasks to control the epidemic.[71] But some people with HIV criticized this program by saying that it focused on epidemiological work rather than providing care to individuals who tested positive.[72] It is true that, overall, treatment was not an early priority of the Peruvian state, as Frasca described: "Dr. Carlos Cáceres, a public health specialist at Lima's Cayetano Heredia University, confirms that in the early years, 'virtually nothing was done about treatment, as if they assumed that in Peru treatment wouldn't happen.' Instead, says Cáceres, 'a good part of the funds went to building the research infrastructure to put together a cohort or participate in vaccine tests.' That was no doubt a worthy project but useless to those encouraged and pressured to find out if they had acquired HIV infection."[73] This perspective would only change in the late 1980s and early 1990s as external aid began to flow to NGOs dedicated to HIV/AIDS in Peru, which then pressured the Peruvian government to provide support to people living with HIV.[74]

By 1996, Cueto argues, the Peruvian state evinced a new commitment to fighting HIV, in part because of the influence of the WHO, and there was a rapid increase in funding to fight the disease.[75] Overall, the Peruvian government's response to the epidemic during this period was impressive. As Cueto describes, the government worked well with NGOs in the field, the total number of reported AIDS cases between 1997 and 2000 actually fell, and Peter Piot (the executive director of UNAIDS) commended Peru for its successes.[76] Peru was able to take pride in its response to the disease:

"Peru's strategy to prevent sexually transmitted infections was heralded as a model for the Andean region, and in 2000 UNAIDS cited Peru's HIV/AIDS prevention program as one of the best in the world. Peru was among the first three countries in Latin America (with Bolivia and Brazil) to adopt syndromic management of sexually transmitted infections and to begin offering prophylaxis to prevent perinatal transmission."[77] But there are some reasons to doubt the government's commitment.

One of the main challenges Peru faces in controlling HIV/AIDS is educating its youth, given that in Peru "43 percent of those sick contracted the virus during their school years."[78] There is a great deal of evidence that many Peruvian adolescents are engaging in unprotected sex. In "Peru, 13 percent of women between the ages of 15 and 19 become mothers, the number of abortions increased by 100,000 since last year, and only 1 out of every 3 adolescents uses any form of birth control in their sexual relationships."[79] One of the government's successes was an effort to address this problem: The Sexual Education Program "was created in 1996, and with $5 million in funding from the U.N. Population Fund, it trained 40,000 teachers— 10 percent of the total teaching staff—and provided them with teaching guides and instructional materials. But since 2000, the Peruvian government has drastically reduced the program's budget. In four years, only 10,000 additional instructors have been trained, and only 4,000 teaching guides have been printed."[80]

Besides questions about Peru's sex education program, there are also concerns about the country's commitment to human rights. On one hand, the head of the nation's AIDS program worked with the congress to pass "Law 26626, which protects the rights of persons living with HIV/AIDS."[81] But the legislation also became a focus of controversy when the congress discussed altering it to mandate the testing of all pregnant women for HIV, a proposal that was condemned by groups such as Human Rights Watch, which argued that in "Peru, a particularly cruel dimension of the proposed reform to law 26626 is how it pits children's rights against women's human rights. The connotation of these arguments, put forward, amongst others, by the president of the congressional health commission, Daniel Robles, is that any woman who values her right to consent or not to HIV testing is failing her moral duties to her future child. This is a false dichotomy. One need not violate a woman's human rights in order to protect those of a child, or to reduce the risk of HIV transmission to infants."[82] The conflict over law 26626 was particularly bitter because of a widespread sense that the government was not concerned with human rights or with upholding agreements that it made in the area of HIV.

This concern came to a head in December 2001 in the midst of a symposium in Lima on access to HIV medications. While some Peruvians are covered by government programs, the vast majority of HIV Peruvians do not have access to these drugs. It was in this context that comments by a government official sparked widespread anger:

> Protesters were enraged by remarks made by Hugo Manrique who represented the Health Ministry at the First Peruvian Symposium on AIDS Treatment Access held on the 11th and 12th of December in Lima's Hotel Jose Antonio. Manrique indicated that the Health Ministry hoped to begin providing anti-retrovirals to 100 children with AIDS in 2002, but that there are no plans to treat more than 8000 adults who have AIDS. When asked about statements supporting universal treatment access made by Peru's Health Minister during the special session of the United Nations on AIDS (UNGASS) in New York, last June, Manrique answered boldly that "we are always signing these international treaties and agreements, but that doesn't mean that we are going to comply." Shocked by Manrique's brazen disregard of commitments made by his own government, Symposium Organizers, including PWA activist Pablo Anamaria, decided on a plan for a demonstration outside Manrique's office the following day. "We are tired of living without the medications that we need, and we are tired of our government's disregard for our health and welfare," commented Anamaria, adding that "this demonstration is the beginning of a new phase of activism here in Peru."[83]

Activists were angered not only by the fact that many people living with HIV were not receiving treatment, but also by the fact that the government seemed to be unconcerned about this. At the same conference that launched this protest, representatives from other Latin American countries discussed "the UNAIDS 'accelerated access' program which has resulted in sharply diminished prices in other Latin American countries including Honduras and Chile. But the UNAIDS representative for Peru, Adriana Gomez, indicated that there were no current plans to promote this initiative in Peru."[84] These were not words likely to mollify the crowd. Many critics remain concerned that in Peru the government has also acquired too much power over the NGOs, which it may use to protect itself from criticism.[85] But this particular event served to galvanize the HIV/AIDS community in Peru.

International groups are trying to fill the gap created by the government's failure to act. Doctors without Borders has launched a program in a "poor suburb of Lima with a population of 350,000."[86] The key idea of the project was to provide decentralized care to people living with HIV, ranging from testing to psychosociological support. Until this point, there had been a mood of hopelessness in the medical community that served this population, as one doctor involved made clear: "Months of preparation and negotiation preceded the program's launch. 'It was a very emotional occasion,' said MSF volunteer John MacRae, MD. 'For years we have seen our patients die around us. Of the group from two years ago, almost nobody is left. Now, finally, we can give them hope that they can continue their lives in relative health.'"[87] There is no questioning the clear successes that Peru has had in its struggle to control HIV.[88] It has been particularly remarkable given the fact that the state in some respects did mount an effective response, even as it was emerging from the violence and chaos caused by the Shining Path and from a cholera epidemic that reflected the generally poor infrastructure that most Peruvians had to endure. The fact that Peru is a drug-producing nation brings the country significant social and political problems that some countries, such as Chile, do not face. Peru also does not have the resources that Brazil has. But Peru has also been slow to take advantage of some programs, such as UNAIDS accelerated access initiative, and to honor its commitments in this area. Peru recently reached an agreement with the Global Fund to Fight AIDS, Tuberculosis, and Malaria that would expand the availability of medications to 90 percent of the Peruvians who needed care. As part of its proposal the Peruvian government promised to assume responsibility for providing these medications in the long term.[89] If it followed through, it would close a hole in what was in other respects a relatively successful program. Peru's experience appears, in many ways, similar to that of its Andean neighbors, which in turn have an epidemiological profile quite different from that of the countries of the Southern Cone.

■ **The Southern Cone**

On the surface the countries of the Southern Cone appear relatively diverse, and the contrast between the economic success of Chile and the compara-

tive weakness of Paraguay is striking. Nonetheless, the nations of this region share a number of commonalities, many of which have their roots in
history. The Spaniards were slower to settle this region, which lacked the
urban civilization, established mines, and fixed populations of the northern
Andes. Instead, the windswept pampas and nomadic Amerindians posed
a formidable obstacle to Spanish expansion and settlement. In Chile, Uruguay, and Argentina much of the indigenous population was exterminated,
assimilated, or swamped by waves of European immigrants, so the region
does not now face the same political contest over indigenous rights that
is defining the experience of Bolivia or Ecuador. Paraguay, unique in the
Southern Cone, has retained a significant cultural heritage from the native
peoples, and Guarani is widely spoken—as an official language—in the
country. Yet Paraguay—from its recent legacy of authoritarian rule to its
integration into Mercosul—has more in common with its southern neighbors than with the Andean region. Among the many shared bonds that
differentiate the nations of this region from those of the Andes is the fact
that none of these countries is a significant producer of illegal narcotics.
Thus they have escaped the violence and social instability associated with
the drug cartels. But the fact that Argentina (and to a lesser extent Uruguay
and Paraguay) is a drug consumer in the global narcotics trade has caused
separate social problems. The HIV/AIDS epidemic in the Southern Cone is
much more fractured than that of the Andes. The particular position of each
country in the drug trade (from Chile, which has minimal involvement, to
Argentina, where drugs are a key factor) has shaped the history of HIV/AIDS
in these countries.

Argentines have long had a strong sense of identity, which was characterized by their distinctness, which they associated with wealth, (European)
culture, and urbanity. Even at independence, much of the new nation's territory was not settled, so the country could be defined as Buenos Aries,
which was equated with civilization, and the rustic beyond, the embodi-
ment of barbarism, as Domingo Faustino Sarmiento described in his classic work on nineteenth-century Argentina.[90] During the nineteenth century
the wars of expansion gradually compressed the territory dominated by
the Mapuche, the nomadic peoples of the pampa. Although these people
still exist, they have been marginalized in the nation's account of its own
history.[91] Instead, Argentines associated their identity with the waves of
Spanish and Italian immigrants who came in the late nineteenth and early
twentieth centuries. The nation enjoyed a long economic boom during this

period, driven by exports in the agricultural sector, in particular wheat and beef. The rise of a working class and enduring social inequalities led the country to adopt populist policies under Juan Domingo Perón, who came to power during World War II and won a free election in 1946. His rise gradually polarized the country into two political camps, and the military eventually seized power in 1976. During the years that followed, Argentina was the site of the famous "Dirty War" memorialized in works such as Jacobo Timerman's *Prisoner without a Name, Cell without a Number.* As Marguerite Feitlowitz's work makes clear, the use of military terror was so pervasive during this period that it even changed the usage of the Spanish language in the country.[92] After the junta made the disastrous decision in March 1982 to invade the Falklands/Malvinas islands, Argentina's subsequent defeat by Britain led to the collapse of the military's legitimacy and a return to democratic rule in 1983.

The nation's history since this time has been shaped not only by the effort to deal with the political legacy of this period but also by the country's relative economic decline. Perón's policies, which favored industrialization over agriculture, contributed to a steady slide in the nation's economic position. Political corruption, military mismanagement, policy errors, and a failed effort to dollarize the economy have led to economic disaster. Nations once much poorer than Argentina elsewhere in the developing world have now far surpassed Argentina's per capita income. This long slide climaxed in December 2001 when Argentina underwent a stunning economic collapse so severe that one successful game show offered the contestants the opportunity to win jobs as retail sales clerks.[93] While in 2004 the Argentine economy rallied, it was a humiliating experience for a country that thought of itself as being distinct in Latin America. These economic hardships, the rise of Brazil (which may win a seat on the United Nations Security Council and has outstripped Argentina as the region's biggest economy), and the country's political turbulence have compelled Argentines to reappraise their national identity. They have also caused immense social suffering and undermined the government's safety net, which has complicated the state's response to AIDS.

Instead, Chile has become South America's economic success, a fact that has generated its own resentments within the region. These tensions are magnified by Chile's history. Chile went to war with its neighbors in 1836–39 and 1879–82. The latter war ended with the nation seizing Bolivia's territory on the Pacific coast, thus isolating Bolivia from access to the sea and giving Chile access to rich resources of guano and mineral deposits. This history continues to poison its relationship with Bolivia into the present. Nonetheless, the nation was both an economic and political success well into the twentieth century. It appeared to have stronger democratic roots than most South American nations, until the political system collapsed in 1973 in a military coup that brought General Augusto Pinochet Ugarte to power. He would govern Chile for seventeen years, only relinquishing power in 1990. During that period he sought to remake Chile, both politically and economically. He turned to the University of Chicago, famous for its conservative economics department, and brought in its graduates to reshape the Chilean regulatory framework. Under their tutelage, all aspects of the Chilean economy, from business regulation to the social security network, were remade. While these economic measures were painful and often unpopular, the political climate of torture and disappearances meant that no Chilean political groups were able to block these reforms. The result was that Pinochet's rule will be remembered for two characteristics: the grave human rights abuses and political terror that have continued to haunt the nation, and Chile's mercurial economic rise.

Chile's success has been so striking as to undermine the arguments of dependency theorists, who were influential in Latin America in the 1970s. Indeed, Chile's example likely helped to inspire many other Latin American nations to adopt neoliberal policies in the 1980s and 1990s. There is now a widespread sense in much of the region that those policies have been a failure, and there is currently a trend to the political left in the region. Yet neoliberal policies continue to work in Chile, although they have generated high levels of inequality, and in 2005 the nation reached free trade agreements with both China and the United States. Its private retirement program even served as an inspiration for the Bush administration's proposal to partially privatize social security in the United States. With its current political stability, economic resources, and active NGO networks, Chile has dealt with the HIV/AIDS epidemic quite effectively. It has been helped in this effort by the fact that Chile has only a minor problem with IV drug use, which in turn may be a reflection of its economic growth over the past three decades. According to UNAIDS, Chile's HIV incidence is 0.3 percent, less than half the rate of Argentina, which is 0.7 percent.[94]

While Chile and Argentina dominate the Southern Cone, there are two smaller states in the region. As Philip Kelly has noted, Paraguay and Uruguay are classic buffer states that to some extent survived because they separated powerful neighbors that shared an interest in their survival.[95] Paraguay is a nation of 5.5 million people that is surrounded by Argentina, Bolivia, and Brazil. Without significant mineral resources, ready access to the ocean, or other forms of natural resources, Paraguay has long faced economic challenges. The nation has also endured bitter wars. The Paraguayan War (also called the War of the Triple Alliance) drew Paraguay into a devastating conflict from 1864 to 1870. Although the origins of the war are complex, the Paraguayan dictator Francisco Solano López began the fighting by invading Brazilian and Argentine territory.[96] The ensuing conflict pitted Brazil, Uruguay, and Argentina against Paraguay in a hopeless struggle. Nonetheless, the Paraguayans had begun to industrialize earlier than their neighbors and had an efficient military, so they enjoyed notable success early in the conflict. But when the tide of war turned against them, as it inevitably did, given the disparity in the material resources available to the two sides, the Paraguayans fought on fanatically. In the end, the conflict may have cost the lives of between 60 and 69 percent of Paraguay's population. The Paraguayans fought so desperately that, by the end of the war, for every man in Paraguay there were four to five women.[97] In the aftermath of the conflict the nation lost some territory, but its losses would have been much more severe were it not for the Brazilian determination to preserve the nation as a buffer against Argentina.[98] The nation then fought a second major war against Bolivia from 1932 to 1935 over its disputed eastern territories. In this case, Paraguay emerged victorious, despite losing 3.5 percent of its population in the fighting.[99]

The nation did not enjoy either economic growth or democratic government in the aftermath of this sacrifice. Instead, General Alfredo Stroessner seized power in 1954. He would govern Paraguay until his overthrow in 1989. Under his regime Paraguay became associated with corruption, and a significant portion of the national income came from smuggling between Argentina and Brazil. Paraguay's subsequent democratization has been a rocky process, with political corruption giving rise to massive scandals, political assassination, and an attempted coup. With the nation's integration into Mercosul, however, the country's reliance on smuggling ended, and Paraguay turned to free-market-oriented policies for economic growth, which have generated widespread political protests. At present there are grave questions about the future of HIV/AIDS in the country, given some studies that suggest the presence of widespread drug use. Nonetheless, the nation's HIV rate of 0.5 percent remains lower than that of Argentina.[100]

SPANISH SOUTH AMERICA

With 3.3 million people, Uruguay is the smallest nation in the Southern Cone. It was once part of the "contested" lands between Argentina and Brazil, which fought an inconclusive war over the region in the early nineteenth century. Uruguay survived as a buffer state that served the interests of both nations and has evolved into a major site for tourism from both its neighbors. With a high rate of literacy and an effective public health service, Uruguay has a strong social safety net, which dates back to the creation of a welfare state under the reformist president José Batlle y Ordóñez, who governed Uruguay from 1903 to 1907 and from 1911 to 1915. Yet Uruguay has endured the same painful history of military rule and human rights abuses as its neighbors. From 1973 to 1985 the country was governed by a military junta, which ultimately lost power in large part due to Uruguay's mounting economic difficulties and rising popular discontent. Since then Uruguay has evolved into a seemingly stable democracy. President Tabare Vazquez, a candidate from the left, was elected in November 2004. With the nation's recent political stability and a strong social safety net, the country has done an excellent job responding to the HIV/AIDS epidemic, and its HIV incidence of 0.3 percent is relatively low.[101]

■ HIV in Chile and Argentina

Given the fact that Argentina and Chile dominate the Southern Cone, both economically and in terms of population, my discussion of AIDS for the Southern Cone will focus on these two countries. This also reflects the fact that little work has been done on HIV in Paraguay and Uruguay. For Chile, one of the best studies has been done by Mauricio Carmona Berríos and Cynthia del Valle Larrañaga, whose work traced the history of the epidemic with a particular focus on the gay community, in a style clearly influenced by Randy Shilts's *And the Band Played On*. Chile's experience is different from Argentina's in that Chile does not have a significant population of IV drug users. Indeed, even now only 5 percent of all HIV cases in Chile are caused by drug usage, despite a slight increase in the percentage of the Chilean population that used injected drugs in the 1990s.[102] Early in the epidemic this fact encouraged Chilean doctors who believed that this characteristic, combined with the geographic isolation of Chile, might help to shield the country from HIV. Indeed, the Andes were described as "a wall that was impossible to cross" for the disease.[103] Chilean authorities sought to make reassuring statements: "Homosexual Chileans—said the then chief of the Programs Department of the Ministry of Health—are not so promiscuous as in the United States. Besides, here there are few intravenous drugs us- ers. All this leads us to think that the situation in Chile is going to be different."[104] Many people in Chile reacted with shock when the disease first arrived, and Carmona Berríos and del Valle Larrañaga describe the flurry of media coverage that surrounded the first AIDS patients in 1984. The second Chilean AIDS patient was kept in isolation, and the newspapers issued daily updates on the state of his health. In the atmosphere of fear and ignorance, many hospital workers were happy when he finally went home.[105]

As Carmona Berríos and del Valle Larrañaga stress, Chile was a major tourist destination in the 1980s, with the levels of tourism reaching historical heights. In this environment, the Andes were no barrier, and many tourists actively participated in the vibrant gay culture in Santiago.[106] There was initially a code of silence surrounding the disease in Chile's gay community. While this rapidly changed, gays continued to have large numbers of sexual partners in Chile even in the mid-1990s, although many gay men adopted safe-sex practices.[107] The concentration of the disease within the gay community perhaps explains a number of characteristics of the epidemic during 1984–94, which we can see in a statistical study carried out by Chile's National Commission on AIDS. The disease was concentrated within Santiago, where the overwhelming majority of cases were men. The disease was centered within the gay male population. In particular, the disease affected men who were professionals and who had a higher level of education than was the norm. Women were more likely than men to be infected by blood transfusions, although IV drug use was also an emerging problem. Interestingly, women were no more likely to be infected if they were professionals. Among people aged thirty-five years and older, 96 percent of HIV cases were acquired through sex.[108] This pattern was very similar to that of the disease elsewhere in South America. In Venezuela, for example, the disease also first appeared in upper-middle-class men who were gay.[109] But in many Latin American countries HIV/AIDS spread rapidly into the heterosexual population. Like its Andean neighbors to the north, Chile is unusual in that the disease has remained relatively concentrated among gay men.[110] This fact may have shaped how the Chilean government responded to the virus.

In some respects, the Chilean state reacted poorly to the HIV/AIDS epidemic, in particular by failing to defend the human rights of gays. There are numerous stories of discrimination from the early years of the epidemic:

At a famous incident in the Chilean port city of Valparaíso in 1990, three hundred patrons of a gay nightclub were taken by police armed with submachine guns to a sexually transmitted disease clinic in the middle of the night and forced to take HIV and syphilis tests on the orders of the city's health authorities. As dawn broke, two were found to be HIV positive. Augusto Pinochet's seventeen-year-old military regime still had one month to go. The raid had been rescheduled from an earlier date when police discovered that the son of a prominent general was in the bar as a patron and decided to avoid problems.[111]

Similar cases of abuses are not hard to find. One HIV-positive gay man was fired from his place of employment because a coworker was friends with someone at the health clinic. This health worker told the coworker that the gay man was HIV-positive, and he was fired.[112] This was illegal; but such cases were frequent, and other gay men found that their employers wanted HIV tests as a condition of employment.[113]

On December 17, 2001, Chile enacted a law designed to protect HIV-positive people from such indignities. But HIV-positive Chileans continue to come forward with stories of such discrimination. One member of Chile's uniformed police (carabineros) filed a grievance against his organization, which he claimed had let him go after eleven years of service after it learned that he was HIV-positive. Alex Cea chose to invoke the law to protect himself, but the outcome was still undecided when his story reached the press. The man, who had a daughter, and whose wife was now HIV-positive, was worried about his family's future, and how without a job he could afford medications.[114]

At the same time, the state's response steadily improved, and there is no denying the progress that has been made. As in much of Latin America, NGOs began to appear in the late 1980s, often with foreign support.[115] These organizations raised the profile of HIV/AIDS, denounced discrimination, and pressured the media to cover the illness in a more balanced manner. The state has also sought to contain the spread of the epidemic, and to mitigate its impact, by means of a number of measures. As Carmona Berríos and del Valle Larrañaga have described, Chile was one of the first Latin American countries to test blood donations. In 1993 the country began to provide AZT free to HIV-positive people. By 1996 this coverage had theoretically expanded to two-drug therapy, despite a heavy drain on government coffers. But the availability of medications remained poor, as Tim Frasca has described: "At the Arriarán Foundation and elsewhere, a few lucky patients were receiving some medicines based on a macabre lottery system. Vargas described how it worked: 'Everyone had fewer than three hundred CD4 cells, they would put our charts in a basket, and whoever was picked, got their meds. I didn't win.' But one day even that system broke down. 'In April of 1997 Dr. Wolff called together the few people who received drugs to tell us that donations of even those few medicines were discontinued. They were out of stock, and there just weren't any more.'"[116] Patients who struggled to obtain their medicines sometimes found the state more of an obstacle than an ally, particularly in the late 1990s when the government cracked down on the importation of AIDS medications into Chile.[117] Many NGOs remained dissatisfied with aspects of Chile's response to the epidemic. Still, "by 2003 coverage for the AIDS combination therapy in Chile's public health system was approaching 100 percent."[118] And Chile has won a major grant from the Global Fund to Fight AIDS, Tuberculosis, and Malaria, which should allow it to greatly strengthen its services for people with HIV.[119]

In some respects Chile is an anomaly. Although IV drug use tends to dominate the spread of the disease in the Southern Cone, in Chile such drug use remains relatively low. One scholar has described Chile as a "country without much of an indigenous injectable drug culture."[120] The nation is neither a major drug user nor consumer. For this reason it has escaped both the violence and instability associated with drug production and the major social problems faced by consuming nations. With an HIV incidence of 0.3 percent, Chile's AIDS epidemic appears to be contained.[121] The virus remains focused among men, who account for nearly 90 percent of all AIDS cases in Chile. In particular studies of pregnant women give reason for hope: "HIV infection among pregnant women in two regions of Chile was almost non-existent during the 1992–1997 time period."[122] Even among people seeking treatment for sexually transmitted infections, there has not been a large incidence of HIV. One study found that in "Antofagasta in the north of the country, HIV prevalence was minimal. Indeed, in 1992, 1993, and 1996–1997, there was no evidence of infection there. In the two other regions, prevalence was at or below 3 percent in all four time periods."[123] There have been some weaknesses in the government's response, in particular in the area of enforcing its own AIDS legislation to prevent discrimination against people living with AIDS, and in making medications accessible. Nonetheless, the response to date has remained effective. Given Chile's relative wealth, however, it could do still more to fight the illness and to serve as a model, much like Brazil, for what a developing nation can do to control the disease.

Argentina's experience of the disease is much more like that of Brazil, in that it has been heavily affected by the nation's position as a consumer in the global narcotics trade. The first case of AIDS appeared in Argentina in 1982 (a year in which three cases were detected) but the disease really began to take off after 1987.[124] The initial pattern of the disease mirrored that of many other Latin American countries, in that it was largely an urban, upper-middle-class phenomenon. In some respects, the state was slow to respond to the disease with a prevention effort, in part because of the influence of the Catholic Church, which wanted HIV education campaigns to stress abstinence.[125] At the same time, it became clear that Argentina would face a particular challenge because of its significant population of IV drug users.

Argentina had begun to be a significant drug consumer in the international market in the 1970s and 1980s, when the HIV epidemic first appeared.[126] In part, the emergence of IV drugs may have been associated with the nation's reaction to military rule, as people interviewed by Frasca suggested: "Around 1986 there was a tremendous fascination, especially among intellectual circles, with intravenous drugs. People wanted to try everything, and I think that it was in some way a result, a legacy of the military dictatorship because during the dictatorship you couldn't do anything. Then when (the military) left, it was like, okay, everything's allowed, so let's do it all."[127] Frasca's interviewees also emphasized the role played by returning exiles, who brought back the need for drugs with them to Argentina: "(Drug experimentation) was also influenced by the people who had left Argentina for Europe during the 1970s, some of them without much of a project for their lives, just to escape (from the dictatorship). They ended up so badly addicted that they came back to Argentina to escape from the heroin."[128] Whatever the origins of Argentina's drug culture, the HIV epidemic in that country soon became intimately associated with drugs in the popular mind.[129]

Cocaine is the most commonly injected drug, and this is doubtless determined by the ready access Argentina has to sources of supply.[130] The rate at which the disease spread within the community of IV drug users was staggering. According to the Ministry of Health the country experienced "a

65-fold increase in reported AIDS cases due to intravenous drug use (IVDU) and a 47-fold increase due to heterosexual transmission between 1987 and 1994."[131] The fact that not only homosexuals but also drug users were the first patients may have undermined the government's will to address the virus during the early history of the disease: "If you admit the size of the problem, you have to take responsibility for doing something about it. And the kind of interventions that were going to be even minimally effective in this case were simply not acceptable in political circles until recently."[132] Indeed, it could be argued that elements of the Argentine state benefited from the drug trade: "During the ten years of the (*Carlos*) Menem government (*1989–1999*), Argentina became a refuge for the laundering of drug money, and wherever the money flows, drug use is close behind."[133] Certainly the Argentine government failed to make drug addiction a major priority, which hampered the nation's plans to fight HIV.

The effort to control HIV in Argentina may also have been hampered because the disease emerged in a context that saw the state play a declining role in public health and other basic governmental activities. In the 1980s and 1990s Argentina underwent a remarkable process of privatization, which transferred many responsibilities from the state to private organizations. This process meant the state was playing a decreasing role in providing services such as public health education. At the same time the number of people living in poverty in Argentina underwent a stunning rise. For example, the "rate of poverty in Buenos Aries increased rapidly, from a minimum of 8% in 1980 to a maximum of 41% during the hyperinflation of 1989."[134] This meant that many people found it more difficult to access health services at the same time they were less likely to be able to afford private health care. There was a clear impact on the provision of care, as "the service in public hospitals deteriorated."[135] The public health service was weakened at the exact moment when resources were most needed to fight an emerging epidemic.

To some extent, NGOs have filled the gap in government-provided services. Most HIV/AIDS organizations in Argentina were founded in the period from 1989 through 1993. Their appearance was a positive step forward, and there are now eighty-three AIDS NGOs in greater Buenos Aries alone. But it also meant that there was a period in which the state was failing to provide many services and the NGOs had not appeared to fill the gap. There are also some remaining concerns about the state/NGO relationship in Argentina, as the work of Kornblit and Petracci suggests. The Argentine state has continued to rely heavily on NGOs, which it has begun to fund in a significant manner. While this funding assists these organizations to provide services, it also raises concerns that these organizations may become too dependent on the government. Another risk is that if the government relies too heavily on NGOs, it may abdicate some of its responsibilities to respond to the epidemic.[136] This is not to downplay the role of NGOs. For example, many Argentines would prefer to test for HIV in an AIDS NGO rather than "the bureaucratic, user-unfriendly public hospitals that also administer the test."[137] But NGOs endure a constant battle to raise funds, and there are some areas where government responsibility is critical.

This is particularly clear in the area of human rights enforcement, where the government's response to the epidemic has sometimes seemed to lack commitment. On one hand, in 2000 the federal government enacted legislation to defend the rights of people who are HIV-positive.[138] Although somewhat late, this legislation was a positive step forward. On the other hand, local, state, and federal governments have a mixed record on implementing past legislation. For example, the Controladuría General Comunal of Buenos Aries, a government organization dedicated to defending citizens' legal rights, issued one study in 1994 that examined its efforts to respond to AIDS. In this document, the organization argued that HIV-positive people who are asymptomatic did not need to be isolated from society. It also recommended that HIV-positive people be integrated into the schools. At the same time, however, the document placed great stress on brothels as a threat to public security and called for energetic action to shut them down. The almost hysterical tone in this section made approaching and working with sex workers a difficult part of an HIV/AIDS education program.[139]

The challenge is that the Argentine government needs to be able to reach out to the most stigmatized members of society, and in particular drug users, in order to fight the disease. There seems to be a sense among HIV-positive people in Argentina that the situation for their counterparts in Brazil is better, as one person infected by IV drug use commented: "In Argentina the people affected are not well treated by the state, which is different from what happens in Brazil, where the state is engaged in prevention and treatment with much greater attention than in this country."[140] Another HIV-positive person decided "to look for work in Brazil 'because it is a country that does not discriminate, for them it's normal, there is more liberty around this issue of illness, in contrast with here where if you have HIV it is more difficult to find work.'"[141] Many people in Argentina with

HIV have faced severe discrimination. Alejandro Freyre "lost his contract for work with an insurance company after it became known that he was HIV positive. His dentist also refused to treat him anymore."[142] Freyre was determined enough to found an AIDS NGO to address discrimination and to obtain funding from a German government grant.[143] But the government also has an essential role to play to fight discrimination.

The Argentine government will have to confront this issue in order to respond successfully to the disease, in particular if it is to address the epidemic among IV drug users. In 1999 there were 16,259 reported cases of AIDS in Argentina, of which 40.4 percent were acquired through injecting drugs and 25.6 percent through unprotected sex between men.[144] While the HIV incidence in the population of men who have sex with men remains high, the proportion of cases in the gay community has steadily fallen, while that among IV drug users has risen.[145] This change took place with great speed: "Since the first AIDS case in a drug injector was reported in 1987, the proportion of cases attributed to drug injection has steadily increased, rising from 11.3% in 1987 to 39% in 1991."[146] While both the gay community and IV drug users are marginalized populations, the drug users are probably even more isolated from society. They suffer from a double stigma in that there is no pride in their identity even within their community, and many Argentines blame them for the spread of the disease into the heterosexual population.[147] It is in fact true that in the Southern Cone, as well as in Brazil, IV drug users have been central to the spread of the epidemic. By the early 1990s, however, it was clear that nowhere else in the region was the problem of IV drug use and HIV as significant as in Argentina.[148] In Argentina the nation's position as a drug consumer and its experience of the HIV/AIDS epidemic cannot be separated.

In Argentina the role of IV drug use in the epidemic's evolution has been so fundamental that it can be seen even biologically. One study found that there "appear to be two HIV-1 epidemics in Argentina: one in heterosexuals and drug users and another in gay men. . . . Biologist María de los Angeles Pando and colleagues at the National Reference Center of AIDS of the University of Buenos Aries recently studied 35 gay HIV positive men and 175 heterosexual HIV positive men and women. They found that 91 percent of gay men had HIV-1 subtype B, while 75 percent of heterosexuals had subtype F, with many of those patients appearing to have a mixture of both subtypes (B/F recombinant forms)."[149] A second study among three populations in Argentina found similar results. As these authors wrote, given "this clear dichotomy between the viruses in the heterosexual community and those in the homosexual community, it is clear that the HIV epidemics in these communities are relatively independent."[150] Within the heterosexual community, drug injection is central to the epidemic.

HIV/AIDS became a major problem in prisons because of IV drug use. One "study conducted in Buenos Aries pointed out that 45% of adolescents lodged in security institutes were drug injectors and presented higher HIV seropositivity (53.5%) than non-drug injectors (2.3%)."[151] Many IV drug users also were forced into sex work to survive, and infection levels in this population rose quickly in the late 1980s. Two studies make this clear. The first "study indicated an HIV seroprevalence of 20% for drug injector prostitutes in 1988. The other, conducted among the same prostitute population during 1989 and 1990, found a seroprevalence of 50% for drug injector prostitutes and 11% for all prostitutes of the same sample."[152] The high rate of HIV among IV drug users may also explain the unusually high rate of mother-to-child transmission in the country. Although the exact figures are debated, according "to Foundation Huesped, another major AIDS organization in Argentina, children under 12 made up a little over 7 percent of all HIV cases in the country, the highest rate in Latin America."[153] HIV has not remained confined to drug injectors.

The Argentine government's effort to deal with this problem has had one clear strength. A Supreme Court decision has compelled the government to provide medications to all HIV-positive people.[154] The government program in charge of fighting AIDS celebrates the fact that in "Latin America and the Caribbean, Argentina occupies the second place after Brazil in the number of treatments available to people living with AIDS."[155] The Argentine state also stresses that the "National Program implements free ARV and non-ARV treatments, tests of viral load and CD-4 counts for all people who did not have other coverage."[156] Since Argentina first began to provide free medications to some people living with HIV in 1993, its coverage has greatly improved, while the state has successfully reduced the price it pays for these drugs.[157]

This effort represented a major commitment by the Argentine government. Still, the coverage has not been complete, and there have been frustrating instances where medications were not available.[158] One study on Argentine women found that the provision of HIV care by the state "is inadequate. Moreover, access to health centers to monitor the course of HIV infection (determination of CD4 and viral load), as well as specific pharmacological treatment, is practically impossible for many women. The immunological monitoring is performed in only a few locations within the Federal District and the medications of the National Program are frequently in short supply."[159] Interruptions in supplies of medications can have significant health effects for people undergoing treatment for HIV. In Argentina "at times, the availability of drugs may be interrupted for as long as fifteen days. In that period, the concentration of HIV in the individual's blood can rise, and the body can develop resistance to the drugs, according to AIDS specialists."[160] The situation was so grave that in 1998 AIDS NGOs took the Ministry of Health to court and argued that it had failed to meet its legal obligations to provide medical services to people living with HIV. The government lost the case as well as a subsequent appeal.[161] Despite this victory, people living with HIV/AIDS in Argentina continue to face a number of obstacles to obtaining the medications they need, not the least of which is a complicated bureaucratic process to obtain the required authorization for treatment. One study "investigated how long it takes to obtain all documentation, and found that a minimum of two to four weeks is required. Considering that this must be repeated every three months, only gathering all paperwork takes from three to four months yearly."[162]

Even within the nation's National AIDS Program there have been questions about the government's commitment to the problem, which has generated frustration at the highest levels of the organization, as events in 2001 made clear:

> Adding to the uncertainty in Argentina's HIV/AIDS arena was Mabel Bianco's resignation last week from her post as director of the National AIDS Program. Among her reasons for leaving, she cited the government's "lack of political will and support" for her efforts. "This lack of support prevents the sustainable development of our activities," Bianco told the fourth Argentine Congress on AIDS, held last week in the western province of Mendoza. She underscored the scant official aid for existing prevention and research programs, and also—though to a lesser degree—the irregularities in the provision of AIDS drugs to the patients.[163]

Of course, many of these difficulties flowed from the generalized economic crisis that overtook Argentina at the end of the millennium, but it is also true that the government seemed to lack the political will to make HIV/AIDS a priority.

The government has often failed to follow its own policies and legislation with regard to the provision of care. For example, in "1991, the Ministry of Health and Social Welfare adopted Resolution 787: Legal Policy related to HIV infection in Federal Prisons. That resolution, in accordance with the AIDS law and its Regulating Decree, established that the HIV test should be voluntary and consented to by the prisoners, and the obligation of the state to provide them with treatment and medicines. However, the majority of prisons do not comply with this law and the prisoners with HIV/AIDS do not enjoy these rights."[164] Enforcement of human rights legislation has been poor, as "Private and Public companies in Argentina usually request the HIV test from their employees or those applying for a job. Not everybody knows that this request is illegal, and those who do know sometimes agree to have the test to avoid losing their jobs or in order to get a new one."[165] Indeed, the government itself violates its international obligations and federal law by mandating HIV tests for "all members of the Armed Forces and Security Forces, including civilians."[166]

The government's response to the epidemic in other respects has been weak. Dr. Sergio Maulen, the president of the Nexo Group, an Argentine AIDS charity, has said that "although the government of Argentina guarantees AIDS medication and treatment through its public hospitals, it is far behind the United States and other countries in education and prevention."[167] The Argentine government is now making a concerted effort to address this problem, but many Argentines remain poorly informed about the virus. Many people seem to have a misguided fear of HIV, given that medical procedures and dentistry seem to be particular sources of anxiety.[168] Argentina is increasing its HIV/AIDS education efforts, but much work remains to be done.

Meanwhile, the epidemic continues its slow evolution. In June 2004 Argentina had reported "26,103 cases of AIDS and 21,967 people infected by HIV."[169] UNAIDS estimates that perhaps 130,000 people (including adults and children) are now living with HIV in Argentina.[170] The disease is found in every province, but it remains a largely urban illness, with two-thirds of cases in either Buenos Aries or its neighboring area.[171] The male-to-female ratio of those infected continues to decline steadily. Women are usually younger than men who are infected. The ratio of women who acquire the disease through sex against those who acquire it through IV drug use is roughly equivalent. The disease is increasingly seen as an illness of poverty.

Even among IV drug users, those of lower socioeconomic status are more likely to become infected with HIV.[172] As Claudio Bloch's work has shown, the level of schooling among those infected has steadily declined with time, although two studies suggest that men who have sex with men may be exempt from this trend.[173] While men who have sex with men also are no longer such a high proportion of people with HIV, this group continues to be heavily affected by the epidemic.[174] There is little evidence that HIV is being brought under control among IV drug users. As UNAIDS has noted, Argentina has a number of advantages in its struggle with HIV/AIDS, because the country "benefits from high quality professionals, with a very strong civil society participation and a good participation of networks of people living with HIV."[175] It will need to take advantage of these strengths, given the financial crisis it has endured and the deep roots that HIV has created among the poorest and most vulnerable members of Argentine society.

■ Conclusion

Spanish South America has the same fractured HIV epidemic as the rest of Latin America. In this region, one factor shaping the epidemic appears to be whether nations are integrated into the regional drug trade and, if so, in what manner. Nations such as Bolivia, Ecuador, Peru, and Colombia, which produce coca or distribute cocaine, have an HIV epidemic dominated by men who have sex with men. The importance of women in the epidemic is increasing in these countries. But IV drug use is only a minor factor at this point. The situation in the Southern Cone is quite different, and the epidemic is complex. Chile is neither a major drug consumer nor a drug producer, and its epidemic remains largely confined to gay men. Elsewhere, however, IV drug use is a significant factor in the transmission of HIV, particularly in Argentina. Indeed, the role of drugs may be even greater than the official figures suggest. As in Brazil, some drug users in the Southern Cone have shifted to crack (or other drugs) because of the stigma of IV drug use and the fear of HIV. While they may no longer acquire HIV from dirty needles, addicts may exchange sex for drugs or money or share homemade crack pipes that leave their lips cut or burned. They may not appear in the statistics as IV drug users, but drugs made them vulnerable to the virus. In this sense, Argentina's experience looks similar to that of major cities in

Brazil, such as São Paulo. While the future of the epidemic in Paraguay and Uruguay is still unclear, drug consumption will remain a key aspect of the disease's evolution in these countries.

At the same time, each country's experience with HIV is shaped more by how it responds to the epidemic than by any predetermined factor, such as the drug trade. Of all the nations in South America, Brazil has the most impressive program to confront HIV. But Argentina and Peru have also made substantial progress, even if their commitments on paper sometimes seem greater than their efforts in the field. Nonetheless, most nations in the region have made significant steps in the effort to control the disease. These nations also generally have the state capacity, and probably the resources, to design their own programs that can be fully as effective as Brazil's. Real progress is being made in areas such as reducing the cost of HIV medications. In this respect, the story of HIV in Spanish South America is as much one of hope as of tragedy.

CONCLUSION

This book has sought to link significant differences in the character of the HIV epidemic in Latin America to international issues. The key role that international forces play in the HIV epidemic was realized early in the epidemic, as the work of Paul Farmer on Haiti makes clear.[1] HIV is a pandemic that affects every aspect of our current world order, from high politics in major global powers to the daily lives of poor farmers in rural Africa or Asia. Indeed, the work of Nicholas Eberstadt suggests that HIV may be one of the factors that most affects the balance of global power in this century, as the disease appears set to devastate Russia if left unchecked, while its future course in the rising powers of India and China remains unclear.[2] In Africa some nations now have HIV rates greater than 40 percent among adults, and the epidemic has become generalized in much of southern Africa. In this international context, perhaps the most compelling question about Latin America's experience is why there been so little spread of HIV.[3] Latin America has widespread poverty, gender inequality, IV drug use, hidden male homosexuality, an extensive sex trade, and evidence from other infectious diseases (resurgent cholera in poor areas and endemic tuberculosis) that the public health system is imperfect. Yet with the exception of Haiti, Guyana, and perhaps Honduras, Latin America has been spared a generalized epidemic. Why? While much epidemiological work remains to be done, understanding the epidemic's history in the region and the international factors that shaped this experience can suggest some initial answers.

To understand Latin America's experience of HIV, it is necessary to consider the epidemic's history. In the case of the Caribbean, what is striking from the perspective of more than two decades is how many aspects of HIV/AIDS have been influenced by international factors, such as sex tourism from Europe and America, the policies of development agencies and the United States, labor migration between the islands and abroad, and developmental issues that have weakened both some Caribbean states and their ability to provide public health services. In the case of Cuba and Haiti, the countries in the Caribbean with the lowest and the highest rates of HIV, respectively, their relationship with the United States affected their initial experience with HIV. Cuba perceived that it needed to provide an alternative to the U.S. model for health, and initially it valued the community's need to control the virus over the rights of individuals. Cuba's pride in its international reputation in the field of public health, its equation of disease with foreign corruption, and its distrust of NGOs (because of their possible links to foreign countries) all led the government to adopt a policy of quarantine to control AIDS. With the collapse of the Soviet Union, Cuba's sanatorium policy became increasingly unaffordable, and at the same time the self-injection movement threatened the island's international support. As the island was becoming increasingly dependent on tourism for its survival, Cuba's HIV/AIDS policy had to be reworked, especially given Cuba's enduring political struggle with the United States. As a result Cuba now has adopted a system more like that of other Latin American nations.

In Haiti the impact of the virus was magnified because of stereotypes in the developed world, which equated the island with voodoo (voudon), zombies, and animal sacrifice. With the initial appearance of HIV, a hysterical overreaction devastated the economy long before the virus itself began to take a heavy toll. This discrimination has continued to facilitate the spread of the disease among transborder labor migrants, not only in Miami or New York but also on the island of Hispaniola itself. Haitians working in Dominican bateyes have proved to be vulnerable to HIV infection not only because of their poverty but also because of a variety of factors related to discrimination: the construction of Haitian and Dominican identities, the political discourses that Dominican leaders have adopted, the perception of race on both sides of the border, and the manner in which religious differences have been portrayed in the two countries. Haiti's experience underlines the fact that HIV—although a disease driven by personal behavior—reflects complex international issues, from the economic issues shaping poverty to the cultural beliefs that define prejudice.

Brazil's experience with HIV highlights the contradictions of globalization, which has perhaps proved to be the dominant global force since the end of the Cold War. If someone had told early activists in the mid-1980s that Brazil would come to the forefront of global efforts to address HIV/AIDS, they likely would have been bemused at the idea. But as Brazil democratized, NGOs, with support from major international charities, successfully pressured the government to fight HIV/AIDS aggressively. After the discovery of an effective therapy for HIV in 1996, the Brazilian government quickly moved to make this treatment available for free to all people living with HIV. This program entailed the construction of a sophisticated system to provide care, which included laboratories to monitor CD-4 counts and viral load, physicians to prescribe and monitor therapy, and a network of dispensaries. On one hand, this program could not have been created without a series of loans from the Word Bank (although this body itself never supported providing free medications to people with HIV). On the other hand, the Brazilian decision to consider producing generic drugs (compulsory licensing) drew the country into a battle with the United States, multinational pharmaceutical companies, and the WTO. With the help of other developing countries and NGOs, Brazil fought a successful legal and diplomatic campaign. Its success has changed the terms of the debate regarding providing medications and care in developing countries, because the program has actually saved the government money, due to a reduction in hospitalizations, hospice care, and new infections.

In Mesoamerica there is a clear distinction between Mexico, in which generally there is a relatively low level of HIV, and its southern neighbors, where HIV rates tend to be higher. The factors behind this are complex, but war and labor migration are two key issues that have shaped the region's diverse experience of HIV. In much of Africa, warfare has clearly increased the spread of HIV. War causes the movement of populations, exposing women to rape or sexual coercion, and provides opportunities for sexual relations between civilians and soldiers, who tend to have a higher level of HIV than the general population. New evidence, however, suggests that sometimes war has the paradoxical effect of slowing the spread of HIV. This

CONCLUSION

appears to be the case in Central America, where Nicaragua was ravaged by war but has had a low prevalence of HIV, while states that did not experience fighting (Panama, Honduras, and Belize) have significantly higher rates of infection.

In general, Mexico appears to have had greater success than most Central American states in containing the virus's spread. Recently, however, the virus has spread into rural areas of Mexico, often from migrant laborers who were infected abroad. The international sex trade, which is bringing women from Central America through Mexico to the United States, is helping to drive the feminization of HIV. Still, several factors have worked to shield Mexico so far, including its low rate of IV drug use and a health-based approach to regulating sex work. But unless the connection between international migration and HIV/AIDS is addressed, the virus will continue its movement into remote areas, where middle-aged married women are being infected in surprising numbers. The experience of both war and migration are thus integral to the virus's movement through the region.

The story of HIV in Spanish South America is particularly complex. To some extent, it makes more sense to examine Latin America in terms of the factors driving the spread of the virus (such as men having sex with men) rather than by region. This idea is supported if we examine one powerful factor shaping the spread of the disease: the international drug trade. In the developed world, we usually think of Latin American countries solely as drug-producing states. But other countries, such as Argentina and Brazil, are major drug markets. There is a third group of countries, such as Chile or Uruguay, that may be neither major producers nor consumers of drugs. How a country functions in terms of the drug trade has implications for its HIV epidemic. In producing states, such as Peru, Bolivia, Ecuador, and Colombia, the HIV epidemic has continued to be dominated by men having sex with men. Nonetheless, the violence and corruption generated by the drug trade has undermined the state's ability to respond to the epidemic and threatens the ability of these countries, especially Colombia, to contain the virus in the long term. Argentina, in contrast, is much more like Brazil in terms of the central role that drugs have played in spreading the virus. Finally, some nations (such as Chile) have not played a major role in the drug trade. In these countries the virus is following a separate, and so far slower, path. The epidemic there tends to be less concentrated among men who have sex with men than in the Andean producer countries, but drugs also have not facilitated the rapid spread of HIV among heterosexuals, as in

Argentina and Brazil. Given these historical accounts, how can we understand the differences between Latin America's experience of the virus and those of other major world regions?

■ The Impact of War

On the surface, Latin America seems to have many risk factors for HIV in common with areas with a high prevalence, from sub-Saharan Africa to Southeast Asia.[4] But in general the virus has not spread in a commensurate manner. Why not? One possible explanation might be the impact of war. Most African states gained their independence during the period from the 1950s through the 1970s. In many cases, independence came only as the result of prolonged conflict with colonial powers. Portuguese Africa was wracked by years of brutal warfare, in countries from Guinea-Bissau to Angola, as five centuries of colonial rule came to an end. In many cases, the fighting did not cease with independence, because new institutions lacked legitimacy, most nations contained multiple ethnic groups with weak allegiances to the state, colonial borders did not reflect African reality, some armed groups wanted to impose their political programs by violence, and the survival of white ruler regimes did not lay the groundwork for peace. Warfare has also plagued many Asian states now heavily affected by HIV, such as Cambodia and Myanmar.[5] Sadly, in the case of Cambodia it even seems that the epidemic may have been driven in part by the activities of United Nations peacekeepers.[6] Warfare associated with the drug trade also seems to be contributing to the spread of the virus.[7]

In contrast, most Latin American countries became independent in the early nineteenth century. Although extensive violence accompanied this experience (with some exceptions, such as Brazil), the region has since come to be perceived as a "zone of peace" in international relations scholarship. The linguistic, cultural, and religious unity of the region has tended to dampen conflict. Although there are notable exceptions (such as the Paraguayan War, 1865–70), in general most conflicts within Latin America have occurred within rather than between states. Most conflicts between states (such as Peru and Ecuador) have been over border issues that led to skirmishes rather than to sustained warfare. Epidemiologists have demonstrated that there is a clear correlation between war and the spread of HIV in some African nations, such as Uganda during the overthrow of Idi Amin.[8]

From this perspective, the absence of sustained warfare in much of Latin America during the latter half of the twentieth century might help to explain the region's relatively low level of HIV/AIDS.

This argument, however, is problematic. Nothing is perhaps more surprising than the complex and contradictory impact that war can have. It appears obvious that war should fuel an HIV epidemic, for reasons that are well known. The displacement of people creates opportunities for the virus to move among communities. Women who are refugees are vulnerable to demands for transactional sex. Rape is often used as a weapon of war. The weakness of the state can make carrying out public health programs difficult. Some regions of nations may be isolated by conflict. People subject to violence may not believe that HIV represents their greatest danger, and they might undertake risky sexual behavior that would not make sense in a more peaceful context. Wandering bands of soldiers in the countryside may carry the virus. Soldiers are particularly likely to have higher rates of HIV than the general population. All these factors have been carefully studied.[9] But as Laurie Garrett notes in a recent article in *Foreign Affairs*, it now appears from a number of cases that war can sometimes have the paradoxical effect of impeding the spread of the virus:

> One counter-intuitive effect of warfare, as the recent histories of Angola, Cambodia, Ethiopia, Namibia, Nigeria, South Africa, and Zimbabwe show, is that it can actually reduce the risk of HIV infection. During wartime, civilians either hunker down in their homes or flee war-torn regions and become refugees. Trade grinds to a halt, borders are locked tight, and social mobility is minimized. Consider Angola, for example. For 27 years, it was wracked by a civil war that left the now-peaceful nation in shambles. War, however, largely kept HIV outside Angola, since most forms of trade and travel, both within the country and across its borders, were essentially shut down for three decades. Since the end of the conflict in 2002, Angola's borders have reopened. Peace has brought greater trade—but also an increased HIV infection rate.[10]

One can see examples in Latin America of both tendencies of war, suggesting that warfare alone cannot account for Latin America's distinctiveness.

The region of Latin America most affected by warfare in the late twentieth century has been Central America. With the exception of Guatemala, the nation most influenced by fighting was Nicaragua. The evidence in this case seems to clearly suggest that the sad and wasteful contra war shielded the country from HIV. In South America the nation most affected by warfare has been Colombia, which has seen major guerrilla groups and fighting during most of the period since the 1950s. In the Colombian case, the violence seems to be driving the virus's spread and hampering efforts to control the disease. But the violence itself makes obtaining good information difficult. Yet it is becoming clear that we need a more complex understanding of war and its impact on women, migration, and HIV. It may not be enough to say that war can be a vector in the spread of the virus. We may need to look at the kind of conflict and how it disrupts the state and affects civilians. Some good work is being begun in this area, but still far too little.[11] Different levels of war and insurrection do not seem to account for disparities in the rates of HIV in Latin America and other regions of the global south.

■ Poverty and Globalization

Another explanation for the region's distinctiveness could focus on poverty. Countries with fewer financial resources might be less able to respond to the virus. Certainly some of the nations most affected by HIV, such as Haiti, are also among the poorest. Latin America began to industrialize during the 1930s, particularly Brazil, Argentina, and Mexico. These three nations account for more than half of the region's population. Clearly, severe inequalities continue to exist within the region, not only in terms of income but also in terms of landholding. Still, some Latin American economies have notable areas of strength, such as Brazil, which is a major exporter of jet airplanes and has great expertise in offshore oil drilling. Tim Frasca notes that Latin America's average per capita income is twice that of Africa.[12] Similarly, many of the countries most heavily affected in Southeast Asia are relatively poor compared with Latin America. Could it be that differences in wealth between Latin America and these regions help to explain why the former has a lower level of HIV?

The relationship between HIV and poverty is complex. One cannot discuss HIV without including issues of international political economy, from structural adjustment programs to international debt, from development programs to the accession terms of the WTO. Paul Farmer has stressed the importance of international factors, such as countries' insertion into the global economy, from the onset of the epidemic.[13] More than this, the link between poverty and HIV has been obvious since the mid-1980s, when people first realized that there was an epidemic among heterosexuals in Africa and Haiti. HIV became associated with impoverishment in the discourse. But as this disease and Susan Sontag have warned us, metaphors can be dangerous.[14] Equating HIV with poverty is not entirely accurate. Early in the epidemic, the disease in developed countries primarily hit well-educated, middle-class, gay men. In Africa and other developing countries it affected this group, too, but it also particularly hit heterosexual civil servants, teachers, soldiers, and doctors[15]—in other words, an urban, educated class. No one was immune. This was part of what made the disease so dreadful, as it particularly targeted people these societies could least do without. With time, the character of the disease in many countries has changed, and as it became increasingly associated with poverty, it has also become progressively more rural. But a nation's poverty, in and of itself, is not a good predictor of how a country will be affected by HIV.[16]

Some poor countries have relatively low rates of HIV, while much more developed countries have been affected heavily. As Barnett and Whiteside make clear, it is mysterious that some countries, such as Sri Lanka and the Philippines, have largely escaped the virus, while other countries at similar levels of development have been heavily affected.[17] This is the case in Latin America. Some countries that are the poorest in the Americas—such as Nicaragua and Bolivia—are among the nations least affected by HIV. Other nations that are much more developed, such as Argentina, have a higher prevalence of the virus. The experience of some poor countries such as Uganda shows that even an impoverished country emerging from civil war can make real progress against the virus. Brazil, which has extreme and destructive social inequality, has a highly effective program to fight HIV. It is difficult to explain the progress of the virus by focusing on development alone, without paying equal attention to politics.

I also am concerned that a focus on poverty can let both national elites and the international community off the hook. National elites can point their fingers at the structural poverty created by failed development plans, structural adjustment programs, unfair terms of trade, and the exploitation of the developed world and fail to act.[18] Yet if anything has become clear from the global experience of HIV, it is that political leadership is a key factor in fighting the virus, perhaps much more significant than the level of

CONCLUSION

economic development alone. This is what has made the spread of the virus so heartbreaking. Russia has been reluctant to fight the virus or to adopt successful models from Africa, perhaps in part from misplaced pride.[19] South Africa has emerged from apartheid and undertaken a major effort to reverse racial and social inequalities. Yet at the same time, the wealthiest country in Africa (with an economy more than four times the size of Nigeria's) has utterly failed to act as HIV has climbed to staggering levels.[20] It now has more cases of HIV than any other country in the world, but it still seems to lack the political will to face the epidemic. The contrast with some poorer nations, which have successfully addressed the epidemic, is painful. While poverty is a key factor, a focus on this issue alone can take attention away from issues that shape the spread of the virus, such as patriarchy, gender inequality, and racial and ethnic discrimination. This may be why addressing the virus may be so difficult politically, because it entails a fundamental questioning of many aspects of society, particularly factors that may benefit national elites.

Similarly, a focus on poverty can also discourage the international community from addressing the disease. If developed countries and international organizations have to first address poverty, the HIV epidemic can appear too daunting a problem to tackle. Fifty years of work in development since World War II have yielded, at best, mixed results. Yet the work of Paul Farmer and Doctors without Borders makes clear that it is possible to provide care for people with HIV in even the most impoverished nations. There are successful models now in both Haiti and Peru.[21] Care is possible with modest funds. The arguments against providing treatment—that people would not comply with drug regimens, that an expensive infrastructure is necessary that cannot be maintained—are proving to be false. The Brazilian example has required a fundamental rethinking about the division between prevention and treatment. If free care can be provided to all in Brazilian slums and rural areas, why can't this be done in other nations? We need much more research on the relationship between poverty and the spread of HIV. There are currently efforts considering how poverty and social inequality shape the spread of the virus in a more sophisticated manner.[22] These efforts have begun to examine broader criteria that influence the virus's impact, such as "social cohesion."[23] But much more work needs to be done, and the questions posed are subtle.

The same situation likely holds true concerning globalization. The relative degree to which major world regions are globalized does not seem to explain the progress of the virus within these areas. Indeed, the experience of HIV is in some sense a tale of the two faces of globalization. On one hand, globalization can create changes that rapidly spread the virus. Structural adjustment programs may undermine public health efforts. Labor migration may expose vulnerable populations to the disease. Traditional communities may be eroded. The WTO and multinational drug companies may deny access to generic drugs. Pressure from the U.S. government may hamper nations' efforts to reach out to sex workers or to teach safe sex as opposed to abstinence. The international sex trade may expose poor Haitians or Brazilians to the virus. Human trafficking can ensnare poor Central American women in the brothels of southern Mexico or the United States. In its current form, the legacy of globalization can appear less as a web of economic interconnections than as a tragic litany of loss.

At the same time, however, globalization brings the expertise of UNAIDS, World Bank loans to fight the disease, the vaccine efforts of the Bill and Melinda Gates Foundation, the financial commitment of the U.S. government, international advocacy for human rights, and pressure for the education and empowerment of women. The excellent work of USAID in Central America and NAMRID in Peru makes clear what the U.S. government can accomplish with the proper policy direction. One of the most positive aspects of the global response to the virus has also been the proliferation of international NGOs. These organizations have fought the pharmaceutical companies, the U.S. government, and the WTO about drug prices; provided funding and expertise for NGOs in developing countries; advanced new ways of thinking about the gay community; funded models such as Paul Farmer's clinic in Haiti; and tried to hold governments to their international obligations. International NGOs have won many critical battles. The only hope for some poor countries that now face a major HIV epidemic comes from the international community and organizations such as these. Poverty and globalization are important parts of the story of HIV. But neither in isolation can explain why Latin America's experience of HIV has so far been distinct.

■ Timing

There are, however, four factors that combined might explain why Latin America's experience has been distinctive. The first of these is timing, as Frasca notes.[24] People first realized that HIV could become a predominately heterosexual epidemic in 1986, when it became clear that many nations in Central Africa were suffering from such an epidemic. Some African countries, such as Uganda, have responded to the virus with alacrity and have either contained or even reduced the level of infection. In doing so, they overcame a far greater challenge than most of Latin America has faced. In 1986, when many African states already had a significant HIV epidemic, absolute numbers of infections were still very low in most Latin American countries, and the disease remained relatively confined within gay communities. This meant that nations from Cuba to Brazil had an opportunity to formulate a response to the virus, to educate the public, to clean up the blood supply, and to make testing available. Most African states did not have this choice. Testing for HIV was not even available in the early years of the epidemic. Part of what drove Latin America's decision to respond to the virus in the late 1980s was the African example, and the fear that without rapid action much of the region would follow the same path. Of course, this explanation does not account for the emerging difference between Latin America and some Asian states. Even more important, within Africa most of southern Africa remained relatively free of the virus until the late 1980s, only to watch the virus climb to staggering levels with astonishing speed during the following decade. South Africa was a clear example of this tragic pattern.[25] Nations that had the opportunity did not always act on it. But Latin America still had a chance that much of Africa did not have, because the virus first emerged on that continent.

■ Migration

Another important factor shaping the HIV epidemic in different regions has been migration, which has been a significant issue in Latin America. In Haiti, for example, farm laborers working in the bateyes of the Dominican Republic may face an increased risk of infection, which they will then bring home with them at the end of the sugarcane season. But the country where HIV rates are most likely to be influenced by migration is Mexico, even though it still has a relatively low rate of HIV. In particular, the return of migrant workers from the United States appears to be a factor driving the spread of the virus in poor, rural communities. Young men from isolated, traditional villages travel to urban areas in the United States and are exposed to sexual opportunities and drugs lacking at home. They experiment, and some become infected with HIV, which they may bring back to their small communities. Migrants from Central America are also terribly vulnerable to exploitation in both Mexico and the United States, where they may face demands for transactional sex or encounter human traffickers.

While recognizing the role of migrants in the epidemic, however, it is also important not to demonize this group. The United States now has a powerful political lobby that targets illegal immigrants and undocumented migrants. CNN's Lou Dobbs has a constant drumbeat of programing about the dangers this group represents.[26] Within Mexico, too, migrants are stigmatized, despite efforts by President Vicente Fox to change the national perception of them. In Mexico, Central Americans are blamed for the spread of HIV in the south, while returning migrants are blamed for the emergence of the virus in rural communities. In Oaxaca, I was shocked by the media coverage given to returning migrants, who were not only blamed for spreading HIV in the region but also described as deviants whose antisocial behavior placed the community at risk in other respects. Much as homophobia hampered early efforts to fight HIV, so, too, does prejudice now limit efforts to work with this group. Migrants are difficult to reach. Many do not speak Spanish; they often come from isolated, rural communities; they are frightened of authority; and they are mobile. Some wonderful work has been done on migration and HIV in Mesoamerica by authors such as Bronfman.[27] But much more work needs to be done, and it will need the cooperation of the migrants themselves.

As significant as migration has been in shaping the HIV epidemic in Latin America, it has likely played a less significant role than in Asia, particularly with regard to the forcible trafficking of women for the sex trade. It is, of course, difficult to find quantitative information on this, because the trade is illicit.[28] But the trafficking of women for the sex trade has been absolutely key to the experience of HIV in South and Southeast Asia, as Chris Beyer's work has described. Of course, a similar trade exists that brings mostly Central American women to the United States through Mexico. But the number of nations involved, the distances traveled by the women, the sophistication of the trafficking networks, and the sheer intensity of the trade seem to be of a different order in South and Southeast Asia than in Latin America.

A brothel in Cambodia may offer women and girls trafficked from Cambodia, Thailand, Vietnam, China or the Philippines. Cambodian women have been trafficked to Singapore, Hong Kong, Malaysia, and Thailand. A brothel in Thailand may have women and girls trafficked from rural Thailand, from Burma, China (Yunnan), Laos and Cambodia. Japan receives most of its trafficked women and girls from Thailand and the Philippines; as many as 50,000 Thai women may work there. India traffics mainly rural and tribal women and girls, as well as large numbers of Nepalese. Malaysia's sex trade has Cambodian, Thai and Burmese women, and Indonesians, in addition to Malaysians. Thai women have been found in sexual slavery in California and in Sweden. Vietnamese women have been found trafficked at sea, traded from ship to ship by pirates, homeless and stateless.[29]

It is possible to measure, perhaps, the impact of this trade on a biological level. For example, Laurie Garrett suggests that Myanmar's role in the evolution of HIV in Asia may have been critical, given recent work examining HIV strains circulating in Asia. The same routes that carry opium poppies also carry women into sexual slavery, with devastating effects: "HIV cases and specific HIV subtypes cluster in poppy-growing regions and then travel along heroin-smuggling routes in Asia. This evidence suggests that Myanmar may be the greatest contributor to new types of HIV in the world. In fact, there has been only one outbreak of HIV in Central Asia that seems to have originated anywhere else."[30]

This stunning fact suggests the extent to which migration and human trafficking can deeply shape a continent's HIV epidemic. Of course, Asia is not unique. In southern Africa, labor migration, particularly during the period of apartheid rule, may have been a key factor in the dispersal of HIV.[31] Most experts on southern Africa's HIV epidemic, such as Barnett and Whiteside, particularly stress the importance of this factor:

Migration and mobility have created patterns of sexual behavior which are perfect for the spread of sexually transmitted diseases. Indeed, we note that migrant-sending countries have higher rates of HIV prevalence than South Africa itself. South Africa is the crucible for HIV transmission in the region. Labour comes into an area of high seroprevalence, where working and living conditions encourage sexual mixing. Infected men return to their home communities where "local" epidemics are established. In the periphery there are neither the resources nor the ability to establish AIDS control programmes. In the longer term it is these communities that bear the cost of increased illness and deaths.[32]

It is possible that in both Africa and Asia migration has played a more essential role in the spread of HIV than has been the case to date in Latin America. Yet their experience perhaps also should serve as a warning, particularly for Mesoamerica.

■ Democracy

Sweeping political changes in Latin America at the same time that HIV emerged in the region also seem to have influenced the course of the epidemic and to have helped to control the spread of the virus.[33] Between 1983, when the Argentine military government collapsed, and 1990, when Pinochet left power in Chile, one authoritarian regime after another fell to popular protest and political exhaustion. There have been exceptions. In 1992 President Fujimori of Peru closed the congress and made himself dictator; he subsequently fled to Japan in shame in 2000. In Mexico the PRI manipulated elections to retain power until 2000, when Vicente Fox of the conservative National Action Party was elected. Throughout the region, however, the overall trend was clear: HIV/AIDS appeared in Latin America during a period that saw rapid growth in civil society as well as a proliferation of grassroots activism dedicated to everything from gay rights to women's issues. From Brazil to Peru, one cannot study the epidemic without being struck by how NGOs played a key role in pressuring the government to respond to HIV, sometimes in the face of scorn or even repression. These organizations quickly became very organized and quite powerful. Health ministers feared them. It is true that some examples contradict this trend. Frasca laments that in Argentina overly close ties between NGOs and the government hindered efforts to fight HIV/AIDS. Sadly, the return to democracy coincided with increased drug use in Argentina. Menem's government not only ignored the spread of the virus but also created a climate of corruption that undermined the work of NGOs.[34] Democracy alone is not enough to guarantee a good response to HIV. But in country after country the popular protests of grassroots activists, often acting with funds from international donors, have led to key policy changes, from the enforcement of human rights provisions to the provision of free treatment to the ill.

CONCLUSION

In Africa during the same period, many countries were under the rule of a strong man or a one-party government or were very weak democracies. The same could be said of some Asian states that were key in the virus's dispersion, such as Myanmar. Countries that were democracies, such as Thailand, seemed to be able to address a serious HIV/AIDS epidemic more effectively.[35] The message may be that democracy matters and can improve the government's response to the epidemic. But there are painful counterexamples, of which the key one is certainly South Africa, in which HIV spread most quickly after the end of apartheid and the establishment of democratic rule.[36] Democracy is not enough to control the virus if political leaders lack the will to do so. States with authoritarian rulers can effectively respond to the virus if the political will exists, as the case of Cuba clearly illustrates. The relationship between democracy and HIV is probably the most understudied question in the field. Based on what I have seen in the region, however, I believe that HIV would have had a far more serious impact on Latin America if it had not been for the flowering of civil society that accompanied the region's democratization.

■ State Capacity

A final factor that may help to explain Latin America's success fighting the virus may be the relative strength of Latin American states, in comparison with some African and Asian counterparts. This has become a key issue in current research because of the realization that poverty is an important factor in explaining the relative spread of HIV, but at the same time not all poor countries are equally affected by the virus.[37] Andrew Price Smith and his colleagues have therefore carried out a careful quantitative study to examine the relative strength of various states and how that strength has influenced the spread of HIV. In their work, economic factors are a key aspect of a state's capacity, but this concept also entails other crucial factors that range from the dedication of government officials to the strength of state institutions. In other words, wealth alone does not define state capacity, although it is a key factor. Their hypothesis is that in cases where state capacity is low, other factors such as "political will and social cohesion" are even more important in explaining whether a country can respond successfully to HIV.[38] Their careful quantitative analysis of fifty countries found that the strength of the state was a major factor in explaining the spread of HIV, although perhaps not the most important one, as the authors were careful to point out: "Additionally, this analysis demonstrates that state capacity alone does not sufficiently explain a nation's ability to generate successful adaptive countermeasures to counter the HIV/AIDS epidemic. The fact that state capacity explains only 38 percent of the variance in adaption suggests that other variables such as political commitment and community mobilization may be of equal or greater importance in determining whether a country adapts successfully."[39]

What does this mean for Latin America? Latin America is stereotyped as a region defined by weak government and political corruption. Having lived in Brazil during the impeachment of President Fernando Collor, having visited Brazil during the scandal that shook President Lula's administration, and having published on military corruption in Brazil, I am well aware of these weaknesses.[40] And yet, what has struck me the most in studying HIV/AIDS in Latin America has been the effectiveness of many states in responding to the epidemic. A relatively poor country, Cuba mobilized the resources of the state to halt HIV and succeeded, although at a high cost to individual rights. Brazil created a structure to provide free medications to all HIV-positive people, which entailed a sophisticated infrastructure of trained doctors, HIV testing, regional laboratories, and medication dispensaries. There are obvious weaknesses and exceptions.[41] But from Mexico to Peru even states in the midst of political turmoil met the challenge of HIV with some success, even if only after widespread popular pressure to do so. Latin American states have created a public health infrastructure, fostered the communications systems that make international collaboration possible, and participated in PAHO. In contrast, the relative weakness of states in key areas of Asia (Myanmar and Cambodia) and Africa (the Democratic Republic of the Congo and Zimbabwe) has compounded other difficulties in fighting HIV/AIDS in these regions. Of course, many states in these areas have success stories, from Thailand to Uganda. But the relative strength of Latin American states may have given this region some advantages in the struggle with HIV/AIDS.

■ Questions

I remain concerned about the future of HIV in Latin America, particularly in rural Mexico and Central America, where patterns of migration may be driving the virus's spread. Much work remains to be done. For authors and epidemiologists who wish to pursue future research, there is a wealth of statistical and qualitative knowledge to draw upon, in particular online. Readers interested in exploring these resources in greater depth will find reams of information to begin their work in the websites described in the following endnote.[42] Some questions in particular seem to demand more attention: the connection between democratization and the ability of a state to respond to HIV/AIDS, the role that the trafficking of women across borders for sex plays in Mesoamerica and the United States, the impact of labor migration on HIV in rural Mexico, the varied impact that war has had on HIV within the region, and the course of the epidemic in Colombia. Some topics will be difficult to work on, such as the Cuban HIV/AIDS epidemic, given the current political climate. But I am struck by how many questions remain, and by how much could be done with the information now available.

My curiosity about HIV/AIDS in Latin America is now more personal. I wonder about the people I met: The Cuban man living with HIV/AIDS who wanted me to help him find shampoo and clippers for his poodle. The Cuban rocker who e-mailed me to ask if I could help him replace his broken glasses—I did not know what to say. The composed transvestite I spoke with in Oaxaca who had remade her life, remained HIV-positive, and now cared for her mother. The leaders of one NGO who did not have enough diapers for all of the HIV-positive babies and were trying to find funds. The many drug users with whom I spoke in Brazil, each of whom had a story of loss and longing. It is hard to care about an issue because of statistics and studies. I have many questions that still trouble me about the course of HIV/AIDS in Latin America. But now I must wonder about the many people whose stories I have heard, and friends with whom I no longer have contact. The privilege of fieldwork is being able to go into another world, which always entails the support of many other people. It's hard to give anything back to these people in a meaningful way, and to me the exchange in the end feels unequal. These people, their stories and challenges, remain in my mind.

CONCLUSION

NOTES

Introduction

1. The term "mosaic of infection" comes from multiple authors, including Cueto, *Culpa e Coraje*, 16. See also de Brito, Ayres de Castilho, and Szwarcwald, "AIDS e Infecção pelo HIV no Brasil," 207.

2. Pan American Health Organization, *AIDS Surveillance*, 7–8.

3. Farmer, *AIDS and Accusation*, 149.

4. Paternostro, *In the Land of God and Man*, provides an excellent survey of sexual practices and beliefs in Latin America from a qualitative perspective. For a list of key works on sexuality in Mexico see Carrillo, *Night Is Young*, 8–9. For one of the best early works on the Mexican case see Izazola, Valdespino, Juárez, Mondragón, and Sepúlveda, "Conocimientos." For sexual beliefs and practices in Peru see Cáceres Palacios, *SIDA en el Perú*, 78, 83, 85–86, 103–4, 109.

5. "Guatemala: AIDS Campaign under Review," *Mesoamérica* 16, no. 12 (December 1997): 1–2.

6. Key and DeNoon, "Nuns Fight AIDS in the Dominican Republic."

7. There are several good works that describe HIV. See in particular Montagnier, *Virus*; Fan, Conner, and Villarreal, *AIDS*; Whiteside and Sunter, *AIDS*, 1–35; Goudsmit, *Viral Sex*.

8. For a comprehensive overview of efforts to develop an HIV vaccine see Cohen, *Shots in the Dark*, and Thomas, *Big Shot*. For a brief treatment of the topic see Goudsmit, *Viral Sex*, 201–18.

9. Cohen, *Shots in the Dark*, 7–13.

10. For a history of the emergence of the disease in the United States see Grmek, *History of AIDS*, 3–20.

11. For the discovery of the virus see ibid., 61–78; Montagnier, *Virus*, 55–69.

12. Hooper, *The River*, 11. See also Grmek, *History of AIDS*, 48; Guest, *Children of AIDS*, 3.

13. Hooper, *The River*, 13. For suggestions that HIV is an older disease than generally believed see Grmek, *History of AIDS*, 110–26. For the primate origins of HIV see Ryan, *Virus X*, 285–86, 292, 295.

14. Grmek, *History of AIDS*, 135; Hooper, *The River*, 29.

15. See Grmek, *History of AIDS*, 175–79. See also Nzilambi et al., "Prevalence of Infection"; Ryan, *Virus X*, 297.

16. Hooper, *The River*, 164.

17. Grmek, *History of AIDS*, 179–81; Hooper, *The River*, 165, 670–75; Goudsmit, *Viral Sex*, 77–110.

18. Hooper, *The River*, 869–70.

19. For a passionate response to these arguments see Hooper's postscript in *The River*, 827–77.

20. Ibid., 175; for similar cases see 669, 862.

21. See Gerry Myer's comments in ibid., 181.

22. The earliest evidence for HIV in Africa dates to the 1960s and early 1970s; see Grmek, *History of AIDS*, 172–75.

23. Barnett and Whiteside, *AIDS in the Twenty-First Century*, 37. For blood transfusions as a possible factor in the emergence of HIV see Hooper, *The River*, 683.

24. Although it is now somewhat dated, Grmek, *History of AIDS*, is still a key source for the early history of the epidemic.

25. Hooper, *The River*, 99, 208; for further genetic evidence that Africa is the homeland of HIV see 178–79. Goudsmit suggests Cameroon as the possible source for HIV I-B; see Goudsmit, *Viral Sex*, 59–76.

26. Hooper, *The River*, 623–43. This argument is strengthened by the case of a Portuguese man who likely contacted HIV-2 in Guinea-Bissau between 1956 and 1966. See Grmek, *History of AIDS*, 131.

27. For the case of the Norwegian sailor see Grmek, *History of AIDS*, 130; Goudsmit, *Viral Sex*, 25–26; Hooper, *The River*, 316–22, 518–22. For the time line for the early course of HIV see Hooper, *The River*, 741; Montagnier, *Virus*, 121–24. Goudsmit, *Viral Sex*, 25–37, presents an alternative time line that posits an early outbreak of HIV in 1930s Germany, which has not found favor in the scholarly community. For the early history of the epidemic in Europe see Grmek, *History of AIDS*, 20–30. For a discussion of the Haitian case see Grmek, *History of AIDS*, 34–36, 153–54.

28. Gómez Gómez, *SIDA en Colombia*, 65–66. The very first Colombian patient was a twenty-three-year-old woman who lived in the port city of Cali, where she served a clientele that included sailors. See Ministerio de Salud, *Plan de Mediano Plazo*, 20.

29. Shilts, *And the Band Played On*, 130, 141, 146–47. See also Grmek, *History of AIDS*, 18–20.

30. Rosenfield and Herbrand, "Part One."

31. Leiner, *Sexual Politics in Cuba*, 131; for the association of the disease internationally with U.S. decadence see 136–37.

32. Carmona Berríos and del Valle Larrañaga, *SIDA en Chile*, 40.

33. For the Mexican experience see Mejía, "SIDA," 17. See also Anderson, "AIDS as an Opportunity," 4–10. For the case of Chile see Carmona Berríos and del Valle Larrañaga, *SIDA en Chile*, 54.

34. Carmona Berríos and del Valle Larrañaga, *SIDA en Chile*, 46–47, 54.

35. Gómez Gómez, *SIDA en Colombia*, 68.

36. Daniel, "AIDS in Brazil," 208.

37. Ibid. For more on discrimination see Parker, "AIDS in Brazil," 22–23; Terto, "A AIDS e o Local de Trabalho no Brasil," 138, 139.

38. For the early perception of AIDS in Brazil see Bastos, *Global Responses to AIDS*, 70–71.

39. See Marins, "Brazilian Policy."

40. Guest, *Children of AIDS*, 65–66, 165–66.

41. Ibid., 7–8; Irwin, Millen, and Fallows, *Global AIDS*, 54.

42. For a discussion of why the African epidemic may be particularly severe, see Barnett and Whiteside, *AIDS in the Twenty-First Century*, 124–56.

43. For a description of the impact of HIV in Africa see Stephanie Nolen's reporting, perhaps the best journalistic account of the continent's epidemic: <http://www.theglobeandmail.com/special/aidsinafrica/>. For an academic account of HIV's impact in the region see Barnett and Whiteside, *AIDS in the Twenty-First Century*, 159–81.

44. For information on Botswana's HIV epidemic see Barnett and Whiteside, *AIDS in the Twenty-First Century*, 119–23. See also <http://www.avert.org/aidsbotswana.htm> as well as the material available at the UNAIDS website: <http://www.unaids.org/en/geographical+area/by+country/botswana.asp>.

45. Youde, "Enter the Fourth Horseman," 199. See also Irwin, Millen, and Fallows, *Global AIDS*, 36; Guest, *Children of AIDS*, 5.

46. Eberstadt, "Future of AIDS," 24–27, 40–41, 43.

47. Garrett, "Lessons," 58. This article also provides a good global overview of the pandemic. For more information on the pandemic, and basic facts pertaining to HIV, see the UNAIDS website: <http://www.unaids.org/NetTools/Misc/DocInfo.aspx?LANG=en&href=http://gva-doc-owl/WEBcontent/Documents/pub/UNA-docs/Q-A_II_en.pdf>.

Chapter 1

1. All quotations are from Norborg and Sand, *Socialism or Death*. I wish to thank Ryan Prout, without whom I would not have found a copy of this work. See Prout, "Jail-House Rock."

2. Ceballos, *Maldita Sea Tu Nombre, Libertad*. I wish to thank Vladimir for providing me with a copy of this work.

3. Cueto, *Culpa e Coraje*, 16.

4. Goodwin, *Global Studies*, 101.

5. Finlinson et al., "Access to Sterile Syringes," 207; the profile of HIV in Puerto Rico is so different that some studies of AIDS in the Caribbean exclude this island. See Inácio Bastos, Strathdee, Derrico, and Fátima Pina, "Drug Use and the Spread of HIV/AIDS," 32, 36; for HIV/AIDS profiles of select Caribbean countries see <http://www.census.gov/ipc/www/hivctry.html>.

6. McEvoy, "Caribbean Crossroads."

7. CIA World Factbook. See also Goodwin, *Global Studies*, 124–25; d'Adesky, *Moving Mountains*, 93.

8. Hunt, *Ideology and U.S. Foreign Policy*, 100.

9. Johnson, *Latin America in Caricature*, 202–3, 144–45. See also Hunt, *Ideology and U.S. Foreign Policy*, 141.

10. Black, *Good Neighbor*, 28; Farmer, *AIDS and Accusation*, 249.

11. Pike, *FDR's Good-Neighbor Policy*, 130.

12. Hunt, *Ideology and U.S. Foreign Policy*, 59; see also the cartoon on p. 63.

13. The best discussion of Haiti's history and how it shaped the island's experience with AIDS is Farmer, *AIDS and Accusation*.

14. Rose and Keystone, "AIDS in a Canadian Woman," 680–81; Hooper, *The River*, 78; Leibowitch, *Strange Virus*, 28; Siegal and Siegal, *AIDS*, 85; Andreani et al., "Acquired Immunodeficiency," 1187–91. For Farmer's skepticism about these cases see *AIDS and Accusation*, 212.

15. Pape et al., "Prevalence of HIV Infection"; Farmer, *AIDS and Accusation*, 129.

16. For a brief discussion of the early history of AIDS in Haiti see Farmer, *AIDS and Accusation*, 125–33; Pape et al., "Characteristics of the Acquired Immunodeficiency Syndrome."

17. For copies of the articles in *Morbidity and Mortality Weekly Report*, see Siegal and Siegal, *AIDS*, 214–15, 231–33, 237–39. See also Shilts, *And the Band Played On*, 167–68; Farmer, *AIDS and Accusation*, 211. For a discussion of AIDS in New York's Haitian community dating to this period see Nicholas et al., "Immune Competence."

18. Leonidas and Hyppolite, "Haiti and the Acquired Immunodeficiency Syndrome," 1020–21; Pitchenik et al., "Opportunistic Infections," 277–84; Teas, "Could AIDS Agent Be a New Variant of African Swine Fever Virus?," 923; Siegal and Siegal, *AIDS*, 86; Sabatier, *Blaming Others*, 45, 62; Farmer, "Exotic and the Mundane," 415–17. See also Farmer, *AIDS and Accusation*, 2–4, 220–28.

19. Greenfield, letter to the editor. See also Hooper, *The River*, 76.

20. Vieira, "Haitian Link," 95.

21. Leibowitch, *Strange Virus*, 41. For the possibility of transmission by insects see also Landesman, "Haitian Connection," 34.

22. Fettner and Check, *Truth about AIDS*, 111.
23. AMA News Release, May 6, 1983, quoted in full in Shilts, *And the Band Played On*, 299.
24. Greco, letter to the editor, 516.
25. Hooper, *The River*, 76; Farmer, *AIDS and Accusation*, 146.
26. Hooper, *The River*, 76.
27. Fettner and Check, *Truth about AIDS*, 117; Sabatier, *Blaming Others*, 47; Farmer, "Exotic and the Mundane," 435.
28. Hooper, *The River*, 76; Farmer, *AIDS and Accusation*, 238.
29. Casper, "AIDS," 201; Farmer, *AIDS and Accusation*, 5, 213–16.
30. Landesman, "Haitian Connection," 35.
31. Sabatier, *Blaming Others*, 46.
32. Bazell, "History of an Epidemic," 14.
33. Siegal and Siegal, *AIDS*, 85.
34. Sabatier, *Blaming Others*, 44.
35. Ibid., 8, 10.
36. Fettner and Check, *Truth about AIDS*, 109–10; Farmer, *Infections and Inequalities*, 104.
37. Hooper, *The River*, 74–75; Farmer, *AIDS and Accusation*, 143–45, 147–48.
38. Sabatier, *Blaming Others*, 45; Fettner and Check, *Truth about AIDS*, 121.
39. Fettner and Check, *Truth about AIDS*, 114.
40. Bazell, "History of an Epidemic," 15, 17; Sabatier, *Blaming Others*, 28; Farmer, *AIDS and Accusation*, 134–40, 225; Pape et al., "Risk Factors Associated with AIDS in Haiti."
41. Farmer, *AIDS and Accusation*, 122, 218–20; Sharif, "Haitians Fight Blood War," 13; d'Adesky, *Moving Mountains*, 101.
42. Pape, "AIDS in Haiti," 228. For this bizarre urban legend see Sabatier, *Blaming Others*, 45, 52. In the developing world, people responded by creating bizarre myths that American women had acquired the disease through sex with dogs. See the comments of a female bar owner in Belize in Kane, *AIDS Alibis*, 55.
43. Hooper, *The River*, 76.
44. Sabatier, *Blaming Others*, 14.
45. For information on Haiti's health care system and how political factors have undermined it see Farmer, "Haiti's Lost Years."
46. Farmer, "Exotic and the Mundane," 421.
47. Sabatier, *Blaming Others*, 28.
48. Boulos et al., "HIV-1 in Haitian Women," 721.
49. Ibid., 723.
50. For a brief history of the early epidemic in Haiti see Farmer, "Exotic and the Mundane," 418–23.

51. Farmer, *AIDS and Accusation*, 8, 11–12, 61–116; Farmer, *Infections and Inequalities*, 158–83; Farmer, "Sending Sickness."

52. Farmer, *AIDS and Accusation*, 113–14, 229–43.

53. Ibid., 228.

54. Boulos, Boulos, and Nichols, "Perceptions and Practices," 322 (emphasis in original).

55. Fitzgerald and Simon, "Commentary," 301–2.

56. Key and DeNoon, "Child Prostitution," 25.

57. Farmer, *AIDS and Accusation*, 78.

58. Fitzgerald and Simon, "Commentary," 303–4; see also d'Adesky, *Moving Mountains*, 102.

59. For the high percentage of Caribbean HIV infections in these two islands see Hawkins, "HIV/AIDS," 19. For more information on AIDS in the Dominican Republic see López Severino and de Moya, *Rutas Migratorias*; Garris et al., "AIDS Heterosexual Predominance."

60. Siegal and Siegal, *AIDS*, 70.

61. Lawrence K. Altman, "The Confusing Haitian Connection to AIDS," *New York Times*, August 16, 1983.

62. López Severino and de Moya, *Rutas Migratorias*, 7–8, 10, 23.

63. Ibid., 22. For the information in this paragraph see ibid., 13, 16–17, 22. For the high rate of HIV infection in tourist areas of the Dominican Republic see Garris et al., "AIDS Heterosexual Predominance," 1174–75.

64. López Severino and de Moya, *Rutas Migratorias*, 24, 30, 33, 34.

65. Fitzgerald and Simon, "Commentary," 307; see also 308.

66. Anne-Marie O'Connor, "Voodoo Priests Hand Out Condoms; Houngans, Mambos Recruited in Fight against AIDS," *Ottawa Citizen*, May 6, 1995.

67. Key and DeNoon, "Nuns Fight AIDS."

68. DeNoon and Key, "Church Leaders Oppose Proposal."

69. Key and DeNoon, "Six Dead in Jamaican Condom Riots."

70. UNAIDS, "AIDS Epidemic Update."

71. Ramsammy, "Are International Pharmaceutical Companies Doing Enough?," 125. These figures for infection rates among those attending clinics to be treated for sexually transmitted diseases are significantly higher than those provided by UNAIDS. See UNAIDS, "AIDS Epidemic Update."

72. UNAIDS, "AIDS Epidemic Update."

73. U.S. State Department, "U.S. President's Emergency Plan."

74. Ibid.

75. Ibid.

76. Ramsammy, "Are International Pharmaceutical Companies Doing Enough?," 125.

77. World Bank, *Project Appraisal Document . . . Guyana*, 3.

78. "AIDS in Haiti."

79. Ibid.; Farmer et al., "Community-Based Approaches to HIV." See also d'Adesky, *Moving Mountains*, 114–15.

80. Some U.S. policies have also negatively affected Haiti. See d'Adesky, *Moving Mountains*, 98–99.

81. Feinsilver, *Healing the Masses*, 14.

82. Ibid., 22; see also 56. My description of the Cuban health care system draws heavily on this work. See also Ubell, "Special Report"; MacDonald, *Developmental Analysis*.

83. Leiner, *Sexual Politics in Cuba*, 131; for the common description of AIDS as the result of U.S. decadence see 136–37.

84. Lumsden, *Machos, Maricones, and Gays*, 165.

85. Ibid.; Santana, Faas, and Wald, "Human Immunodeficiency Virus," 174.

86. Healton and Bayer, "Controlling AIDS in Cuba," 1022.

87. Rosenfield and Herbrand, "Part One."

88. Rosenfield and Herbrand, "Part Three"; Scheper-Hughes, "AIDS, Public Health, and Human Rights."

89. Scheper-Hughes, "AIDS, Public Health, and Human Rights," 965–66. See also Leiner, *Sexual Politics in Cuba*, 122.

90. Pérez-Stable, "Cuba's Response," 563. See also MacDonald, *Developmental Analysis*, 163. Healton and Bayer, "Controlling AIDS in Cuba," 1023, provided a lower figure of 3 million Cubans having been tested by 1989.

91. Leiner, *Sexual Politics in Cuba*, 117.

92. Ibid., 118.

93. This point was stressed by a health care worker who contracted HIV through sexual contact with his partner and was informed of his HIV-positive status in 1988. This man said that any refusal to enter the sanatoriums would have led to a conflict with the health authorities, who would have taken him to court. See Rosenfield and Herbrand, "Part One." Leiner, *Sexual Politics in Cuba*, 122, 125, discusses the psychological factors that made resistance difficult. For a further discussion of the issue see also Healton and Bayer, "Controlling AIDS in Cuba," 1024; MacDonald, *Developmental Analysis*, 167.

94. See the footage of the sanatoriums in John Marshall Law School, *Aspects of Criminalization*. For the existence of more restrictive sanatoriums see Mac-Donald, *Developmental Analysis*, 168.

95. Lumsden, *Machos, Maricones, and Gays*, 163. I toured Los Cocos on June 14, 2004, as a member of Cuba AIDS Project, and our tour guide (a subdirector at the sanatorium) described the early history of the facility.

96. Rosenfield and Herbrand, "Part One." For a further description of the sanatoriums see Leiner, *Sexual Politics in Cuba*, 117–21.

97. Leiner, *Sexual Politics in Cuba*, 31. For homophobia and Cuba's AIDS policy see d'Adesky, *Moving Mountains*, 82.

98. Leiner, *Sexual Politics in Cuba*, 21. My discussion of homosexuality in Cuba is based on Leiner, *Sexual Politics in Cuba*, and Lumsden, *Machos, Maricones, and Gays*.

99. Lumsden, *Machos, Maricones, and Gays*, 12.

100. Leiner, *Sexual Politics in Cuba*, 2. For a thoughtful critique of quarantine as a policy see also d'Adesky, *Moving Mountains*, 76–77.

101. Leiner, *Sexual Politics in Cuba*, 2.

102. Santana, Faas, and Wald, "Human Immunodeficiency Virus," 185.

103. Elizabeth Aguilera, "Cuba's Low HIV Rate Belies the Stigma, Ignorance Many Face," *Denver Post*, February 10, 2003. Accessed through LexisNexis.

104. See the correspondence concerning "Controlling AIDS in Cuba," and Bayer and Healton's response, in *New England Journal of Medicine*, September 21, 1989, 829–30. The debate was begun by Healton and Bayer's article "Controlling AIDS in Cuba," April 13, 1989. See also Lumsden, *Machos, Maricones, and Gays*, 162.

105. Leiner, *Sexual Politics in Cuba*, 133–34. See also Healton and Bayer, "Controlling AIDS in Cuba," 1022; Hansen and Groce, "From Quarantine to Condoms," 261; Prout, "Jail-House Rock," 426.

106. Leiner, *Sexual Politics in Cuba*, 121.

107. Enríquez, "Economic Reform," 203.

108. MacDonald, *Developmental Analysis*, 269, 277. The CDC and PAHO believed the outbreak to have been caused by malnutrition, but some authors have wondered if there could have been an unknown virus present in Cuba. See Farmer, *Pathologies of Power*, 77.

109. Enríquez, "Economic Reform," 204.

110. Feinsilver, *Healing the Masses*, 34, 51. See also Tim Golden, "Health Care, Cuba's Pride, Falls on Hard Times," *New York Times*, October 30, 1994; MacDonald, *Developmental Analysis*, 231–232.

111. MacDonald, *Developmental Analysis*, 288.

112. Guillermoprieto, *Looking for History*, 101.

113. Swanson, Gill, Wald, and Swanson, "Comprehensive Care and the Sanatoria."

114. Key and DeNoon, "Cuba Sees AIDS Rise Linked to Tourism Growth."

115. Acosta, "Health-Cuba." For more on prostitution in Cuba after the fall of the Soviet Union see Guillermoprieto, *Looking for History*, 96, 111–25.

116. Pérez-Stable, "Cuba's Response," 565. For the importance of tourism to the Cuban economy see Jackiewicz, "Working World," 374. Most Cubans who become infected with HIV do so as a result of unprotected sex with other Cubans, not foreigners; lecture for members of Cuba AIDS Project, Los Cocos sanatorium, June 17, 2004.

117. Hansen and Groce, "From Quarantine to Condoms," 271.

118. There was some bias in this measure, in that homosexual men were the least likely to be released, but it represented a significant change to the program. See Leiner, *Sexual Politics in Cuba*, 120–21. I was told at Los Cocos sanatorium that this policy was introduced in December 1993.

119. Prout, "Jail-House Rock," 426.

120. Leiner, *Sexual Politics in Cuba*, 129; Healton and Bayer, "Controlling AIDS in Cuba," 1023; Quinn, Zacarias, and St. John, "AIDS in the Americas."

121. Leiner, *Sexual Politics in Cuba*, 143–44.

122. For a defense of the Cuban policy, based on cultural relativism, see Santana, Faas, and Wald, "Human Immunodeficiency Virus," 193.

123. John Marshall Law School, *Aspects of Criminalization*.

124. Such divisions among the sanatorium residents have been found by others. See Santana, Faas, and Wald, "Human Immunodeficiency Virus," 188.

125. See the comments of Dr. Jorge Pérez Ávila in Norborg and Sand, *Socialism or Death*.

126. Malcomson, "Socialism or Death?," 48. See also Ceballos, *Maldita Sea Tu Nombre, Libertad*.

127. Norborg and Sand, *Socialism or Death*.

128. Ibid.

129. According to Prout, Cuban government officials did harshly criticize Norborg and Sand's video after a screening in Mexico City; they also successfully pressured Mexican officials not to screen the video on public television. See Prout, "Jail-House Rock," 431–32.

130. Malcomson, "Socialism or Death?," 46; for the government's indifference see also 47.

131. Katel, "Cuba"; Malcomson, "Socialism or Death?"

132. For the film's origins see Malcomson, "Socialism or Death?," 48.

133. Ceballos, *Maldita Sea Tu Nombre, Libertad*. Translation by Luis Rivera. The following quotations (until the next endnote) are from this film.

134. Maggie O'Kane, "Deadly Quest for Paradise," *Ottawa Citizen*, October 1, 1994. All subsequent quotations regarding this story are from this source.

135. Norborg and Sand, *Socialism or Death*. All subsequent quotations referring to the documentary are taken from this source. For a thoughtful analysis of this film and a description of its content, see Prout, "Jail-House Rock."

136. Ichaso, *Bitter Sugar*.

137. Prout, "Jail-House Rock," 427.

138. Ryan, "One Who Burns Herself."

139. Ichaso, *Bitter Sugar*.

140. Ryan, "One Who Burns Herself," 29.

141. Conversation with roquero, June 2004, Cuba.

142. While the Cuban government never denied that self-injection took place, it has sought to conceal information about this problem in every way possible. For example, Cuba never included figures for self-injection in its official HIV statistics. Instead, Cuban AIDS figures "show that 99 percent of HIV cases have been the result of infection through unprotected sex." This figure seems unlikely if even a fraction of the people who claimed to have self-injected were telling the truth. See Acosta, "Health-Cuba." Cuba also claims not to have a problem with IV drug use, despite the fact that many roqueros described their drug habits in the documentaries of Ceballos and Norborg.

143. Torres Peña and Abreu, "Acerca del Programa."

144. Lecture for members of Cuba AIDS Project, Los Cocos sanatorium, June 17, 2004.

145. Hansen and Groce, "From Quarantine to Condoms," 261.

146. For information on these changes see Rosenfield and Herbrand, "Part Three."

147. Hansen and Groce, "From Quarantine to Condoms," 266.

148. The Cuban government has managed to largely prevent the vertical transmission of AIDS. To date, there have only been seventeen cases in Cuba of mothers infecting their babies; lecture, Los Cocos sanatorium, June 17, 2004.

149. Father Fernando de la Vega, talk to members of Cuba AIDS Project, Havana, June 17, 2004. For more information on this church's work see d'Adesky, *Moving Mountains*, 83.

150. Father Fernando de la Vega, talk to members of Cuba AIDS Project, Havana, June 17, 2004.

151. Personal conversation with Dr. Barksdale, Havana, June 17, 2004.

152. Ibid.

153. Conversation with support group member, Havana, June 17, 2004. For information on the Pedro Kourí Institute see d'Adesky, *Moving Mountains*, 85.

154. This information is taken from a lecture at Los Cocos sanatorium on June 17, 2004; a lecture by Dr. Jorge Pérez Ávila at Instituto Pedro Kourí on June 18, 2004; and conversations with doctors at the institute on the same date.

155. Lecture, Los Cocos Sanatorium, June 17, 2004.

156. See Barksdale, *HIV/AIDS in Cuba*, 2. For an internee's critique of the sanatoriums see d'Adesky, *Moving Mountains*, 78–79.

157. Guillermoprieto, *Looking for History*, 116.

158. Ibid., 122.

159. Hansen and Groce, "From Quarantine to Condoms," 270–72.

160. MacDonald, *Developmental Analysis*, 280.

161. See the comments of Monica Ruiz: Clive Cookson, "Cuba Leads Way on AIDS Treatment and Prevention," *Financial Times* (London), February 17, 2003; Farmer, *Pathologies of Power*, 75.

162. Farmer, *AIDS and Accusation*, 10, 149–50, 261; d'Adesky, *Moving Mountains*, 71, 92. MacDonald, *Developmental Analysis*, 171, contrasts Cuba's experience with that of the Dominican Republic.

163. Goudsmit, *Viral Sex*.

164. See Gibbs, "Cuba to Help Caribbean Fight AIDS."

165. Farmer, *AIDS and Accusation*, 149.

Chapter 2

1. All material in this opening section is from Cypriano, *Odô Yá*.

2. Bill Clinton, "Credit Where It's Due," *Wall Street Journal*, November 20, 2003.

3. Mark Schoofs, "South Africa Reverses Course on AIDS Drugs," *Wall Street Journal*, November 20, 2003.

4. Jim Yardley, "AIDS Care in Rural China Now Better Than Nothing," *New York Times*, November 21, 2003.

5. "Brazil Fights for Affordable Drugs," 332.

6. For a description of the Brazilian government's AIDS program see Marins, "Brazilian Policy." See also Quesada, "IDB News," 47–48.

7. David Brown, "World AIDS Day a Reminder of the Disease's Toll," *Oregonian*, December 1, 2003.

8. For the perception of Brazilian sexuality abroad see Larvie, "AIDS and the New Brazilian Sexuality," 290–92; d'Adesky, *Moving Mountains*, 28.

9. For a chronology of Brazilian HIV/AIDS see Galvão, *1980–2001*. For the early perception of AIDS in Brazil see Galvão, *AIDS no Brasil*, 48–55.

10. For the early perception of AIDS in Brazil see Bastos, *Global Responses to AIDS*, 70–71. See also Moraes and Carrara, "AIDS"; Larvie, "AIDS and the New Brazilian Sexuality," 297.

11. Bastos, *Global Responses to AIDS*, 72.

12. Daniel, "AIDS in Brazil," 201. See also Daniel, "Bankruptcy of Models," 34; Parker, "AIDS in Brazil," 9; Teixeira, "Políticas Públicas," 49–50.

13. Parker, "AIDS in Brazil," 21–23.

14. Daniel, "AIDS in Brazil," 202; for similar examples of government negligence regarding AIDS see 209.

15. For Brazilian sexual identities and how they were perceived to impede organizing efforts against HIV/AIDS see Larvie, "AIDS and the New Brazilian Sexuality," 301–4.

16. Daniel, "AIDS in Brazil," 200.

17. Parker, "'Within Four Walls,'" 80; for more on this attitude see Daniel and Parker, "Third Epidemic," 50.

18. The material that follows on this case is taken from Wiik, "Contact, Epidemics, and the Body."

19. Ibid., 402.

20. Ibid., 403.

21. Ibid., 403.

22. Ibid., 404.

23. Inácio Bastos, Barcellos, Lowndes, and Friedman, "Co-Infection"; Inciardi, Surratt, and Telles, *Sex, Drugs, and HIV/AIDS*, 36–38; Daniel and Parker, *Sexuality, Politics, and AIDS*, 19.

24. Varella, *Estação Carandiru*, 67–68.

25. Ibid., 68. This practice is called "booting." For a full description of this practice see Inciardi, Surratt, and Telles, *Sex, Drugs, and HIV/AIDS*, 8–9.

26. Varella, *Estação Carandiru*, 69.

27. Ibid. "Virological studies have indicated that HIV can survive in ordinary tap water for extended periods of time" (Inciardi, Surratt, and Telles, *Sex, Drugs, and HIV/AIDS*, 8).

28. Inácio Bastos, Barcellos, Lowndes, and Friedman, "Co-Infection," 1166.

29. Parker, *Bodies, Pleasures, and Passions*, 95.

30. Ibid., 145.

31. Ibid., 146.

32. For a sophisticated discussion of Brazilian sexual roles, in particular the michê and transvestites, see Parker, "'Within Four Walls'"; see also Parker, "Negotiation of Difference." For a thorough discussion of transvestism see Inciardi, Surratt, and Telles, *Sex, Drugs, and HIV/AIDS*, 88–99.

33. Inciardi, Surratt, and Telles, *Sex, Drugs, and HIV/AIDS*, 99.

34. Graham, *House and Street*, 10–27.

35. Inciardi, Surratt, and Telles, *Sex, Drugs, and HIV/AIDS*, 98.

36. Ibid., 110.

37. Parker, "Negotiation of Difference," 87; Inciardi, Surratt, and Telles, *Sex, Drugs, and HIV/AIDS*, 91; Varella, *Estação Carandiru*, 65.

38. Parker, "Negotiation of Difference," 87–88.

39. Galvão, *1980–2001*, 9.

40. De Brito, Ayres de Castilho, and Szwarcwald, "AIDS e Infecção pelo HIV no Brasil," 208. The epidemiological information that follows is based on this source as well as Szwarcwald, Landmann, Inácio Bastos, Esteves, and Tavares de Andrade, "A Disseminação," and Ayres de Castilho, "Epidemiologia do HIV/AIDS." See also World Bank AIDS II, *Project Appraisal Document*, 4–5.

41. Parker, "AIDS in Brazil," 12.

42. De Brito, Ayres de Castilho, and Szwarcwald, "AIDS e Infecção pelo HIV no Brasil," 210–11; Szwarcwald, Landmann, Inácio Bastos, Esteves, and Tavares de Andrade, "A Disseminação," 10.

43. Szwarcwald, Landmann, Inácio Bastos, Esteves, and Tavares de Andrade, "A Disseminação," 15.

44. Parker, "AIDS in Brazil," 7.

45. Telles Pires Dias and Fonseca Nobre, "Análise dos Padrões," 1175; Ayres de Castilho, "Epidemiologia do HIV/AIDS," 18.

46. De Brito, Ayres de Castilho, and Szwarcwald, "AIDS e Infecção pelo HIV no Brasil," 207. See also Parker, "AIDS in Brazil," 20.

47. Szwarcwald, Landmann, Inácio Bastos, Esteves, and Tavares de Andrade, "A Disseminação," 11.

48. De Brito, Ayres de Castilho, and Szwarcwald, "AIDS e Infecção pelo HIV no Brasil," 212; Ayres de Castilho, "Epidemiologia do HIV/AIDS," 24–25.

49. Szwarcwald, Landmann, Inácio Bastos, Esteves, and Tavares de Andrade, "A Disseminação," 9–10; de Brito, Ayres de Castilho, and Szwarcwald, "AIDS e Infecção pelo HIV no Brasil," 209.

50. Parker, "AIDS in Brazil," 10.

51. Ibid., 11.

52. Ibid., 15–16; Bastos, Global Responses to AIDS, 59.

53. Parker, "AIDS in Brazil," 17–18.

54. Ibid., 23.

55. Information accessed December 12, 2002, from <http:www.aids.org.br/ smartsite.asp?PaginaID=52>. See also Galvão, 1980–2001, 7–8, 13.

56. For an overview of this topic see Galvão, "As Respostas das Organizações," 69–108; Parker, "AIDS in Brazil," 25.

57. Parker, "Introdução," 9–10. See also Galvão's summary of Parker's chronology in Galvão, AIDS no Brasil, 29.

58. Parker, "Introdução," 11–12; Bastos, Global Responses to AIDS, 73.

59. Galvão, AIDS no Brasil, 64–65. See also Galvão, "As Respostas das Organizações," 94–95; for the importance of the Ford Foundation see also 97. For a sophisticated look at this issue see also Abadía-Barrero, "Cultural Politics."

60. Bastos, Global Responses to AIDS, 84.

61. Galvão, AIDS no Brasil, 98–100, 118, 124.

62. World Bank AIDS III, Project Appraisal Document, 10. For more information on this topic see also Larvie, "AIDS and the New Brazilian Sexuality," 298–99; World Bank AIDS II, Project Appraisal Document, 3–4. The Brazilian AIDS program itself has been reorganized a bewildering number of times. See Galvão, AIDS no Brasil, 118–19.

63. Daniel, "AIDS in Brazil," 208. I have taken the idea to contrast the lives of two men, Cazuza and Lauro Corona, from Bastos, Global Responses to AIDS, 175 n. 20. Her work is essential to any understanding of AIDS in Brazil; despite great effort I have been unable to obtain the following source, which examines the media coverage surrounding the deaths of Cazuza and Lauro Corona: Antônio Fausto Neto, "AIDS: Um Discurso das Mídias," Centro Cultural Banco

do Brasil, *Veredas*, Rio de Janeiro (1997): 28–29, in the bibliography of Galvão, *AIDS no Brasil*, 237.

64. Daniel, "AIDS in Brazil," 208. For more on discrimination see Parker, "AIDS in Brazil," 22–23; Terto, "A AIDS e o Local de Trabalho no Brasil," 138, 139.

65. Bastos, *Global Responses to AIDS*, 175 n. 20; Biaggio, "Cazuza Mostra a Sua Cara," 1, 3. For media treatment of people with AIDS in Brazil during the 1980s see Daniel, "AIDS in Brazil," 199.

66. Borges, *Como Evitar a AIDS*.

67. Grupo de Apoio á Prevenção á AIDS, *Brasil*.

68. See Grupo pela Vidda, *Conquistas*; see also Grupo pela Vidda, *Direitos*. For a document that describes political organization among prostitutes in Vila Mimosa, an old downtown area of Rio de Janeiro, see ABIA, *Ação anti-AIDS*.

69. Galvão, *AIDS no Brasil*, 65. For a broad discussion of religion and AIDS in Brazil see Galvão, "As Respostas Religiosas," 109–34.

70. Galvão, "As Respostas Religiosas," 119.

71. Quesada, "Fruits of Foresight," 48; Galvão, *AIDS no Brasil*, 71, 73, 87–88. See also Teixeira, "Políticas Públicas," 51–52; d'Adesky, *Moving Mountains*, 35.

72. Galvão, "As Respostas Religiosas," 121, 130–31; Parker, "Politics of AIDS Education," 119; Bastos, *Global Responses to AIDS*, 173 n. 93.

73. Interview with Paulo Roberto Teixeira.

74. Wadia, "Brazil's AIDS Policy."

75. For a broad discussion of religion in Brazil see Levine, *Brazilian Legacies*, 120–40; Eakin, *Brazil*, 122–32. For material on African religions see Voeks, *Sacred Leaves*, 51–68, 147–68. For the difficulty in calculating the number of houses (*terreiros*) of African religion in Brazil see Galvão, "As Respostas Religiosas," 111.

76. For information on Brazil's musical history see Appleby, *Music of Brazil*.

77. Cypriano, *Odô Yá*. Initially the Afro-Brazilian community was reluctant to address the issue of AIDS; see Galvão, "As Respostas Religiosas," 115, 129; also 127–28.

78. Cypriano, *Odô Yá*; Galvão, "As Respostas Religiosas," 127. For more information see da Silva and Chagas Guimarães, "Odô-Yá Project."

79. Cypriano, *Odô Yá*.

80. Ibid. See also this source for the changes to the practice of ritual shaving as well as the creation of AIDS education materials.

81. Ibid.

82. "Candomblé—Saúde—Axé."

83. For the growing importance that the evangelical movement has placed on fighting AIDS, see Burkhalter, "Politics of AIDS," 7–14.

84. For a concise critique of the World Bank see Ellwood, *No-Nonsense Guide*, 38–52.

85. Araújo de Mattos, Terto, and Parker, *As Estratégias do Banco Mundial*, 7–14; Parker, "Introdução," 13; Galvão, *AIDS no Brasil*, 135–36. For a good overview of the World Bank's loans to Brazil for AIDS work see Galvão, *AIDS no Brasil*, 113–64.

86. UNAIDS, *Integrated Plan*, 46.

87. World Bank AIDS II, *Project Appraisal Document*. For a brief history of the World Bank loans to fight AIDS in Brazil see World Bank AIDS III, *Project Appraisal Document*, 6. See also Galvão, *AIDS no Brasil*, 113–49. For an overview of AIDS I see Galvão, *AIDS no Brasil*, 146–47.

88. World Bank AIDS II, *Project Appraisal Document*, 7. World Bank Documents on AIDS II and AIDS III are available at the institution's website. When I contacted the World Bank in March 2004, however, it refused to release the program report on AIDS I, because this was "an internal bank document."

89. Galvão, "As Respostas das Organizações," 99–101.

90. World Bank AIDS II, *Project Appraisal Document*, 8. For more on the role of NGOs in AIDS I see Boyd and Garrison, "NGO Participation"; Larvie, "AIDS and the New Brazilian Sexuality," 308. For more recent figures on NGOs see World Bank AIDS III, *Project Appraisal Document*, 58.

91. Galvão, *AIDS no Brasil*, 113–14, 142, 152, 157–59.

92. Interview with Paulo Roberto Teixeira.

93. Ibid.

94. Daniel, "AIDS in Brazil," 209. Galvão, *AIDS no Brasil*, 124, gives the year as 1990.

95. For the chronology of the government's provision of AZT see Galvão, *1980–2001*, 10, 12.

96. Interview with "Jean," GIV leader; interview with "Getúlio."

97. For a description of the Brazilian government's AIDS policy and its successes see Pio Marins, "Brazilian Policy"; Quesada, "IDB News," 45–46; Boyd and Garrison, "NGO Participation," 2; World Bank AIDS III, *Project Appraisal Document*, 60; d'Adesky, *Moving Mountains*, 30, 36.

98. World Bank AIDS III, *Project Appraisal Document*, 11, 13.

99. Ibid., 60.

100. "Brazil Fights for Affordable Drugs," 333. The best single sources on this issue are Galvão, "Access to Antiretroviral Drugs in Brazil"; Passarelli and Terto, "Good Medicine." See also Ahmad, "Brazil and USA at Loggerheads." For an international context for this debate see Elizabeth Becker, "International Business: Trade Talks Fail to Agree on Drugs for Poor Nations," *New York Times*, December 21, 2002; Boulet, Perriens, and Renaud-Thery, *Patent Situation*. For a look at the TRIPS provision of the WTO see Barton et al., "Integrating."

101. Benatar, Daar, and Singer, "Global Health Ethics," 110.

102. Cullet, "Patents and Medicines," 143.

103. Sell and Prakash, "Using Ideas Strategically," 164.

104. Cullet, "Patents and Medicines," 147; Sell and Prakash, "Using Ideas Strategically," 161. For a good description of the debate see d'Adesky, *Moving Mountains*, 21–25.

105. For more information see Curti, "WTO Dispute Settlement."

106. Cohen and Lybecker, "AIDS Policy and Pharmaceutical Patents," 13.

107. Rosenburg, "Look at Brazil."

108. Key and DeNoon, "Anti-AIDS Free Distribution"; Jennifer L. Rich, "Roche Reaches Accord on Drug with Brazil," *New York Times*, September 1, 2001.

109. Sell and Prakash, "Using Ideas Strategically," 162.

110. Ashraf, "USA and Brazil End Dispute"; see also Gottlieb, "US Concedes."

111. Passarelli, "As Patentes e os Remédios contra a AIDS," 8.

112. Jennifer L. Rich, "Brazil Welcomes Global Move on Drug Patents," *New York Times*, November 16, 2001; Sell and Prakash, "Using Ideas Strategically," 167.

113. "Brazil to Share AIDS Drugs," *New York Times*, 9 July 2002.

114. Cohen, "FTAA Summit." For an outline of the issues concerning intellectual property rights in the draft copy of the Free Trade Area of the Americas proposal see FTAA, "Draft Agreement."

115. NGOs have done a great deal of intellectual work on this issue. See, for example, Health Gap, "Medical Apartheid." See also Health Gap, "Meeting Report"; Consumer Project et al., "NGO Letter." For the role of intergovernmental organizations see Cullet, "Patents and Medicines," 149.

116. Cohen and Lybecker, "AIDS Policy and Pharmaceutical Patents," 13.

117. Cullet, "Patents and Medicines," 153; Abadía-Barrero, "Cultural Politics."

118. Sell and Prakash, "Using Ideas Strategically," 149, 165.

119. Chequer, "Atenção."

120. Interview with "João." João believed that HIV was an ancient disease modified by U.S. scientists in a lab with the support of the Church as a means to control population growth.

121. Interview with "Jean," GIV leader.

122. World Bank AIDS II, *Project Appraisal Document*, 5. For an overview of the World Bank's thoughts on Brazil's provision of free medications see Araújo de Mattos, Terto, and Parker, *As Estratégias do Banco Mundial*, 16–18; Galvão, *AIDS no Brasil*, 198.

123. World Bank AIDS II, *Project Appraisal Document*, 10.

124. Ibid., 18–19. For a document briefly describing (in three pages) the program see World Bank, *Brazil—Second AIDS and STD Control Project*.

125. World Bank AIDS III, *Project Appraisal Document*, 6.

126. Ibid., 4.
127. Ibid., 6.
128. Ibid., 9. See also Parker, "Desafios para o Futuro: Questões-chave para a Política," in Daniel and Parker, *Sexuality, Politics, and AIDS*, 179–180.
129. World Bank AIDS III, *Project Appraisal Document*, 5.
130. Ibid., 7.
131. Szwarcwald, Landmann, Inácio Bastos, Esteves, and Tavares de Andrade, "A Disseminação."
132. For the situation in the Amazon see also Linn et al., "HIV Prevention," 1010.
133. Ibid.
134. World Bank, *Indigenous Peoples*, 1.
135. Parker, "Politics of AIDS Education," 123–24. For an example of a successful education program see Hearst, Lacerda, Gravato, Hudes, and Stall, "Reducing AIDS Risk."
136. Telles Pires Dias and Fonseca Nobre, "Análise dos Padrões."
137. Interview with "Jean," GIV leader.
138. "Brazil Fights for Affordable Drugs."
139. Passarelli, "As Patentes e os Remédios contra a AIDS," 7; Galvão, *AIDS no Brasil*, 162–63.
140. Andrew Downie, "Brazil Shares AIDS-Fight Blueprint," *Christian Science Monitor*, August 8, 2002; in 2003 Brazil and the U.S. agreed to cooperate on this program. See d'Adesky, *Moving Mountains*, 29.
141. Russell, *Health Gap Global Access Project*.
142. Interview with Paulo Roberto Teixeira.
143. Interview with "Drauzio."
144. BBC News Website, "Brazil Turns Down US AIDS Funds," <http://news.bbc.co.uk/2/hi/americas/4513805.stm>, accessed May 4, 2005. For more information on this topic see Mensagem encaminhada de Imprensa. This service issues daily bulletins on AIDS news in Brazil.
145. Michael M. Phillips (Washington) and Matt Moffett (Rio de Janeiro), "Brazil Refuses U.S. AIDS Funds due to Antiprostitution Pledge," *Wall Street Journal*, May 2, 2005.
146. Interview with "Edison."
147. Support group meeting, Municipal Health Program (CRT), São Paulo, Tuesday, July 19, 2005.
148. Personal communication from Senora "C," São Paulo, Wednesday, July 20, 2005.
149. Interview with "Gabriela."
150. Interview with "Juscelino."
151. Interview with "João."
152. Interview with "Celso."

237

153. Interview with "Paulo."

154. Interview with members of Projeto Esperança; interview with "Juscelino"; interview with "Paulo"; interview with "Claudio."

155. Interview with "Paulo."

156. Interview with "Eduardo."

157. Interview with "Oswaldo."

158. Interview with "Alberto." I did hear, however, some drug users say that they were still able to lead normal lives under the influence of their drug. For example, "Juscelino" still used cocaine, and he believed that it helped him to function better in his work; interview with "Juscelino."

159. Interview with "Juscelino."

160. Ibid. He also said that injecting drug use was also uncommon in prison because it was too expensive, and it was dangerous to create debts in prison, a place where "there is no pardon." His comments on crack were echoed by "Paulo," who had also spent time in Carandiru. Paulo said that crack was easy to smuggle, since it was small and could easily be brought in concealed in goods such as fruit. But it was unpopular in prison because it led to paranoia and "destroyed people." Paulo was an injecting drug user when he was arrested, and he continued to use injecting drugs after his incarceration; interview with "Paulo."

161. Interview with "Juscelino."

162. Interview with "Paulo"; interview with "Claudio."

163. Interview with "Paulo."

164. Tour of GIV, São Paulo, Thursday, July 21, 2005.

165. Interview with members of Projeto Esperança.

166. Interview with Paulo Roberto Teixeira.

167. Ibid.

168. Ibid.

169. Donald G. McNeil, "Plan to Battle AIDS Worldwide Is Falling Short," *New York Times*, March 28, 2004, <http://www.nytimes.com/2004/03/28/international/28 AI...>, accessed March 29, 2004.

170. Sell and Prakash, "Using Ideas Strategically," 147.

171. For a look at the impact of Brazil's program on the international debate see Rosenburg, "Look at Brazil."

Chapter 3

1. Interview with "Eva." I have changed Eva's name, as with almost all of my interviewees in this book, as required by the Human Subjects Review Board of Portland State University. I conducted the interview with the help of research assistant Liliana Sanchez. For more information on transvestite subculture

in Oaxaca see Higgins and Coen, *Streets, Bedrooms, and Patios,* 108–65. I wish to give particular thanks to Michael Higgins as well as Bill Wolf of Frente Común Contra el SIDA. Bill, in particular, gave me leads that led me to many of the people that I interviewed.

2. Nuñez, Flores, Forsythe, and Sweat, *Impacto Socioeconómico,* 6; Figueroa, *El SIDA en Honduras,* 1; "Honduras," *Mesoamérica* 18, no. 8 (August 1999): 5; see the comments of Kofi Annan in "Honduras Is Haven for AIDS," *Mesoamérica* 21, no. 4 (April 2002): 7.

3. Information from the UNAIDS website, <www.unaids.org>, accessed September 23, 2004. See "Mexico: Epidemiological Fact Sheets on HIV/AIDS and Sexually Transmitted Diseases." The fact sheets for the United States and Central American countries were accessed on the same date from the same website. For the fact that Mexico's HIV rate is lower than the rate for either most Central American countries or the United States see del Rio and Sepúlveda, "AIDS in Mexico," 1445. The information on the total number of HIV-positive people in Mexico comes from a handout from Frente Común Contra el SIDA titled "Casos Reportados de SIDA y Estimaciones de Infección de VIH en México."

4. For a description of the different Oaxacan peoples see Whipperman, *Moon Handbooks,* 58–67.

5. Dr. José Antonio Izazola quoted in Frasca, *AIDS in Latin America,* 73.

6. Del Rio and Sepúlveda, "AIDS in Mexico," 1445.

7. Mejía, "SIDA," 17. See also Anderson, "AIDS as an Opportunity," 4–10.

8. Mejía, "SIDA," 30–47.

9. For a discussion of the Mexican press coverage of the epidemic see Pamplona, "El SIDA."

10. Anderson, "AIDS as an Opportunity," 7. Anderson herself based this on material from González Ruiz, *Cómo Propogar el SIDA,* 90. See also Carrillo, *Night Is Young,* 13–14.

11. Wilson, *Hidden in the Blood,* 61.

12. Ibid., 150.

13. Valdespino, García, and Izazola, "Distribución de la Epidemia del Sida," 271.

14. Del Rio and Sepúlveda, "AIDS in Mexico," 1449. For an early history of the epidemic see Minichiello, Magis, Uribe, Anaya, and Bertozzi, "Mexican HIV/AIDS Surveillance System," 14. Much of the information in this paragraph is based on these two articles.

15. Del Rio and Sepúlveda, "AIDS in Mexico," 1449.

16. Ibid., 1450–52.

17. For a history of this effort see Stover and Bravo, "Impact of AIDS," 61–62.

18. Carrillo, *Night Is Young,* 219.

19. Stover and Bravo, "Impact of AIDS," 61.

20. Castro and Leyva, "Mexico," 147–48; Stover and Bravo, "Impact of AIDS," 61–62.

21. Castro and Leyva, "Mexico," 151–52.

22. Carrillo, *Night Is Young*, 338 n. 27.

23. Ibid., 217–18.

24. "Baja en el País Mortalidad por Sida Tras Uso de Antirretrovirales, Revela Informe," *La Jornada*, August 25, 2004, 24.

25. D'Adesky, *Moving Mountains*, 133.

26. Jennifer Mena, "Mercy Smugglers Help Alleviate AIDS in Mexico," *Los Angeles Times*, September 16, 2000.

27. Frasca, *AIDS in Latin America*, 97.

28. Minichiello, Magis, Uribe, Anaya, and Bertozzi, "Mexican HIV/AIDS Surveillance System," 14.

29. D'Adesky, *Moving Mountains*, 127.

30. For a brief history of the epidemic see Minichiello, Magis, Uribe, Anaya, and Bertozzi, "Mexican HIV/AIDS Surveillance System," 14. For the geography of the epidemic see Castro and Leyva, "Mexico," 139–40; Carrillo, *Night Is Young*, 215. For statistical information on AIDS from early in the Mexican epidemic see Valdespino, García, and Izazola, "Distribución de la Epidemia del Sida," 275–77.

31. Valdespino, García, and Izazola, "Distribución de la Epidemia del Sida," 279.

32. González Block and Liguori, *El SIDA*, 11, 13, 34, 53.

33. This figure comes from a handout from Frente Común Contra el SIDA titled, "De los 72,864 Casos Reportados de SIDA en México." The figures in turn came from the director general of CENSIDA, Jorge Saavedra López, as they were reported in *La Jornada*, June 2, 2004.

34. For a list of key works see Carrillo, *Night Is Young*, 8–9. For one of the best early works on the topic see Izazola, Valdespino, Juárez, Mondragón, and Sepúlveda, "Conocimientos."

35. For a discussion of machismo see Carrillo, *Night Is Young*, 23–25; for men losing their virginity to prostitutes see 106–7. Carrillo's work is perhaps the best single study of Mexican sexuality.

36. Beyrer, *War in the Blood*, 132, 167. For a discussion of a transvestite subculture in urban Oaxaca see Higgins and Coen, *Streets, Bedrooms, and Patios*, 109–65. For the fact that young men in the rural isthmus region of Oaxaca often lose their virginity to *muxe*, a form of transvestite, see Pecheur, "Third Gender." For information on transvestite life in Mexico City see Prieur, *Mema's House*. For a broader discussion of the role that transvestites play in Latin sexual culture see Paternostro, *In the Land of God and Man*, 108–95. One can overestimate the tolerance for Mexican transvestites. One Mexican town, Tecate,

banned cross-dressing as a measure to fight AIDS. See Anna Gorman, "Baja City Can't Skirt This Issue," *Los Angeles Times*, November 26, 2002.

37. Beyrer, *War in the Blood*, 163–69.

38. Pecheur, "Third Gender."

39. Ibid.

40. See ibid.; D'Adesky, *Moving Mountains*, 130.

41. Higgins and Coen, *Streets, Bedrooms, and Patios*, 169.

42. Anderson, "AIDS as an Opportunity," 15.

43. Ibid., 16.

44. Ibid., 14–15; see also d'Adesky, *Moving Mountains*, 124.

45. The statistics are contained in the handout "Panorama Epidemiologico de VIH-SIDA en el Estado de Oaxaca, 1986–2004," Servicios de Salud de Oaxaca, June 30, 2004. They are repeated in a handout from Frente Común Contra el SIDA, "De los 2,298 Casos Reportados en Oaxaca."

46. Anderson, "AIDS as an Opportunity," 26.

47. Interview with employee at MEXFAM. In accordance with the terms of the Human Subjects Review Board at Portland State University, I do not use the names of any interviewees unless they have asked me to do so.

48. Interview with "Maria."

49. For examples of the Church opposing sex education efforts and condom use see Carrillo, *Night Is Young*, 218, 220, 241. For the fact that most Mexicans ignore the Church's teachings on family planning see ibid., 166.

50. Interview with Bill Wolf, August 26, 2004. I use Wolf's name with his permission.

51. Anderson, "AIDS as an Opportunity," 31–33.

52. For the strength of Guadalajara's HIV/AIDS program see Frasca, *AIDS in Latin America*, 80, 83–85.

53. Interview with Bill Wolf, August 23, 2004.

54. I wish to thank COESIDA in Oaxaca City for cooperating with my work. The information that follows is based on multiple interviews with COESIDA employees in a range of positions during interviews carried out in August 2004. See also d'Adesky, *Moving Mountains*, 130–32.

55. Interview with "Maria."

56. Interview with "Paula." Patients needing hospitalization would be sent either to the hospitals for the Instituto de Servicios Sociales a los Trabajadores del Estado (ISSTE) or to the Instituto Mexicano del Seguro Social (IMSS).

57. For a look at the familial impact of AIDS see Castro, Orozco, Aggleton, Eroza, and Hernández, "Family Responses to HIV/AIDS."

58. Interview with Dr. Q.

59. Carrillo, *Night Is Young*, 217.

60. Castro and Leyva, "Mexico," 148–49; for a brief history and description of these organizations see 148–51.

61. Most of the information on this organization comes from my interviews with Bill Wolf, August 23, 26, 2004.

62. This same argument was made in a press bulletin by Miguel Ángel Ramírez Almanza titled "Como Interpretar las Estadísticas de la Secretaria de Salud Sobre el SIDA." This document had not yet been released to the press when I received a copy in August 2004.

63. Interview with Dr. Q.

64. There are also tensions among AIDS NGOs, due in part to the competition for resources. See Castro and Leyva, "Mexico," 152–53.

65. Press Bulletin by Miguel Ángel Ramírez Almanza, "Como Interpretar las Estadísticas de la Secretaria de Salud Sobre el SIDA."

66. "Encuesta de Pacientes del COESIDA—Marzo de 2002," Frente Común Contra el SIDA, Oaxaca, A.C. This handout mistakenly referred to 145 people surveyed. The correct number was 153.

67. D'Adesky, *Moving Mountains*, 131.

68. Handout from Frente Común, "De los 72,864 Casos Reportados de SIDA en México." This handout cites as its source Jorge Saavedra López, Director General, CENSIDA, in *La Jornada*, June 2, 2004.

69. Interview with members of Vinni Gaxhea. The organization has a website: <http://groups.msn.com/OAXACAGAYSYBIS>.

70. Interview with "Julio."

71. Uhlig, "Prostitutes in Mexico."

72. World Bank, *Confronting AIDS*, 121.

73. Uhlig, "Prostitutes in Mexico." For more information on the early history of AIDS and sex workers in Mexico see Valdespino, García, and Izazola, "Distribución de la Epidemia del Sida," 283–84.

74. Interview with Dr. Q. The statistics are contained in the handout "Panorama Epidemiologico de VIH-SIDA en el Estado de Oaxaca, 1986–2004," Servicios de Salud de Oaxaca, June 30, 2004.

75. Bellis, *Hotel Ritz*, x. For possible reasons why U.S. sex workers are more at risk see 3–5.

76. Ibid., 26.

77. Ibid., 72.

78. Ibid., 74.

79. Ibid., 85.

80. Bronfman, "Mexico and Central America," 625.

81. Ibid., 612.

82. For information on migration patterns see Bronfman, Camposortega, and Medina, "Migración Internacional," 443–49.

242

83. Juan Antonio Zuñiga and Roberto Gonzalez Amador, "El Dinero de Migrantes Pagó el Total de los Intereses de la Deuda Externa," *La Jornada*, August 25, 2004, 23.

84. Bronfman, "Mexico and Central America," 613.

85. The statistical information on migrants in the opening of this paragraph is drawn from Mishra, Conner, and Magaña, *AIDS Crossing Borders*, 6–15.

86. Castro and Leyva, "Mexico," 145; Bronfman, "Mexico and Central America," 625–28; Mishra, Conner, and Magaña, *AIDS Crossing Borders*, 33–34, 85, 87.

87. Mishra, Conner, and Magaña, *AIDS Crossing Borders*, 81.

88. Ibid., 66.

89. McQuiston and Gordon, "Timing," 277.

90. Peragallo, "Latino Women and AIDS Risk," 217.

91. Mishra, Conner, and Magaña, *AIDS Crossing Borders*, 15, 144.

92. Ibid., 65.

93. Interview with Dr. "Rodrigo."

94. Interview with Dr. Q. The sociologist Jose Luis Romero has also found that Central American migrants are important to the understanding of the epidemiology of AIDS in Jalisco. See Monica Medel, "Transit of Central Americans Raising AIDS Rates in Mexico," June 14, 2002, EFE News Services, accessed through LexisNexis. See also Key, DeNoon, and Boyles, "Coordinating Anti-AIDS Measures in Border Areas."

95. Angeles Mariscal, Ernesto Martinez, and Claudio Bañnales, "SSA: El VIH Se Extiende por las Zonas Rurales de Chiapas vía Indocumentados Centroamericanos," *La Jornada*, December 3, 2003, 47. For more information on Central American migrants in Mexico and AIDS see Bronfman, "Mexico and Central America," 616–17.

96. Magdalena Avilo, "Indocumentos, los Principales Portadores del SIDA, Aseguran," *Noticias*, December 23, 2003. For another account of AIDS among migrants in the Mixteca see Francisco Martínez, "La Migración, Principal Causa de SIDA," *Imparcial*, December 3, 2003.

97. Jorge Vega Aguilar, "Se Prostituyen 50% de Personas que Emigran a EU," *El Tiempo*, February 4, 2003. NGOs are working to reduce the stigma that migrants face. See Monica Castañeda, "No Satanizar a Migrantes como Transmisores," *El Gráfico*, May 19, 2003.

98. Interview with "Maria." For the national government's efforts to reach out to this population see Hernandez, "Mexican Government Programs."

99. Interview with "Celia."

100. Bronfman, "Mexico and Central America," 625.

101. Mishra, Conner, and Magaña, *AIDS Crossing Borders*, 37.

102. Anderson, "AIDS as an Opportunity," 14. I draw on Anderson's work for much of the information on women that follows in this paragraph.

103. Ibid., 16–17. See also d'Adesky, *Moving Mountains*, 137–39.

104. Anderson, "AIDS as an Opportunity," 17.

105. Ibid., 35–36.

106. Silvia Chavela Rivas, "Afecta Principalmente a Migrantes: Se Propega el SIDA entre Amas de Casa," *Noticias*, July 21, 2003.

107. Alejandro Villegas, "Afecta SIDA en Mayor Grado a Amas de Casa y Migrantes," *El Tiempo*, April 24, 2003.

108. Eaton, "Eso Es Lo Que Me Chinga Más," 33.

109. Ibid., 1.

110. Ibid., 2.

111. For more information on migration and women in Oaxaca see ibid., 15–18.

112. Sepúlveda, "AIDS in Mexico," 18. See also Mishra, Conner, and Magaña, *AIDS Crossing Borders*, 51; Bronfman, Camposortega, and Medina, "Migración Internacional."

113. Bronfman, "Mexico and Central America," 609.

114. Mena, "AIDS Now a Migrant."

115. Javier Peralta, "Promueven Campaña contra SIDA," *Reforma*, December 16, 2002, A-16. Other states have fit a similar pattern for some time. In 1992, of "the 323 cases of AIDS and HIV infection that have been reported in Michoacán, for instance, 110, or 34 percent, have been people who said they had lived in the United States" (Tim Golden, "AIDS Is Following Mexican Migrant Workers Back Home," *New York Times*, March 8, 1992).

116. Bronfman, "Mexico and Central America," 616.

117. Interview with Dr. Q.

118. AIDS Weekly Editors, "Sex Workers in Mexico-U.S. Border Regions Potential Source for HIV/AIDS Spread," *AIDS Weekly*, January 13, 2003, 9. Accessed through LexisNexis.

119. James Smith, "U.S. Mexico Team Up on Health Care," *Los Angeles Times*, October 17, 2001; Mishra, Conner, and Magaña, *AIDS Crossing Borders*, 201–8.

120. Mena, "AIDS Now a Migrant."

121. Sam Dillon, "Mexico: AIDS Cases Rise 14 Percent," *New York Times*, January 14, 1999.

122. Sandra Ramos Rojas, "VIH-SIDA se Femeniza por Migración y Bisexualidad," *El Imparcial*, March 16, 2003.

123. For a history of these uprisings and their origins see LaFaber, *Inevitable Revolutions*.

124. Booth and Walker, *Understanding Central America*, 50, 70–71.

125. Paris, *At War's End*, 112.

126. <www.usaid.gov/our_work/global_health/aids/countries/lac/caregion.pdf>, accessed April 20, 2003.

127. Beyrer, *War in the Blood*, 198–99.
128. Irwin, Millen, and Fallows, *Global AIDS*, 35–37; see also Elbe, "HIV/AIDS and the Changing Landscape," and Mock et al., "Conflict and HIV." The latter work is a careful study that creates a useful typology of the factors in war that influence the spread of HIV and suggests that the character of the conflict may be important to this process.
129. Irwin, Millen, and Fallows, *Global AIDS*, 36.
130. Youde, "Enter the Fourth Horseman," 199.
131. Beyrer, *War in the Blood*, 140, 145.
132. World Bank, *Confronting AIDS*, 161.
133. Hooper, *The River*, 42–51.
134. For examples of the use of rape as a weapon (and even the intentional transmission of HIV) see Youde, "Enter the Fourth Horseman," 200.
135. Beyrer, *War in the Blood*, 63–65.
136. Ibid., 199.
137. "Honduras," *Mesoamérica* 21, no. 12 (December 2002): 4.
138. "Honduras," *Mesoamérica* 18, no. 8 (August 1999): 5.
139. Timothy Griffiths, "Honduras: Vicious HIV Virus Subtype in Honduras," *Mesoamérica* 15, no. 3 (March 1996): 5.
140. "AIDS in Central America: '95 Update," *Mesoamérica* 15, no. 1 (January 1996): 3. A year earlier Honduras's figures had been even more striking. See Van Wichen, Largaespada, Ormel, and Montesdeoca, *Es Tiempo de Actuar*, 11.
141. "Honduras: AIDS' Rapid Growth," *Mesoamérica* 13, no. 5 (May 1994): 10.
142. García Trujillo, Paredes, and Sierra, *VIH/SIDA*, 31.
143. <www.usaid.gov/our_work/global_health/aids/countries/lac/caregion.pdf>, accessed April 20, 2003.
144. García Trujillo, Paredes, and Sierra, *VIH/SIDA*, 34.
145. Chelala, "Central America," 154.
146. AIDSCAP, *Estudio de Conocimientos*, 17.
147. Zapata et al., "Perfil Epidemiologico," 23. For more on the presence of U.S. military forces as a possible source for the virus see Low et al., "AIDS in Nicaragua," 697.
148. Mendez Ordoñez, *Mujer y SIDA*, 8.
149. Figueroa, *El SIDA en Honduras*, 10; see also 70. It still remains true that the gay community was heavily affected, with more than a third of gay men in the city of San Pedro Sula testing positive for HIV in the mid-1990s. See García Trujillo, Paredes, and Sierra, *VIH/SIDA*, 36.
150. *Estudio Multicéntrico*, 5.
151. Ibid., 3.
152. Figueroa, *El SIDA en Honduras*, 17. See also García Trujillo, Paredes, and Sierra, *VIH/SIDA*, 21.

153. Summerfield, "Nicaragua," 967.

154. Figueroa, *El SIDA en Honduras*, 66. For maps of the prevalence of AIDS in Honduras see García Trujillo, Paredes, and Sierra, *VIH/SIDA*, 25–26.

155. Mendez Ordoñez, *Mujer y SIDA*, 9; for a careful breakdown of AIDS cases by city in Honduras see 55. See also Figueroa, *El SIDA en Honduras*, 61. For a brief analysis of the epidemiology of the Honduran AIDS epidemic see "Antecedentes de la Epidemicia en Honduras," <www.pasca.org/nograficas/situacion/antecedentes.honduras.pdf>, accessed April 20, 2003.

156. Low et al., "AIDS in Nicaragua," 693.

157. Low, Smith, Gorter, and Arauz, "AIDS and Migrant Populations in Nicaragua," 1593.

158. García Trujillo, Paredes, and Sierra, *VIH/SIDA*, 29.

159. Low et al., "AIDS in Nicaragua," 688. For a highly critical look at changes to the Nicaraguan health care system after the Sandinista defeat see Hopkinson and Chalmers, "Nicaragua."

160. Van Wichen, Largaespada, Ormel, and Montesdeoca, *Es Tiempo de Actuar*, 12.

161. Low et al., "AIDS in Nicaragua," 694.

162. Summerfield, "Nicaragua."

163. For the above facts see Van Wichen, Largaespada, Ormel, and Montesdeoca, *Es Tiempo de Actuar*, 50, 57–58, 63, 68.

164. Ibid., 7.

165. Ibid., 13.

166. Ibid., 19.

167. See the Nicaragua heading, <http//unaids.org/hivaids/statistics/fact_sheets/index_ehn.h>, accessed April 6, 2003.

168. *Estudio Multicéntrico*, 2, 4.

169. Low et al., "AIDS in Nicaragua," 698.

170. For statistics on HIV/AIDS in Central America see "Children and the Impact of HIV/AIDS," *Mesoamérica* 21, no. 8 (August 2002): 6.

171. García Trujillo, Paredes, and Sierra, *VIH/SIDA*, 13.

172. Nuñez, Flores, Forsythe, and Sweat, *Impacto Socioeconómico*, 10. For a discussion of the fortunate error in this prediction see García Trujillo, Paredes, and Sierra, *VIH/SIDA*, 39.

173. For the problems the government faced in confronting the Honduran AIDS epidemic see García Trujillo, Paredes, and Sierra, *VIH/SIDA*, 47.

174. "HIV/AIDS in Honduras and USAIDS Involvement," <http://www.usaid.gov/regions/lac/>, accessed April 11, 2003.

175. See <www.pasca.org/nograficas/ambiente/matriz.pdf>, accessed December 10, 2004.

176. "Honduras Is Haven for AIDS," *Mesoamérica* 21, no. 4 (April 2002): 7.

177. See <http://hivinsite.ucsf.edu/global?page+cr05-00-00>, accessed April 13, 2003.

178. From the Honduras heading, <http//unaids.org/hivaids/statistics/fact_sheets/index_ehn.h>, accessed April 4, 2003.

179. Ibid.

180. From the Belize heading, <http//unaids.org/hivaids/statistics/fact_sheets/index_ehn.h>, accessed April 4, 2003.

181. "Costa Rica," *Mesoamérica* 21, no. 12 (December 2002): 11.

182. "Costa Rica: PANI-Covenant House Report on Street Kids," *Mesoamérica* 21, no. 10 (December 2002): 9.

183. Mata and Herrera, "AIDS and HIV," 182.

184. Ibid., 181.

185. Pana, *SIDA*, 12.

186. Schifter, *La Formacion de una Contracultura*, 268–69, 271–77.

187. Frasca, *AIDS in Latin America*, 106.

188. Ibid., 116.

189. From the Costa Rica heading, <http//unaids.org/hivaids/statistics/fact_sheets/index_ehn.h>, accessed April 4, 2003.

190. Mata and Herrera, "AIDS and HIV," 175.

191. Frasca, *AIDS in Latin America*, 105, 112–13.

192. From the El Salvador heading, <http//unaids.org/hivaids/statistics/fact_sheets/index_ehn.h>, accessed April 4, 2003.

193. "HIV/AIDS in El Salvador and USAIDS Involvement," <http://www.usaid.gov/regions/lac/>, accessed April 11, 2003.

194. *Estudio Multicéntrico*, 2.

195. See <www.pasca.org/nograficas/ambiente/matriz.pdf>, accessed December 10, 2004. For a discussion of human rights in the region see Cuadra-Hernández, Magali, Leyva-Flores, Hernández-Rosete, and Bronfman-Pertzovsky, "Derechos Humanos."

196. From the Panama heading, <http//unaids.org/hivaids/statistics/fact_sheets/index_ehn.h>, accessed April 18, 2004.

197. Moreno Castillo, *El SIDA*, 41, 58.

198. Vázquez, *El SIDA y el Trabajo*, 56.

199. See <www.pasca.org/nograficas/ambiente/matriz.pdf>, accessed December 10, 2004.

200. Ibid.

201. "Guatemala: AIDS Campaign under Review," *Mesoamérica* 16, no. 12 (December 1997): 1–2.

202. Frasca, *AIDS in Latin America*, 129; see also 130.

203. *Estudio Multicéntrico*, 2, 5.

204. "HIV/AIDS in El Salvador and USAIDS involvement," <http://www.usaid.gov/regions/lac/>, accessed April 11, 2003.

205. See <www.pasca.org/nograficas/ambiente/matriz.pdf>, accessed December 10, 2004. For information on AIDS in Central America the best single source is the PASCA website: <http://www.pasca.org/index2.htm>.

206. Frasca, *AIDS in Latin America*, 137–38.

207. Jordan, "AIDS Orphans' Numbers Grow."

208. See the headings for Guatemala, Belize, Nicaragua, El Salvador, and Costa Rica at <http//unaids.org/hivaids/statistics/fact_sheets/index_ehn.h>, all accessed April 2003.

209. See Aguilar, Nuñez, and Stover, *Proyecciones*. Accessed August 18, 2004, at <www.pasca.org/docs/projecciones_gt.pdf>.

210. See <www.usaid.gov/our_work/global_health/aids/countries/lac/caregion.pdf>, accessed April 20, 2003. Truck drivers may play an important role in spreading the virus. See Pana, *Al Vaivén de un Cabezal*.

211. Bronfman, "Mexico and Central America," 629.

212. Bronfman, Leyva, Negroni, and Rueda, "Mobile Populations," 45.

213. Chúa, Almendáres, Matute, and Velásquez, *VIH-SIDA*, 10, 14.

214. Bronfman, Leyva, Negroni, and Rueda, "Mobile Populations," 47; see also 46.

215. See <www.usaid.gov/our_work/global_health/aids/countries/lac/caregion.pdf>, accessed April 20, 2003.

216. Ian MacBean, "Happy Hour for the AIDS Cocktail," *Mesoamérica* 22, no. 2 (February 2003): 12.

217. Nicholas D. Kristof, "Death by Dividend," *New York Times*, November 22, 2003.

218. "Central America, Drug Companies Reach Agreement."

219. Opuni et al., "Resource Requirements," 62.

220. Jordan, "AIDS Orphans' Numbers Grow."

221. Chequer, Cuchi, Mazin, and García Calleja, "Access to Antiretroviral Treatment," 51.

222. Ibid., 52.

Chapter 4

1. Cueto, *Culpa e Coraje*, 123.

2. Pan American Health Organization, *AIDS Surveillance*, 7.

3. Ibid., 8.

4. Ibid., 7.

5. Ibid., 7–8.

6. Hansis, *Latin Americans*, 5.

7. Starn, "Missing the Revolution."

8. For information on Peru's cholera epidemic see Cueto, "Stigma and Blame during an Epidemic." For more information on the multi-drug-resistant tuberculosis in Peru see Farmer, *Infections and Inequalities*, 190–93, 235–40, 242–44, 273–78, 280.

9. See Giraldo, *Colombia*.

10. Brinkley, "Anti-Drug Gains."

11. David S. Cloud, "Clinton Not Expected to Certify Colombia as a Drug-Fighting Ally," *Oregonian*, February 26, 1997.

12. Human Rights Watch, *Colombia's Killer Networks*.

13. Agence France Press announcement, March 23, 1998, as reported on the Colombia Support Network, <http://www.igc.org/csn>, accessed March 25, 1998.

14. Juanita Darling and Ruth Morris, "U.S. Military Presence in Colombia Grows," *Oregonian*, August 1, 1999.

15. "Colombian Air Force Plane Found Smuggling Cocaine," *Oregonian*, November 11, 1998.

16. Quill Lawrence, "World: Americas, Colombian Air Force Drugs Arrests," *BBC News: BBC Online Network*, November 13, 1998, <http://news2.thls.bbc.co.uk/hi/english/world/americas/newsid_213000/213483.stm>, accessed November 13, 1998; also "World: Americas, Cocaine on Colombian Air Force Plane" (dates unknown), <http://news2.thls.bbc.co.uk/hi/english/world/americas/newsid_211000/211869.stm>; "Colombian Defense Minister Resigns," *Oregonian*, March 17, 1997. See also Scott and Marshall, *Cocaine Politics*, 190.

17. Brinkley, "Anti-Drug Gains." Also see this source for the extent of U.S. financing for Plan Colombia.

18. Murillo de la Rocha, "Relaciones Boliviano-Chilenas."

19. Alvaro Zuazo, "Bolivia's Natural Gas Find Unleashes Political Divisions," *Oregonian*, July 15, 2004.

20. Juan Forero, "Bolivians Support Gas Plan and Give President a Lift," *New York Times*, July 19, 2004.

21. Scott and Marshall, *Cocaine Politics*, 44–46.

22. Gerlach, *Indians, Oil, and Politics*.

23. DEA website, "Statement of Asa Hutchison, Administrator, Drug Enforcement Administration before the Senate Caucus on International Narcotics Control," <http://www.usdoj.gov/dea/pubs/cngrtest/ct091702html>, accessed March 27, 2005.

24. See the statistics for Ecuador in table 3 of Pan American Health Organization, *AIDS Surveillance*, 18.

25. Tabet et al., "HIV, Syphilis, and Heterosexual Bridging."

26. Magis Rodríguez, Marques, and Touzé, "HIV and Injection Drug Use."

27. Tabet et al., "HIV, Syphilis, and Heterosexual Bridging," 1274; Paternostro, *In the Land of God and Man*, 27.

28. Paternostro, *In the Land of God and Man*, 28.

29. Ibid., 38–42.

30. Ibid., 110.

31. Ibid., 127.

32. Ibid., 117.

33. Bautista et al., "Seroprevalence and Risk Factors."

34. Garcia Calleja et al., "Status of the HIV/AIDS Epidemic," 3.

35. Geeta Rao Gupta, "Vulnerability and Resilience: Gender and HIV/AIDS in Latin America and the Caribbean," <www.iadb.org/sds/doc/Vulnerability.pdf>, accessed May 12, 2005.

36. U.S. Census Bureau, "HIV/AIDS Profile: Colombia," International Programs Center, Population Division, U.S. Census Bureau, HIV/AIDS Surveillance Data Base, June 2000, <www.census.gov/ipc/hiv/colombia.pdf>, accessed February 17, 2005.

37. Perez and Dabis, "HIV Prevention in Latin America," 78.

38. Ibid., 77.

39. Ministerio de Salud, *Plan de Mediano Plazo*, 20; BBC News, "Colombia"; Gómez Gómez, *SIDA en Colombia*, 173.

40. Gómez Gómez, *SIDA en Colombia*, 65–66.

41. Ibid., 68.

42. Ibid., 69, 72.

43. Ibid., 79.

44. Ministerio de Salud, *Plan de Mediano Plazo*, 20, 25; for a chart with information on HIV/AIDS from 1983 through 1993 see Olivos Lombana, *Amor e SIDA*, 108, 111.

45. Gómez Gómez, *SIDA en Colombia*, 115–26.

46. Olivos Lombana, *Amor e SIDA*, 101–4.

47. Gómez Gómez, *SIDA en Colombia*, 172.

48. Olivos Lombana, *Amor e SIDA*, 147.

49. Ibid., 115.

50. Ibid., 112–13.

51. BBC News, "Colombia."

52. Juan O. Tamayo, "Experts See Jump in Heroin Use, Cases of HIV among Colombia's Young, Poor," *Miami Herald*, June 20, 1999, accessed through EBSCO Host, accession number 4N78671571720483.

53. BBC News, "Colombia."

54. The Global Fund, "Portfolio of Grants in Colombia," <www.theglobalfund.org/search/portfolio.aspx?countryID=COL&lang=>, accessed April 14, 2005.

55. BBC News, "Colombia."

56. Ibid.

57. UNAIDS, Country Report, Colombia, <www.unaids.org>, accessed May 17, 2005.

58. Cueto, *Culpa e Coraje*, 39.

59. Ibid., 40.

60. Cáceres Palacios, *SIDA en el Perú*, 40–44. For a list of works addressing the HIV epidemic in Peru see Cueto, *Culpa e Coraje*, 49.

61. Cáceres Palacios, *SIDA en el Perú*, 87, 100–101.

62. Ibid., 96.

63. Ibid., 97.

64. Ibid., 83, 97–101.

65. Cueto, *Culpa e Coraje*, 45.

66. Cáceres Palacios, *SIDA en el Perú*, 78, 83, 85–86, 103–4, 109; Cueto, *Culpa e Coraje*, 55. The following paragraph paraphrases Cueto's work in a brief fashion.

67. Cueto, *Culpa e Coraje*, 52–53, 59–60.

68. Ibid., 61.

69. Frasca, *AIDS in Latin America*, 45.

70. Ibid., 38.

71. For the compulsory testing of gay men in Lima see Cueto, *Culpa e Coraje*, 62. For information on NAMRID, on which this passage is based, see ibid., 63–70.

72. Frasca, *AIDS in Latin America*, 58–59.

73. Ibid., 61.

74. Cueto, *Culpa e Coraje*, 74, 77, 88. Frasca's work suggests that the Peruvian state still prioritizes research and testing over support; see Frasca, *AIDS in Latin America*, 64–65.

75. Cueto, *Culpa e Coraje*, 107–8, 113.

76. Ibid., 107–13, 124, 128. For cooperation between the government and NGOs see also Frasca, *AIDS in Latin America*, 56.

77. USAID, Country Profile, HIV/AIDS, Peru, <www.usaid.gov>, accessed May 7, 2005. See also Cueto, *Culpa e Coraje*, 117–18.

78. Brousek, "Analysis."

79. Ibid.

80. Ibid.

81. USAID, Country Profile, HIV/AIDS, Peru, <www.usaid.gov>, accessed May 7, 2005.

82. Human Rights Watch, "HIV/AIDS Tests: Published in El Comercio on May 8, 2004," <//hrw.org/english/docs/2004/05/14/peru8584.htm>, accessed May 16, 2005.

83. Richard Stern, "In Peru, People Living with HIV/AIDS Demand Treatment Access," December 14, 2001, <www.cptech.org/ip/health/aids/peru12142001.html>, accessed May 16, 2005.

84. Ibid.

85. Frasca, *AIDS in Latin America*, 66.

86. Doctors without Borders, Field News, "AIDS Treatment in Peru," September 15, 2004, <www.doctorswithoutborders-usa.org/news/2004/0915-2004.cfm>, accessed May 16, 2005.

87. Ibid.

88. Cueto, *Culpa e Coraje*, 114–17, 124–29.

89. The Global Fund, "Portfolio of Grants in Peru," <www.theglobalfund.org/search/portfolio.aspx?countryID=PER&lang=>, accessed April 14, 2005. See also the material in the full proposal, grant agreement, and grant performance report, which may be found on this site.

90. Faustino Sarmiento, *Life in the Argentine Republic*.

91. See Senderowicz, "Towards a Discourse of Mestizaje."

92. Timerman, *Prisoner without a Name*; Feitlowitz, *Lexicon of Terror*.

93. *Empty ATM*.

94. UNAIDS epidemiological fact sheets, 2004 update, <www.unaids.org>, accessed February 26, 2005.

95. Kelly, *Checkerboards and Shatterbelts*, 39.

96. Smallman, *Fear and Memory*, 10.

97. Whigham and Potthast, "Paraguayan Rosetta Stone," 185.

98. Monteoliva Doratioto, "A Ocupação Político-Militar."

99. Hughes, "Logistics and the Chaco War," 412.

100. UNAIDS epidemiological fact sheets, Paraguay, 2004 update, <www.unaids.org>, accessed February 26, 2005.

101. UNAIDS epidemiological fact sheets, Uruguay, 2004 update, <www.unaids.org>, accessed February 26, 2005.

102. Magis Rodríguez, Marques, and Touzé, "HIV and Injection Drug Use," 35–36.

103. Carmona Berríos and del Valle Larrañaga, *SIDA en Chile*, 54. For the belief that the low rate of drug use and the nation's geographic isolation could shield the country from HIV see 36. For the fact that HIV was not perceived as much of a threat see 40.

104. Ibid., 40. See also Frasca, *AIDS in Latin America*, 215.

105. Carmona Berríos and del Valle Larrañaga, *SIDA en Chile*, 46–47, 54.

106. Ibid., 60–61.

107. Ibid., 19–27, 71, 83. See also Frasca, *AIDS in Latin America*, 249.

108. Comision Nacional del SIDA, *Perfil del VIH/SIDA*, 1–3, 11–12, 25–30, 54. For

the concentration of the disease in Santiago see also Smith, "On the Limited Utility," 3.

109. Consejo Episcopal Latinoamerica, *SIDA*, 54.

110. Frasca, *AIDS in Latin America*, 214.

111. Ibid., 214.

112. Carmona Berríos and del Valle Larrañaga, *SIDA en Chile*, 103–5, 129.

113. Ibid., 105–6, 129–30.

114. Victor Hugo Robles, "SIDA, Orden y Patria," *El Periodista*, July 6, 2003, 32.

115. Carmona Berríos and del Valle Larrañaga, *SIDA en Chile*, 114, 125–28.

116. Frasca, *AIDS in Latin America*, 243.

117. This paragraph is based on information from Carmona Berríos and del Valle Larrañaga, *SIDA en Chile*, 144, 148, 161–63.

118. Frasca, *AIDS in Latin America*, 244.

119. Ibid., 251.

120. Smith, "On the Limited Utility," 3.

121. UNAIDS factsheet, epidemiological fact sheets, Chile, 2004 update, <www.unaids.org>, accessed February 26, 2005. For more statistics on HIV/AIDS in Chile see also CONASIDA, "Memoria Anual."

122. U.S. Census Bureau, "HIV/AIDS Profile: Chile," International Programs Center, Population Division, U.S. Census Bureau, HIV/AIDS Surveillance Data Base, June 2000, <www.census.gov/ipc/hiv/chile.pdf>, accessed February 17, 2005.

123. Ibid.

124. Bloch, "El Sida," 26, 37.

125. For the influence of the Catholic Church on Argentina's AIDS policy see Kornblit and Petracci, "Las ONGs," 389.

126. Bloch, "El Sida," 83.

127. Alejandra Trossero, quoted in Frasca, *AIDS in Latin America*, 164.

128. Ibid., 165.

129. Frasca, *AIDS in Latin America*, 165.

130. Libonatti et al., "Role of Drug Injection," 137.

131. Betts, Astarloa, Bloch, Zacarias, and Chelala, "Changing Face of AIDS," 94.

132. Graciela Touzé, quoted in Frasca, *AIDS in Latin America*, 166.

133. Lisandro Orlov, quoted in ibid., 167.

134. Touzé, "Obstacles," 372.

135. Bianco et al., *Human Rights*, 4; see also 7.

136. This information on AIDS NGOs in Argentina is taken from Kornblit and Petracci, "Las ONGs," 387–400, and Pecheny, "Los Jóvenes." For the transfer of responsibilities from the public sector to the private see Kornblit and Petracci, "Las ONGs," 387; for the number of AIDS NGOs in greater Buenos

Aries see 391; for the fact that these organizations rely heavily on government support see 399. For the Argentine state's increasing reliance on AIDS NGOs see Pecheny, "Los Jóvenes," 424.

137. Walsh, "Argentine AIDS Agencies Blossom."

138. Pecheny, "Los Jóvenes," 423. For a broad survey of AIDS legislation in Argentina see Hamilton, "Septiembre/Octubre 2004." See also <http://www.laccaso.org/pdfs/Rep_Argentina.pdf>.

139. Controladuría General Comunal, *El Flagelo del SIDA*, 4–17, 31–32.

140. Kornblit, "Personas Afectadas," 215. For more information on HIV and drug users see Moscatello, Campello, and Benetucci, "Bloodborne and Sexually Transmitted Infections."

141. Kornblit and Mendes Diz, "Personas Afectadas," 344.

142. Walsh, "Argentine AIDS Agencies Blossom."

143. Ibid.

144. Kornblit et al., *SIDA*, 9.

145. Bloch, "El Sida," 45.

146. Libonatti et al., "Role of Drug Injection," 136.

147. Kornblit, "Personas Afectadas," 187; Kornblit et al., "SIDA y Conductas Sexuales," 28–29.

148. Libonatti et al., "Role of Drug Injection," 135–36.

149. Matías A. Loewy, "HIV-1 Subtype Linked to Transmission in Argentina," *Reuters Health*, April 18, 2003, <www.thebody.com/cdc/news_updates_archive/2003/apr18_03/hiv_transmission.html>, accessed January 7, 2005.

150. Avila et al., "Two HIV-1 Epidemics," 425.

151. Libonatti et al., "Role of Drug Injection," 138.

152. Ibid.

153. Walsh, "Argentine AIDS Agencies Blossom." See also de los Angeles Pando et al., "High Human Immunodeficiency Virus." For information that Argentina is sixth in the Americas in terms of reported HIV cases among children see Fallo et al., "Clinical and Epidemiological Aspects." For information on Foundation Huesped see the organization's website at <www.huesped.org.ar>.

154. Frasca, *AIDS in Latin America*, 170.

155. Hamilton, "Septiembre/Octubre 2004."

156. Ibid.

157. Dr. Arnoldo Victor Castillo, National Secretary for Health Care, Address to the 26th Special Session of the General Assembly on HIV/AIDS, New York, June 27, 2001, <www.un.org/ga/aids/statements/docs/argentinaE.html>, accessed April 14, 2005. For a detailed analysis of how Argentina provides these medications see Bianco et al., *Human Rights*, 19–27.

158. Pecheny, "Los Jóvenes," 424. It is also true, however, that the Argentine government continued to provide these medications even after the 2001 economic collapse. See Frasca, *AIDS in Latin America*, 171.

159. Center for Reproductive Law and Policy, *Women's Reproductive Rights*, 13.

160. Valente, "Argentina."

161. Bianco et al., *Human Rights*, 12.

162. Ibid., 23; see also 26.

163. Valente, "Argentina."

164. Bianco et al., *Human Rights*, 9.

165. Ibid., 10.

166. Ibid.

167. Walsh, "Argentine AIDS Agencies Blossom."

168. Kornblit et al., "SIDA y Conductas Sexuales," 37–41.

169. Hamilton, "Septiembre/Octubre 2004."

170. UNAIDS, "Argentina," <www.unaids.org>, accessed April 14, 2005.

171. Bloch, "El Sida," 37.

172. Libonatti et al., "Role of Drug Injection," 138.

173. For AIDS as an illness of poverty in Argentina see Bloch, "El Sida," 30–35; for AIDS and education see 39. For the fact that education level does not seem to influence the risk of HIV among men who have sex with men, see de los Angeles Pando et al., "High Human Immunodeficiency Virus," 737; see also Avila et al., "Two HIV-1 Epidemics," 424. For general statistics on HIV and Argentina see U.S. Census Bureau, "HIV/AIDS profile: Argentina," <www.census.gov/ipc/hiv/argentin.pdf>, accessed May 10, 2005; see also Bloch, "El Sida," 26–28.

174. De los Angeles Pando et al., "High Human Immunodeficiency Virus."

175. UNAIDS, "Argentina," <www.unaids.org>, accessed April 14, 2005.

Conclusion

1. Farmer, *AIDS and Accusation*, 149.

2. Eberstadt, "Future of AIDS." See also d'Adesky, *Moving Mountains*, 206–22. For information on China's epidemic see Clyde B. McCoy, Douglas Feldman, Lisa R. Metsch, Robert S. Anwyl, Shenghan Lai, and Xue-ren Wang, "China," in McElrath, *HIV and AIDS*, 69–86. In January 2006 new information emerged to suggest that China may have 650,000 people living with HIV, considerably lower than many previous estimates. See Jim Yardley, "New Estimate in China Finds Fewer AIDS Cases," *New York Times*, January 26, 2006.

3. Frasca has argued that because Africa has a higher rate of infection than Latin

America, the latter region is "rarely on the radar in discussions of AIDS" (*AIDS in Latin America*, 253).

4. For a brief description of Asia's epidemic see Barnett and Whiteside, *AIDS in the Twenty-First Century*, 14; Irwin, Millen, and Fallows, *Global AIDS*, 8–10.
5. Beyrer, *War in the Blood*, 57–58, 140–46.
6. Ibid., 63–65.
7. Ibid., 197–203.
8. Smallman-Raynor and Cliff, *War Epidemics*, 550–63; Hooper, *The River*, 42–51, 767–71.
9. Elbe, "HIV/AIDS and the Changing Landscape"; Garrett, "Lessons," 54–56.
10. Garrett, "Lessons," 57.
11. Mock, "Conflict and HIV."
12. Frasca, *AIDS in Latin America*, 7.
13. Farmer, *AIDS and Accusation*, 149.
14. Sontag, *AIDS and Its Metaphors*.
15. Barnett and Whiteside, *AIDS in the Twenty-First Century*, 311–12.
16. For a sophisticated discussion of HIV and poverty, in a global context, see ibid.
17. Ibid., 88.
18. Price-Smith, Tauber, and Bhat, "State Capacity," 159.
19. Eberstadt, "Future of AIDS," 24–27.
20. According to the CIA World Factbook (accessed June 29, 2005, at <www.cia.gov/cia/publications/factbook/>) the relative size of African economies in 2004 was as follows: Egypt, $314 billion; Nigeria, $125.7 billion; and South Africa, $491.4 billion.
21. Farmer, "Global AIDS."
22. Barnett and Whiteside, *AIDS in the Twenty-First Century*, 88–97.
23. Ibid., 98–123.
24. Frasca, *AIDS in Latin America*, 5.
25. Whiteside and Sunter, *AIDS*, 49–52.
26. Rachel L. Swarns, "Dobb's Outspokenness Draws Fans and Fire," *New York Times*, February 15, 2006.
27. Bronfman, "Mexico and Central America."
28. For one list of resources on this topic see <http://www.daywalka.org/resourcecenter.htm>, accessed May 17, 2006.
29. Beyrer, *War in the Blood*, 128; see also 59–60, 129–35.
30. Garrett, "Lessons," 58.
31. Whiteside and Sunter, *AIDS*, 62–64.
32. Barnett and Whiteside, *AIDS in the Twenty-First Century*, 152–53. See also Epstein, "Hidden Cause of AIDS."
33. See Frasca, *AIDS in Latin America*, 11–13.
34. Ibid., 164–69, 173–80.

35. For the contrast between Thailand and South Africa, see Guest, *Children of AIDS*, 9. For a broader look at the Thai experience see Beyrer, *War in the Blood*, 16–35, 113–14; Barnett and Whiteside, *AIDS in the Twenty-First Century*, 334–35.

36. For the failure of the government's response in South Africa, and in particular the role of Thabo Mbeki, see Mattes, "South Africa," 27–28; Guest, *Children of AIDS*, 3; Behrman, *Invisible People*, 201–5; Barnett and Whiteside, *AIDS in the Twenty-First Century*, 297–98.

37. Price-Smith, Tauber, and Bhat, "State Capacity," 149–50.

38. Ibid., 151.

39. Ibid., 159.

40. Smallman, "Shady Business."

41. For activists involved in the day-to-day struggle against HIV, the failings of government efforts are easier to note than the successes. See Frasca, *AIDS in Latin America*, 253–54.

42. For epidemiological information on individual Latin American countries see the country profiles at <www.unaids.org>. PAHO also has a wealth of quantitative information: <http://www.paho.org/english/ad/fch/ai/aids.htm>. The Population Reference Bureau has many useful studies: <http://www.prb.org/>. A great deal of information can also be found at <http://www.usaid.gov/locations/latin_america_caribbean/>. For news reports from the region on HIV see <http://www.thebody.com/whatis/demo_latinam.html>. For general information on Latin America's HIV epidemic see also <http://www.laccaso.org/>. One NGO with a wealth of research on HIV in Brazil is the ABIA; their website allows browsers to access manuscripts and theses: <www.abiaids.org.br>. For the website of Brazil's National Program to fight STDs and AIDS see <http://www.aids.gov.br/data/Pages/LUMISFDF29F77PTBRIE.htm>. With the help of USAID, Central America has created the most impressive collection of electronic resources on HIV/AIDS in the region. See <http://www.pasca.org/index2.htm>. For HIV/AIDS statistics in Oaxaca, and a critical interpretation, the following website is helpful: <http://www.frentecomunoaxaca.org/en012.htm>. For information on international access to medications see <http://www.healthgap.org/>. The links from these various resources should lead researchers to a wealth of other useful sites.

BIBLIOGRAPHY

Interviews

All interviews were conducted by the author.
"Alberto," member of Projeto Esperança. São Paulo, July 20, 2005.
Bill Wolf. Oaxaca City, August 23, 26, 2004.
"Celia," a COESIDA employee. Oaxaca City, August 24, 2004.
"Celso," former IV drug user. São Paulo, July 18, 2005.
"Claudio," crack user. São Paulo, July 18, 2005.
"Drauzio," HIV-positive man. São Paulo, July 19, 2005.
Dr. Q. Oaxaca City, August 27, 2004.
Dr. "Rodrigo," Secretary of Health. Oaxaca City, August 24, 2004.
"Edison," crack addict. São Paulo, July 19, 2005.
"Eduardo," injecting drug user. São Paulo, July 20, 2005.
Employee at MEXFAM. Oaxaca City, August 25, 2004.
"Eva." Oaxaca City, August 26, 2004.
"Gabriela." São Paulo, July 20, 2005.
"Getúlio," GIV leader. São Paulo, July 21, 2005.
"Jean," GIV leader. São Paulo, July 21, 2005.
"João," HIV-positive man. São Paulo, July 19, 2005.
"Julio." Oaxaca City, August 23, 2004.
"Juscelino," drug user. São Paulo, July 18, 2005.
"Maria," a COESIDA employee. Oaxaca City, August 24, 2004.
Members of Vinni Gaxhea. Oaxaca City, August 25, 2004.
Members of Projeto Esperança. São Paulo, July 20, 2005.
"Oswaldo," drug user. São Paulo, July 20, 2005.
"Paula," a nurse and COESIDA employee. Oaxaca City, August 24, 2004.
"Paulo," ex–drug user. São Paulo, July 18, 2005.
Paulo Roberto Teixeira, Consultor Sênior, Programa Estadual, DST, AIDS-SP.
    São Paulo, July 19, 2005.

Even though there are gaps in the literature, there are far too many works available on AIDS in Latin America to include all of them here. As a result, this is a select bibliography of useful sources that I consulted in writing this book. The fact that a work is not included in this bibliography is not a judgment of its quality.

Abadía-Barrero, César Ernesto. "The Cultural Politics of the Brazilian AIDS Social Movement: A Local and Global Revolution." Paper presented at the meeting of the Latin American Studies Association, Dallas, Texas, March 27–29, 2003.

ABIA [Associação Brasileira Interdisciplinar de AIDS]. *Ação anti-AIDS*, no. 15. Rio de Janeiro: ABIA, 1991. Pamphlet. Princeton University Microfilm Collection, Supplement no. 3, "Socioeconomic Conditions in Latin America." Roll 1, Subsection Brazil, Scholarly Resources.

Acosta, Dalia. "Health-Cuba: Sex Workers Shun Condoms, Risking Disease." *Inter Press Service*, October 16, 2002. Accessed through LexisNexis, May 28, 2003.

Aguilar, Sergio, César Nuñez, and John Stover. *Proyecciones sobre la Magnitud de la Epidemia de VIH-SIDA en Guatemala, 1980–2010*. Guatemala City: PASCA, 1999.

Ahmad, Khabir. "Brazil and USA at Loggerheads over Production of Generic Anti-retrovirals." *Lancet*, February 10, 2001, 453.

AIDSCAP. *Estudio de Conocimientos, Creencias, Actitudes y Prácticas sobre Sexualidad y ETS/VIH/SIDA en Grupos de Población Específicos*. Tegucigalpa, Honduras: Proyeto USAID/AIDSCAP, 1997.

"AIDS in Haiti: H is for Hope." *Economist*, June 19, 2004, 39.

Anderson, Paula Jean. "AIDS as an Opportunity for Compassion and Growth through Dialogue." M.A. thesis, Portland State University, 2003.

Andreani, Tony, R. Modigliani, Y. le Charpentier, A. Galian, J. C. Brouet, M. Liance, J. R. Lachance, B. Messing, and B. Vernisse. "Acquired Immunodeficiency with Intestinal Cryptosporidiosis: Possible Transmission by Haitian Whole Blood." *Lancet*, May 28, 1983, 1187–91.

Aperecida Nappo, Solange, Zila van der Meer Sanchez, Lúcio Garcia de Olivereria. *Comportomento de Risco de Mulheres Usuárias de Crack em Relação às DST/AIDS*. São Paulo: CEBRID, n.d.

Appleby, David P. *The Music of Brazil*. Austin: University of Texas Press, 1983.

Araújo de Mattos, Ruben, Veriano Terto Jr., and Robert Parker. *As Estratégias do Banco Mundial e a Resposta à AIDS no Brasil*. Rio de Janeiro: ABIA, 2001.

Ashraf, Haroon. "USA and Brazil End Dispute over Essential Drugs." *Lancet*, June 30, 2001, 2112.

Avila, María M., María A. Pando, Gladys Carrion, Liliana Martinez Peralta,

Horacio Salomón, Manuel Gomez Carrillo, José Sanchez, Sergio Maulen, Jesse
Hierholzer, Mark Marinello, Mónica Negrete, Kevin L. Russell, and Jean K. Carr.
"Two HIV-1 Epidemics in Argentina: Different Genetic Subtypes Associated
with Different Risk Groups." *Journal of Acquired Immune Deficiency Syndromes*
29 (2002): 422–26.

Ayres de Castilho, Euclides. "Epidemiologia do HIV/AIDS no Brasil." In *Políticas, Instituições e AIDS: Enfrentando a Epidemia no Brasil,* edited by Richard G.
Parker, 17–42. Rio de Janeiro: ABIA: Jorge Zahar, 1997.

Barksdale, Byron. *HIV/AIDS in Cuba: From Vigilant Quarantine to Vaccine Quest.*
Pamphlet. Cuba AIDS Project.

Barton, John, Daniel Alexander, Carlos Correa, Ramesh Mashelkar, Gill Samuels,
and Sandy Thomas. "Integrating Intellectual Property Rights and Development Policy." *Report of the Commission on Intellectual Property Rights* (chap. 2).
London. September 2002, <http://www.iprcommission.org>. Accessed January
28, 2003.

Barnett, Tony, and Alan Whiteside. *AIDS in the Twenty-First Century.* New York:
Palgrave MacMillan, 2002.

Bastos, Cristiana. *Global Responses to AIDS: Science in Emergency.* Bloomington:
Indiana University Press, 1991.

Bautista, C. T., J. L. Sanchez, S. M. Montano, V. A. Laguna-Torres, J. R. Lama, J.
L. Sanchez, L. Kusunoki, H. Manrique, J. Acosta, O. Montoya, A. M. Tambare,
M. M. Avila, J. Viñoles, N. Aguayo, J. G. Olson, and J. K. Carr. "Seroprevalence
and Risk Factors for HIV-1 Infection among South American Men Who Have
Sex with Men." *Sexually Transmitted Infections* 80, no. 6 (December 2004):
498–504.

Bazell, Robert. "The History of an Epidemic." *New Republic,* August 1, 1983, 14.

BBC News. "Colombia: AIDS Gender Gap Shrinking as More Women Become
Infected." From Cambio website, Bogotá, October 7, 2003. Accessed through
LexisNexis. October 8, 2003.

Behrman, Greg. *Invisible People.* New York: Free Press, 2004.

Bellis, David J. *Hotel Ritz: Comparing Mexican and U.S. Street Prostitutes—Factors
in HIV/AIDS Transmission.* New York: Haworth Press, 2003.

Benatar, Solomon R., Abdallah S. Daar, and Peter A. Singer. "Global Health Ethics:
The Rationale for Mutual Caring." *International Affairs* 79, no. 1 (January 2003):
107–38.

Betts, Claude D., L. Astarloa, C. Bloch, F. Zacarias, and C. Chelala. "The Changing
Face of AIDS in Argentina." *Journal of the American Medical Association,* July 10,
1996, 94–96.

Beyrer, Chris. *War in the Blood: Sex, Politics, and AIDS in Southeast Asia.* New York:
Zed Books, 1998.

Biaggio, Jaime. "Cazuza Mostra a Sua Cara." *O Globo*, June 16, 2002, 1–3.

Bianco, Mabel, Maria Ines Re, Laura Pagani, and Estela Barone. *Human Rights and Access to Treatment for HIV/AIDS in Argentina.* Toronto: LACCASO, 1998. Available at <http://www.laccaso.org/pdfs/argeng.pdf>.

Black, George. *The Good Neighbor.* New York: Pantheon, 1988.

Bloch, Claudio. "El Sida, una Nueva Enfermedad de la Pobreza." In *El Sida en Argentina: Epidemiología, Subjetividad y Ética Social,* by Pedro Cahn, Claudio Bloch, and Silvana Weller, 21–95. Buenos Aries: Arkhetypo, 1999.

Booth, John A., and Thomas W. Walker. *Understanding Central America.* 2nd ed. Boulder, Colo.: Westview Press, 1993.

Borges, José Francisco. *Como Evitar a AIDS.* Literatura de cordel pamphlet. Av. Major Aprigio da Fonseca, 420 CEP. 55660-000 Bezerros PE.

Boulet, P., J. Perriens, and F. Renaud-Thery. *Patent Situation of HIV/AIDS-Related Drugs in 80 Countries.* Geneva: UNAIDS/WHO, 2000.

Boulos, Michaelle L., Reginald Boulos, and Douglas J. Nichols. "Perceptions and Practices Relating to Condom Use among Urban Men in Haiti." *Studies in Family Planning* 22, no. 5 (September–October 1991): 322.

Boulos, Reginald, N. A. Halsey, E. Holt, A. Ruff, J. R. Brutus, T. C. Quinn, M. Adrien, and C. Boulos. "HIV-1 in Haitian Women, 1982–1988." *Journal of Acquired Immune Deficiency Syndromes* 3 (1990): 721–28.

Boyd, Barbara, and John Garrison. "NGO Participation in HIV/AIDS Control Project in Brazil Achieves Results." *Social Development Notes* 47 (May 1999): 1–4.

"Brazil Fights for Affordable Drugs against HIV/AIDS." *Revista Panamerica de Salud Pública/PanAmerican Journal of Public Health* 9, no. 5 (2001): 331–37.

Brinkley, Joel. "Anti-Drug Gains in Colombia Don't Reduce Flow to the United States." *New York Times,* April 28, 2005.

Bronfman, Mario. "Mexico and Central America." *International Migration* 36, no. 4 (December 1998): 609–42.

Bronfman, Mario, Sergio Camposortega, and Hortencia Medina. "La Migración Internacional y el SIDA: El Caso de México y Estados Unidos." *AIDS* 16, no. 3 (December 2002): 435–56.

Bronfman, Mario N., René Leyva, Mirka J. Negroni, and Celina M. Rueda. "Mobile Populations and HIV/AIDS in Central America: Research for Action." *AIDS* 16, no. 3 (December 2002): 42–49.

Brousek, David. "Analysis: Peru Must Face Its AIDS Epidemic." UPI, July 16, 2004, <www.upi.com/view.cfm?StoryID=20040715-15424-4978r>. Accessed May 16, 2005.

Burkhalter, Holly. "The Politics of AIDS: Engaging Conservative Activists." *Foreign Affairs* 83, no. 1 (January/February 2004): 7–14.

Cáceres Palacios, Carlos. *SIDA en el Perú: Imagenes de Diversidad*. Lima: Universidad Peruana Cayetano Heredia, 1998.

Cahn, Pedro, Claudio Bloch, and Silvana Weller. *El Sida en Argentina: Epidemiología, Subjetividad y Ética Social*. Buenos Aries: Arkhetypo, 1999.

"Candomblé—Saúde—Axé." Centro Baiano Anti-Aides poster. Rua Frei Vicente, 24—Pelourinho—Fone: (71) 321–1848 Apoio: Ministerio da Saúde Unesco—Sesab—SMS—Kimeta Society Agradecimentos: Artista Gil Abelha, Brascard Nordeste Edições de Postais Ltda, Fotógrapo Lúcio Mendes (2/2001).

Carlini, E. A. "Redução de Danos: Uma Visão Internacional." *Jornal Brasileiro de Psiquiatria* 52, no. 5 (2003): 335–39.

Carlini, E. A., and José Carlos F. Galduróz. "Revisão—Perfil de Uso de Cocaína no Brasil." *Jornal Brasileiro de Psiquiatria* 44, no. 6 (1995): 287–303.

Carlini, E. A., José Carlos F. Galduróz, Ana Regina Noto, and Solange A. Nappo. *I Levantamento Domiciliar Sobre o Uso de Drogas Psicotrópicas no Brasil, 2001*. São Paulo: CEBRID: Secretaria Nacional Antidrogas, 2001.

Carlini, E. A., Ana Regina Noto, José Carlos F. Galduróz, and Solange A. Nappo. "Visão Histórica Sobre o Use de Drogas: Passado e Presente; Rio de Janeiro e São Paulo." *Jornal Brasileiro de Psiquiatria* 45, no. 4 (1996): 227–36.

Carlini, E. A., Eliana Rodrigues, and José Carlos F. Galduróz, eds. *Cannabis Sativa L. e Substâncias Canabinóides em Medicina*. São Paulo: CEBRID/Secretaria Nacional Antidrogas, 2004.

Carmona Berríos, Mauricio, and Cynthia del Valle Larrañaga. *SIDA en Chile: La Historia Desconicida*. Santiago de Chile: Editorial Andrés Bello, 2000.

Carrillo, Hector. *The Night Is Young: Sexuality in Mexico in the Time of AIDS*. Chicago: University of Chicago Press, 2002.

Casper, Virginia. "AIDS: A Psychosocial Perspective." In *The Social Dimensions of AIDS*, edited by Douglas A. Felman and Thomas M. Johnson, 197–209. New York: Praeger, 1986.

Castro, Roberto, and René Leyva. "Mexico." In *HIV and AIDS: A Global View*, edited by Karen McElrath, 137–58. Westport, Conn.: Greenwood Press, 2002.

Castro, Roberto, Emanuel Orozco, Peter Aggleton, Enrique Eroza, and Juan Jacobo Hernández. "Family Responses to HIV/AIDS in Mexico." *Social Science and Medicine* 47, no. 10 (1998): 1473–84.

Ceballos, Vladimir. *Maldita Sea Tu Nombre, Libertad*. VHS documentary. Video Zurnon, I.S.A., and Brown University, 1994.

Center for Reproductive Law and Policy. *Women's Reproductive Rights in Argentina: A Shadow Report*. New York: Center for Reproductive Law and Policy, 2000.

"Central America, Drug Companies Reach Agreement to Lower Cost of AIDS Drugs." *AIDS Weekly*, 17 February 2003, 38.

Chelala, César A. "Central America: The Cost of War." *Lancet*, January 20, 1990, 153–54.

Chequer, Pedro. "Atenção a Saúde de Pessoas com HIV/AIDS: Experiências na América Latina e no Caribe." *Boletim ABIA* 46 (July–September 2001): 2.

Chequer, Pedro, Paloma Cuchi, Rafael Mazin, and Jesus M. García Calleja. "Access to Antiretroviral Treatment in Latin American Countries and the Caribbean." *AIDS* 16, no. 3 (December 2002): 50–57.

Chúa, Carlos, Ernesto Almendáres, Jorge Matute, and Adilis Velásquez. *VIH-SIDA en la Zona 6 de la Ciudad de Guatemala*. Guatemala City: Universidad de San Carlos de Guatemala, 1999.

CIA. CIA World Factbook, <http://www.cia.gov/cia/publications/factbook/geos/ha.html>. Accessed July 27, 2003.

Cohen, Jillian Clare, and Kristina M. Lybecker. "AIDS Policy and Pharmaceutical Patents: Brazil's Strategy to Safeguard Public Health." Paper presented at the meeting of the Latin American Studies Association, Dallas, Texas, March 27–29, 2003.

Cohen, Jon. *Shots in the Dark*. New York: Norton, 2001.

Cohen, Jonathan. "FTAA Summit: Reject Tighter Patents on AIDS Drugs." Human Rights Watch, October 29, 2002, <http://www.hrw.org/press/2002/10/ftaa1029.htm>. Accessed January 15, 2003.

Comision Nacional del SIDA, Chile. *Perfil del VIH/SIDA en Cifras, Chile, 1984–1994*. Santiago: Ministry of Health, 1995.

CONASIDA, Chile. "Memoria Anual de CONASIDA." *Revista Chilena de Infectología* 21, no. 2 (2004): 126–50.

Consejo Episcopal Latinoamericano. *SIDA*. Bogotá: CELAM, 1989.

Consumer Project on Technology, Essential Action, Médecins Sans Frontières, Oxfam International, Health GAP Coalition, and the Third World Network to the World Trade Organization's TRIPS Council. "NGO Letter on Compulsory Licensing and Exports." January 28, 2002, <http://www.globaltreatmentaccess.org>. Accessed January 27, 2003.

Controladuría General Comunal, Buenos Aries. *El Flagelo del SIDA*. Buenos Aries: Controladuría General Comunal/Prevención del SIDA de la Secretaría de Educación de la Municipalidad de la Ciudad de Buenos Aries, 1994.

Cuadra-Hernández, Silvia Magali, René Leyva-Flores, Daniel Hernández-Rosete, and Mario N. Bronfman-Pertzovsky. "Los Derechos Humanos en las Normas sobre el VIH/SIDA en México y Centroamérica, 1993–2000." *Salud Pública de México* 44, no. 6 (November–December 2002): 508–18.

Cueto, Marcos. *Culpa e Coraje: Historia de las Políticas sobre el VIH/Sida en el Perú*. Lima: Consorcio de Investigación Económica y Social, 2001.

———. "Stigma and Blame during an Epidemic: Cholera in Peru, 1991." In

Disease in the History of Modern Latin America: From Malaria to AIDS, edited by Diego Armus, 268–89. Durham: Duke University Press, 2003.

Cullet, Phillipe. "Patents and Medicines: The Relationship between TRIPS and the Human Right to Health." *International Affairs* 79, no. 1 (January 2003): 139–60.

Curti, Andrea. "The WTO Dispute Settlement Understanding: An Unlikely Weapon in the Fight against AIDS." *American Journal of Law and Medicine* 27 (2001): 469–85.

Cypriano, Tânia. *Odô Yá: Life with AIDS*. VHS video. New York: Brazil Image/8 Viva! Pictures, 1997.

d'Adesky, Anne-Christine. *Moving Mountains: The Race to Treat Global AIDS*. New York: Verso, 2004.

Daniel, Herbert. "AIDS in Brazil." In *AIDS: The Politics of Survival*, edited by Nancy Krieger and Glen Margo, 197–211. Amityville, N.Y.: Baywood, 1994.

———. "The Bankruptcy of Models: Myths and Realities of AIDS in Brazil." In *Sexuality, Politics, and AIDS in Brazil: In Another World?*, edited by Herbert Daniel and Richard Parker, 33–48. London: Falmer Press, 1993.

Daniel, Herbert, and Richard Parker, eds. *Sexuality, Politics, and AIDS in Brazil*. London: Falmer Press, 1993.

———. "The Third Epidemic: An Exercise in Solidarity." In *Sexuality, Politics, and AIDS in Brazil: In Another World?*, edited by Herbert Daniel and Richard Parker, 49–62. London: Falmer Press, 1993.

da Silva, José Marmo, and Marco Antonio Chagas Guimarães. "Odô-Yá Project: HIV/AIDS Prevention in the Context of Brazilian Religion." *Journal of Health Communication* 5 (2000): 119–122.

de Brito, Ana Maria, Euclides Ayres de Castilho, and Célia Landmann Szwarcwald. "AIDS e Infecção pelo HIV no Brasil: Uma Epidemia Multifacetada." *Revista da Sociedade Brasileira de Medicina Tropical* 34, no. 2 (March–April 2000): 207–17.

de los Angeles Pando, Maria, Sergio Maulen, Mercedes Weissenbacher, Rubén Marone, Ricardo Duranti, Liliana Martínez Peralta, Horacio Salomón, Kevin Russell, Monica Negrete, Sergio Sosa Estani, Silvia Montano, José L. Sanchez, and Maria Mercedes Ávila. "High Human Immunodeficiency Virus Type 1 Seroprevalence in Men Who Have Sex with Men in Buenos Aries, Argentina: Risk Factors for Infection." *International Journal of Epidemiology* 32, no. 5 (October 2003): 735–40.

del Rio, Carlos, and Jaime Sepúlveda. "AIDS in Mexico: Lessons Learned and Implications for Developing Countries." *AIDS* 16, no. 11 (July 26, 2002): 1445–57.

DeNoon, Daniel J., and Keith K. Key. "Church Leaders Oppose Proposal to Give Prisoners Condoms." *AIDS Weekly Plus*, February 3, 1997, 19.

Eakin, Marshal. *Brazil: The Once and Future Country*. New York: St. Martin's Griffin, 1998.

Eaton, Victoria May. "Eso Es Lo Que Me Chinga Más: Social Changes Experienced by HIV-Positive Women in Oaxaca, Mexico." Undergraduate thesis, Pacific University, 2005.

Eberstadt, Nicholas. "The Future of AIDS: Grim Toll in Russia, China, and India." *Foreign Affairs* 81, no. 6 (November/December 2002): 22–45.

Elbe, Stefan. "HIV/AIDS and the Changing Landscape of War in Africa." *International Security* 27, no. 2 (Fall 2002): 159–77.

Ellwood, Wayne. *The No-Nonsense Guide to Globalization*. London: Verso, 2003.

The Empty ATM. Directed by Angus McQueen. PBS, Wide Angle. VHS tape. New York: PBS/Ford Foundation, 2003.

Enríquez, Lara J. "Economic Reform and Repeasantization in Post-1990 Cuba." *Latin American Research Review* 38, no. 1 (February 2003): 203–4.

Epstein, Helen. "The Hidden Cause of AIDS." *New York Review of Books*, May 9, 2002, 43–49.

Estudio Multicéntrico Centroamericano de Prevalencia deVIH/ITS y Comportamientos en poblaciones específicas en Honduras, <www.pasca.org/estudio/informes/ni/revista_emc_ho.pdf>. Accessed April 14, 2003.

Fallo, Aurelia A., Wanda Dobrzanski-Nisiewicz, Nora Sordelli, Maria Alejandra Cattaneo, Gwedolyn Scott, and Eduardo L. Lopez. "Clinical and Epidemiological Aspects of Human Immunodeficiency Virus-1 Infected Children in Buenos Aries, Argentina." *International Journal of Infectious Diseases* 6, no. 1 (March 2002): 9–16.

Fan, Hung Y., Ross F. Conner, and Luis P. Villarreal. *AIDS: Science and Society*. 4th ed. Sudbury, Mass.: Jones and Bartlett, 2004.

Farmer, Paul. *AIDS and Accusation: Haiti and the Geography of Blame*. Berkeley: University of California Press, 1992.

———. "The Exotic and the Mundane: Human Immunodeficiency Virus in Haiti." *Human Nature* 1, no. 4 (1990): 415–46.

———. "Global AIDS." *Perspectives in Biology and Medicine* 48, no. 1 (Winter 2005): 10–16.

———. "Haiti's Lost Years: Lessons for the Americas." *Current Issues in Public Health* 2 (1996): 143–51.

———. *Infections and Inequalities*. Los Angeles: University of California Press, 1999.

———. *Pathologies of Power: Health, Human Rights, and the New War on the Poor*. Berkeley: University of California Press, 2003.

———. "Sending Sickness: Sorcery, Politics, and Changing Conceptions of AIDS in Rural Haiti." *Medical Anthropology Quarterly* 4, no. 1 (1990): 6–27.

Farmer, Paul, Fernet Léandre, Joia S. Mukherjee, Marie Sidonise Claude, Patrice

Nevil, Mary C. Smith-Fawzi, Serena P. Koenig, Arachu Castro, Mercedes C. Becerra, Jeffrey Sachs, Amir Attaran, and Jim Yong Kim. "Community-Based Approaches to HIV Treatment in Resource-Poor Settings." *Lancet*, August 4, 2001, 404–9.

Faustino Sarmiento, Domingo. *Life in the Argentine Republic in the Days of Tyrants; or, Civilization and Barbarism*. New York: Hafner, 1960.

Fausto, Boris. *A Concise History of Brazil*. New York: Cambridge University Press, 1999.

Fausto Neto, Antônio. "AIDS: Um Discurso das Mídias." Centro Cultural Banco do Brasil, *Veredas*, Rio de Janeiro (1997): 28–29.

Fee, Elizabeth, and Daniel M. Fox, eds. *AIDS and the Burdens of History*. Berkeley: University of California Press, 1988.

Feinsilver, Julie Margot. *Healing the Masses: Cuban Health Politics at Home and Abroad*. Los Angeles: University of California Press, 1993.

Feitlowitz, Marguerite. *A Lexicon of Terror: Argentina and the Legacies of Torture*. New York: Oxford Univesity Press, 1998.

Fettner, Ann Giudici, and William A. Check. *The Truth about AIDS: Evolution of an Epidemic*. New York: Holt, Rinehart and Winston, 1984.

Figueroa, Faizury. *El SIDA en Honduras*. Tegucigalpa, Honduras: Centro de Documentacion de Honduras, 1993.

Finlinson, H. Ann, Héctor M. Colón, Rafaela R. Robles, Sherry Deren, Mayra Soto López, and Aileen Muñoz. "Access to Sterile Syringes by Injection Drug Users in Puerto Rico." *Human Organization* 58, no. 2 (Summer 1999): 207.

Fitzgerald, Daniel W., and Toby B. Simon. "Commentary: Telling the Stories of People with AIDS in Rural Haiti." *AIDS Patient Care and STDs* 15, no. 6 (2001): 301–8.

Frasca, Tim. *AIDS in Latin America*. New York: Palgrave Macmillan, 2005.

FTAA—Free Trade Area of the Americas. "Draft Agreement, Chapter on Intellectual Property Rights," <http://www.ftaa-alca.org/ftaadraft/eng/ngipe_1.asp>. Accessed January 15, 2003.

Galduróz, José Carlos F., Ana Regina Noto, and E. A. Carlini. "A Situação do Consumo e Controle de Drogas Psicotrópicas no Brasil: Comentários Gerais." *Temas* 53 (1997): 1–9.

Galduróz, José Carlos F., Ana Regina Noto, Arilton Martins Fonseca, and E. A. Carlini. *V Levantamento Nacional Sobre O Consumo de Drogas Psicotrópicas Entre Estudantes do Ensino Fundamental e Médio da Rede Pública de Ensino nas 27 Capitais Brasileiras, 2004*. São Paulo: CEBRID/Secretaria Nacional Antidrogas, 2004.

Galduróz, José Carlos F., Ana Regina Noto, Solange A. Nappo, and E. L. Carlini. "First Household Survey on Drug Abuse in São Paulo, Brazil, 1999: Principal Findings." *São Paulo Medical Journal* 121, no. 6 (2003): 231–37.

Galduróz, José Carlos F., Ana Regina Noto, Solange A. Nappo, and E. A. Carlini. "Household Survey on Drug Abuse in Brazil: Study Involving the 107 Major Cities of the Country—2001." *Addictive Behaviors* 30 (2005): 545–56.

Galvão, Jane. *1980–2001: Uma Cronologia da Epidemia de HIV/AIDS no Brasil e no Mundo*. Rio de Janeiro: ABIA, 2002.

———. "Access to Antiretroviral Drugs in Brazil." *Lancet*, December 7, 2002, 1862–66.

———. *AIDS no Brasil*. Rio de Janeiro: ABIA/Editora 34, 2000.

———. "As Respostas das Organizações Não-governamentais Brasileiras Frente à Epidemia de HIV/AIDS." In *Políticas, Instituições, e AIDS: Enfrentando a Epidemia no Brasil*, edited by Richard Parker, 69–108. Rio de Janeiro: ABIA: Jorge Zahar, 1997.

———. "As Respostas Religiosas Frente á Epidemica de HIV/AIDS no Brasil." In *Políticas, Instituições, e AIDS: Enfrentando a Epidemia no Brasil*, edited by Richard Parker, 109–34. Rio de Janeiro: ABIA: Jorge Zahar, 1997.

Garcia Calleja, Jesus M., Neff Walker, Paloma Cuchi, Stefano Lazzari, Peter D. Ghys, and Fernando Zacarias. "Status of the HIV/AIDS Epidemic and Methods to Monitor It in the Latin American and Caribbean Region." *AIDS* 16, no. 3 (December 2002): 3–12.

García Trujillo, Odalys, Mayté Paredes, and Manuel Sierra. *VIH/SIDA: Análisis de la Evolución de la Epidemia in Honduras*. Tegucigalpa, Honduras: Fundación Fomento en Salud, 1998.

Garrett, Laurie. "The Lessons of HIV/AIDS." *Foreign Affairs* 84, no. 4 (July/August 2005): 51–65.

Garris, Ivelisse, Evelyn M. Rodríguez, E. Antonio de Moya, Ernesto Guerrero, Clotilde Peña, Elizardo Puello, Elizabeth Gómez, Edgar R. Monterroso, Mercedes Weissenbacher, and Sten H. Vermund. "AIDS Heterosexual Predominance in the Dominican Republic." *Journal of Acquired Immune Deficiency Syndromes* 4 (1991): 1173–78.

Gerlach, Allen. *Indians, Oil, and Politics: A Recent History of Ecuador*. Wilmington, Del.: Scholarly Resources Books, 2003.

Gibbs, Stephen. "Cuba to Help Caribbean Fight AIDS." *BBC News*, <http://news.bbc.co.uk/2/hi/americas/3899657.stm>. Accessed June 16, 2004.

Giraldo, Javier. *Colombia: The Genocidal Democracy*. Monroe, Maine: Common Courage Press, 1996.

Gómez Gómez, Sonia. *SIDA en Colombia*. 2nd ed. Medellín, Colombia: Editorial Colina, 1989.

González Block, Miguel Angel, and Ana Luisa Liguoiri. *El SIDA en los Estratos Socioeconómicos de México*. Morelos, Mexico: Instituto Nacional de Salud Pública, 1992.

González Ruiz, Edgar. *Cómo Propogar el SIDA: Conservadorism y Sexualidad.* Mexico City: Cal y Arena, 1994.

Goodwin, Paul B. *Global Studies: Latin America.* 8th ed. Guilford, Conn.: Dushkin/McGraw-Hill, 1998.

Gottlieb, Scott. "US Concedes on Cheaper Drug Production in Brazil." *British Medical Journal,* July 7, 2001, 12.

Goudsmit, Jaap. "Malnutrition and Concomitant Herpesvirus Infection as a Possible Cause of Immunodeficiency Syndrome in Haitian Infants. (With reply by LaPoint Normand, Zave Chad, Gilles Delage, et al.)." *New England Journal of Medicine,* September 1, 1983, 554–55.

———. *Viral Sex: The Nature of AIDS.* New York: Oxford University Press, 1997.

Graham, Sandra Lauderdale. *House and Street: The Domestic World of Servants and Masters in Nineteenth-Century Rio de Janeiro.* Austin: University of Texas Press, 1995.

Greco, Ralph S. Letter to the editor. *Lancet,* August 27, 1983, 516.

Greenfield, William R. Letter to the editor. *Journal of the American Medical Association,* July 4–December 26, 1986, 2199.

Grmek, Mirko D. *History of AIDS: Emergence and Origin of a Modern Pandemic.* Translated by Russell C. Maulitz and Jacalyn Duffin. Princeton: Princeton University Press, 1990.

Grupo de Apoio á Prevenção á AIDS—Bahia (GAPA-BA). *Brasil, Terra dos Prazeres.* Salvador: GAPA-BA, n.d. Pamphlet. Princeton University Microfilm Collection, Supplement no. 3, "Socioeconomic Conditions in Latin America." Roll 1, Subsection Brazil, Scholarly Resources.

Grupo pela Vidda. *Conquistas.* Rio de Janeiro: Grupo pela Vidda/R.J., n.d. Pamphlet.

———. *Direitos das Pessoas Vivendo com HIV e AIDS.* Rio de Janeiro: Grupo Pela Vidda, 1994. Pamphlet. Princeton University Microfilm Collection, Supplement no. 3, "Socioeconomic Conditions in Latin America." Roll 1, Subsection Brazil, Scholarly Resources.

Guest, Emma. *Children of AIDS: Africa's Orphan Crisis.* London: Pluto Press, 2001.

Guillermoprieto, Alma. *Looking for History: Dispatches from Latin America.* New York: Random House, 2001.

Hamilton, Dra Gabriela. "Septiembre/Octubre 2004, Informe de Gestión." Programa Nacional de Lucha contra los R.H., VIH/SIDA y ETS. <www.msal.gov.ar/htm/site/Lusida/frIndex.htm>. Accessed March 10, 2005.

Hansen, Helena, and Nora Ellen Groce. "From Quarantine to Condoms: Shifting Policies and Problems of HIV control in Cuba." *Medical Anthropology* 19 (2001): 261–72.

Hansis, Randall. *The Latin Americans: Understanding Their Legacy.* New York: McGraw Hill, 1997.

Hawkins, Denise B. "HIV/AIDS: A Predator in Paradise." *Black Issues in Higher Education*, January 30, 1995, 19.

Health Gap. "Medical Apartheid: Patents, Public Health, and Access to Medicines," <http://www.healthgap.org>. Accessed January 27, 2003.

———. "Meeting Report: Strategy Session on the Free Trade Area of the Americas (FTAA), Intellectual Property Rights & Access to Medicines," October 3, 2002, <http://www.healthgap.org>. Accessed January 27, 2003.

Healton, Cheryl, and Ronald Bayer. "Controlling AIDS in Cuba: The Logic of Quarantine." *New England Journal of Medicine*, April 13, 1989, 1022–23.

Hearst, Norman, Regina Lacerda, Neide Gravato, Esther Sid Hudes, and Ron Stall. "Reducing AIDS Risk among Port Workers in Santos, Brazil." *American Journal of Public Health* 89, no. 1 (January 1999): 76–78.

Hernandez, Grisela. "Mexican Government Programs for Migrant Health: The National HIV/AIDS Program in Mexico." *Journal of Multicultural Nursing and Health* 8, no. 2 (Summer 2002): 40.

Higgins, Michael James, and Tanya L. Coen. *Streets, Bedrooms, and Patios: The Ordinariness of Diversity in Oaxaca*. Austin: University of Texas Press, 2000.

Hooper, Edward. *The River: A Journey to the Source of HIV and AIDS*. New York: Little, Brown, 2000.

Hopkinson, Amanda, and Frank Chalmers. "Nicaragua: The First 100 Days." *Lancet*, August 4, 1990, 300–301.

Hughes, Matthew. "Logistics and the Chaco War: Bolivia versus Paraguay, 1932–1935." *Journal of Military History* 69, no. 2 (April 2005): 411–37.

Human Rights Watch. *Colombia's Killer Networks: The Military-Paramilitary Partnership with the United States*. New York: Human Rights Watch, 1996.

Hunt, Michael H. *Ideology and U.S. Foreign Policy*. New Haven: Yale University Press, 1987.

Ichaso, Leon. *Bitter Sugar*. DVD film, English subtitles, 102 minutes. Azucar films, 1996.

Inácio Bastos, Francisco, C. Barcellos, C. M. Lowndes, and S. R. Friedman. "Co-Infection with Malaria and HIV in Injecting Drug Users in Brazil: A New Challenge to Public Health?" *Addiction* 94, no. 8 (1999): 1165–74.

Inácio Bastos, Francisco, Steffanie A. Strathdee, Monica Derrico, and Maria de Fátima Pina. "Drug Use and the Spread of HIV/AIDS in South America and the Caribbean." *Drugs: Education, Prevention, and Policy*, 6, no. 1 (Spring 1999): 29–49.

Inciardi, James A., Hilary L. Surratt, and Paulo R. Telles. *Sex, Drugs, and HIV/AIDS in Brazil*. Boulder, Colo.: Westview Press, 2000.

Irwin, Alexander, Joyce Millen, and Dorothy Fallows. *Global AIDS: Myths and Facts*. Cambridge, Mass.: South End Press, 2003.

Izazola, José Antonio, José Luis Valdespino, Luis Guillermo Juárez, Manuel Mondragón, and Jaime Sepúlveda. "Conocimientos, Actitudes y Práticas Relacionadas con El SIDA: Bases para el Diseño de Programas Educativos." In *SIDA, Ciencia y Sociedad en México*, edited by Jaime Sepúlveda Amor, Mario N. Bronfman, Guillermo M. Ruiz Palacios, Estanislao C. Stanislawski, and José Luis Valdespino, 297–336. Mexico City: Fondo de Cultura Económica: Instituto Nacional de Salud Pública, 1989.

Jackiewicz, Edward L. "The Working World of the Paladar: The Production of Contradictory Space during Cuba's Period of Fragmentation." *Professional Geographer* 55, no. 3 (August 2003): 372–82.

John Marshall Law School. *Aspects of Criminalization: Cuba's HIV-AIDS Quarantine.* VHS tape. Chicago: John Marshall Law School, 1993.

Johnson, John J. *Latin America in Caricature.* Austin: University of Texas Press, 1980.

Jordan, Mary. "AIDS Orphans' Numbers Grow in Guatemala." *Oregonian,* November 30, 2003.

Kane, Stephanie. *AIDS Alibis: Sex, Drugs, and Crime in the Americas.* Philadelphia: Temple University Press, 1998.

Katel, Paul. "Cuba: Did Some Youths Get AIDS on Purpose?" *Newsweek,* May 16, 1994, 42.

Kelly, Philip. *Checkerboards and Shatterbelts: The Geopolitics of South America.* Austin: University of Texas Press, 1997.

Key, Keith K., and Daniel J. DeNoon. "Anti-AIDS Free Distribution Cocktail Begins in Brazil." *AIDS Weekly Plus,* November 25, 1996, 15.

———. "Child Prostitution Spreads AIDS among Young Haitians." *AIDS Weekly Plus,* September 23, 1996, 25.

———. "Cuba Sees AIDS Rise Linked to Tourism Growth." *AIDS Weekly Plus,* December 23, 1996, 12.

———. "Nuns Fight AIDS in the Dominican Republic." *AIDS Weekly Plus,* April 3, 1995, 22–23.

Key, Sandra, and Daniel DeNoon. "Six Dead in Jamaican Condom Riots." *AIDS Weekly Plus,* September 8, 1997, 17.

Key, Sandra W., Daniel DeNoon, and Salynn Boyles. "Coordinating Anti-AIDS Measures in Border Areas." *AIDS Weekly Plus,* June 28–July 5, 1999, 8.

Kornblit, Ana Lía. "Las Personas Afectadas por el Consumo de Drogas." In *SIDA: Entre el Cuidado y el Riesgo: Estudios en Población General y en Personas Afectadas,* edited by Ana Lía Kornblit et al., 173–238. Buenos Aries: Alianza Editorial, 2000.

Kornblit, Ana Lía, and Ana María Mendes Diz. "Las Personas Afectadas por Práticas Heterosexuales." In *SIDA: Entre el Cuidado y el Riesgo: Estudios en Población General y en Personas Afectadas,* edited by Ana Lía Kornblit et al., 293–355. Buenos Aries: Alianza Editorial, 2000.

Kornblit, Ana Lía, and Mónica Petracci. "Las ONGs Que Trabajan en el Campo del VIH/SIDA: Una Tipología." In *SIDA: Entre el Cuidado y el Riesgo: Estudios en Población General y en Personas Afectadas*, edited by Ana Lía Kornblit et al., 385–411. Buenos Aries: Alianza Editorial, 2000.

Kornblit, Ana Lía, et al. "SIDA y Conductas Sexuales." In *SIDA: Entre el Cuidado y el Riesgo: Estudios en Población General y en Personas Afectadas*, edited by Ana Lía Kornblit et al. Buenos Aries: Alianza Editorial, 2000.

Kornblit, Ana Lía, Ana María Mendes Diz, Mónica Petracci, Mario Pecheny, Jorge Vujosevich, Liliana Giménez, Malena Verardi, and Fabián Beltramino, eds. *SIDA: Entre el Cuidado y el Riesgo: Estudios en Población General y en Personas Afectadas*. Buenos Aries: Alianza Editorial, 2000.

LaFaber, Walter. *Inevitable Revolutions*. New York: Norton, 1983.

Landesman, Sheldon H. "The Haitian Connection." In *The AIDS Epidemic*, edited by Kevin Cahill, 28–37. New York: St. Martin's Press, 1983.

Larvie, Patrick. "Nation, Science, and Sex: AIDS and the New Brazilian Sexuality." In *Disease in the History of Modern Latin America: From Malaria to AIDS*, edited by Diego Armus, 290–313. Durham, N.C.: Duke University Press, 2003.

Leibowitch, Jacques. *A Strange Virus of Unknown Origin*. Translated by Richard Howard. New York: Ballantine, 1985.

Leiner, Marvin. *Sexual Politics in Cuba: Machismo, Homosexuality, and AIDS*. San Francisco: Westview Press, 1994.

Leonidas, Jean-Robert, and Nicole Hyppolite. "Haiti and the Acquired Immunodeficiency Syndrome." *Annals of Internal Medicine*, June 1983, 1020–21.

Levine, Robert M. *Brazilian Legacies*. Armonk, N.Y.: M. E. Sharpe, 1997.

Libonatti, O., E. Lima, A. Peruga, R. Gonzalez, F. Zacarias, and M. Weissenbacher. "Role of Drug Injection in the Spread of HIV in Argentina and Brazil." *International Journal of STD and AIDS* 4, no. 3 (May–June 1993): 135–41.

Linn, J. Gary, L. Garnelo, B. A. Husaini, C. Brown, A. A. Benzaken, and Y. N. Stringfield. "HIV Prevention for Indigenous People of the Amazon Basin." *Cellular and Molecular Biology* 47, no. 6 (2001): 1009–15.

López Severino, Irene, and E. Antonio de Moya. *Rutas Migratorias de Haití a República Dominicana: Implicaciones para el VIH/SIDA y los Derechos Humanos de las Personas Infectados*. Buenos Aires: Laccaso Onusida, 1999.

Low, Nicola, George Davy Smith, Anna Gorter, and Rita Arauz. "AIDS and Migrant Populations in Nicaragua." *Lancet*, December 22–29, 1990, 1593–94.

Low, Nicola, Matthias Egger, Anna Gorter, Peter Sandiford, Alcides González, Johanna Pauw, Jane Ferrie, and George Davey Smith. "AIDS in Nicaragua: Epidemiological, Political, and Sociocultural Perspective." *International Journal of Health Services* 23, no. 4 (1993): 685–702.

Lumsden, Ian. *Machos, Maricones, and Gays: Cuba and Homosexuality*. Philadelphia: Temple University Press, 1996.

MacDonald, Scott B. *Dancing on a Volcano: The Latin American Drug Trade*. New York: Praeger, 1988.

MacDonald, Theodore H. *A Developmental Analysis of Cuba's Health Care System since 1959*. Lewiston, N.Y.: Edwin Mellen Press, 1999.

Magis Rodríguez, Carlos, Luiz Fernando Marques, and Graciela Touzé. "HIV and Injection Drug Use in Latin America." *AIDS* 16, no. 3 (December 2002): 34–41.

Malcomson, Scott. "Socialism or Death?" *New York Times Magazine*, September 25, 1994, 44–49.

Marins, José Ricardo Pio. "The Brazilian Policy on Free and Universal Access to Antiretroviral Treatment for People Living with HIV and AIDS." Powerpoint presentation, Regional Forum of the Latin American and Caribbean Regional Health Sector Reform, Ocho Rios, St. Ann, Jamaica, February 20–22, 2002.

Mata, Leonardo, and Gisela Herrera. "AIDS and HIV Infection in Costa Rica— A Country in Transition." *Immunology and Cell Biology* 66 (1988): 175–83.

Mattes, Robert. "South Africa: Democracy without the People?" *Journal of Democracy* 13, no. 1 (January 2002): 22–36.

McElrath, Karen, ed. *HIV and AIDS: A Global View*. Westport, Conn.: Greenwood Press, 2002.

McEvoy, Peggy. "Caribbean Crossroads." *Washington Quarterly* 24, no. 1 (2000): 229–30.

McQuiston, Chris, and Ann Gordon. "The Timing Is Never Right: Mexican Views of Condom Use." *Health Care* 21 (2000): 277–90.

Mejía, Max. "SIDA: Historias Extraordinarias del Siglo XX." In *El SIDA en Mexico: Los Efectos Sociales*, edited by Francisco Galván Díaz, 17–60. Azcapotzalco, Mexico: Ediciones de Cultura Popular/Universidade Autónoma Metropolitano, 1988.

Mena, Jennifer. "AIDS Now a Migrant to Mexico: US Workers Bring Disease Back to Rural Villages." *Los Angeles Times*, September 15, 2000.

Mendez Ordoñez, Maria Elena. *Mujer y SIDA en Honduras*. Tegucigalpa, Honduras: Centro de Estudios de la Mujer, Honduras, 1995.

Mensagem encaminhada de Imprensa—Programa Nacional de DST e AIDS, May 3, 2005.

Minichiello, Shanthi Noriega, Carlos Magis, Patricia Uribe, Luis Anaya, and Stefano Bertozzi. "The Mexican HIV/AIDS Surveillance System." *AIDS* 16, no. 3 (December 2002): 13–17.

Ministerio de Salud, Colombia. *Plan de Mediano Plazo para la Prevención y el Control del SIDA, Plan a Mediano Plazo, 1990–1993*. Bogotá: Ministerio de Salud, 1990s.

Mishra, Shiraz I., Ross Conner, and J. Raul Magaña. *AIDS Crossing Borders.* Boulder, Colo.: Westview Press, 1996.

Misir, Prem. "The National Battle against HIV/AIDS in Guyana: Deficiencies in Epidemiological Profile Abound." *Guyana Chronicle,* September 10, 2003, n.p.

Mock, Nancy B. "Conflict and HIV: A Framework for Risk Assessment to Prevent HIV in Conflict-Affected Settings in Africa." *Emerging Themes in Epidemiology,* October 29, 2004, <http://www.ete-online.com/content/1/1/6>. Accessed June 29, 2005.

Mock, Nancy B., Sambe Duale, Lidanne F. Brown, Ellen Mathys, Heather C. Maonaigh, Nina K. L. Abul-Husn, and Sterling Elliott. "Conflict and HIV: A Framework for Risk Assessment to Prevent HIV in Conflict-Affected Settings in Africa." *Emerging Themes in Epidemiology* 1, no. 6 (2004), accessed on-line by BioMed Central Ltd., January 24, 2005.

Montagnier, Luc. *Virus.* Translated by Stephen Sartarelli. New York: Norton, 2000.

Monteoliva Doratioto, Francisco Fernando. "A Ocupação Político-Militar Brasileira do Paragauai (1869–1876)." In *Nova História Militar Brasileira,* edited by Celso Castro, Vitor Izecksohn, and Hendrik Kraay, 209–36. Rio de Janeiro: FGV/Editora Bom Texto, 2004.

Moraes, Claudia, and Sérgio Carrara. "AIDS: Um Vírus Só Não Faz a Doença." *Comunicações do ISER* 17 (1985): 5–19.

Morena Castillo, José Luis. *El SIDA: Una Realidad en Panama.* 5th ed. Panama City: Ministerio de Educación, 1997.

Moscatello, Graciela, Patricia Campello, and Jorge A. Benetucci. "Bloodborne and Sexually Transmitted Infections in Drug Users in a Hospital in Buenos Aries, Argentina." *Clinical Infectious Diseases* 37 (2003): 343–47.

Murillo de la Rocha, Javier. "Relaciones Boliviano-Chilenas: A 100 Años del Tratado de Paz y Amistad." *Foreign Affairs en Español* 4, no. 3 (2004): 43–58.

Nappo, Solange A. "Cocaine Use: Key Informant (KY) Report from São Paulo—Brasil." *Jornal Brasileiro de Psiquiatria* 49, no. 5 (2000): 149–66.

Nappo, Solange A., José Carlos Galduróz, Marcelo Raymundo, and Elisaldo A. Carlini. "Changes in Cocaine Use as Viewed by Key Informants: A Qualitative Study Carried Out in 1994 and 1999 in São Paulo, Brazil." *Journal of Psychoactive Drugs* 33, no. 3 (July–September 2001): 241–53.

Nicholas, P., J. Masci, J. deCatalogne, S. Solomon, J. G. Bekesi, and I. J. Selikoff. "Immune Competence in Haitians Living in New York." *New England Journal of Medicine,* November 10, 1983, 1187–88.

Norborg, Bengt, and Bo Sand. *Socialism or Death.* VHS documentary, English subtitles, 48 minutes. SVT News & Current Affairs, 1995.

Noto, Ana R., Solange A. Nappo, José C. F. Galduróz, Rita Mattei, and E. A. Carlini. "Use of Drugs among Street Children." *Journal of Psychoactive Drugs* 29, no. 2 (April–June 1997): 185–92.

Nuñez, Cesar Antonio, Mario Flores, Steven Forsythe, and Michael D. Sweat. *El Impacto Socioeconómico del VIH/SIDA en Tegucigalpa y San Pedro Sula, Honduras.* Tegucigalpa: Ministerio de Salud Publica de Honduras, 1995.

Nzilambi, N., K. M. De Cock, D. N. Forthal, H. Francis, R. W. Ryder, I. Malebe, J. Getchell, M. Laga, P. Piot, and J. B. McCormick. "The Prevalence of Infection with Human Immunodeficiency Virus over a Ten-Year Period in Rural Zaire." *New England Journal of Medicine*, February 4, 1988, 276–79.

Olivos Lombana, Andrés. *Amor e SIDA.* Bogotá: Paulinas, 1994.

Opuni, Marjorie, Stefano Bertozzi, Lori Bollinger, Juan-Pablo Gutierrez, Ernest Massiah, William McGreevey, and John Stover. "Resource Requirements to Fight HIV/AIDS in Latin America and the Caribbean." *AIDS* 16, no. 3 (December 2002): 58–65.

Pamplona, Francisco. "El SIDA en la Prensa de México: Análisis del Discurso Periodístico." In *SIDA, Ciencia y Sociedad en México*, edited by Jaime Sepúlveda Amor, Mario N. Bronfman, Guillermo M. Ruiz Palacios, Estanislao C. Stanislawski, and José Luis Valdespino, 391–411. Mexico City: Fondo de Cultura Económica: Instituto Nacional de Salud Pública, 1989.

Pana, Johnny Madrigal. *Al Vaivén de un Cabezal.* San José, Costa Rica: Editorial ILPES, 1998.

———. *SIDA: Un Ensayo Evaluativo sobre Conocimiento y Actitud en la Mujer.* San José, Costa Rica: Asociación Demográfica Costarricense, 1988.

Pan American Health Organization and the World Health Organization. *AIDS Surveillance in the Americas, Biannual Report, 2002.* Washington, D.C.: Pan American Health Organization, 2002.

Pape, Jean W. "AIDS in Haiti, 1980–1996." In *The Caribbean AIDS Epidemic*, edited by Glenford Howe and Alan Cobley, 226–42. Kingston, Jamaica: University of West Indies Press, 2000.

Pape, Jean W., B. Liautaud, F. Thomas, J. R. Mathurin, M. M. St. Amand, M. Boncy, V. Pean, M. Pamphile, A. C. Laroche, and W. D. Johnson. "Characteristics of the Acquired Immunodeficiency Syndrome (AIDS) in Haiti." *New England Journal of Medicine*, October 20, 1983, 945–50.

———. "Risk Factors Associated with AIDS in Haiti." *American Journal of the Medical Sciences* 291, no. 1 (January 1986): 4–7.

Pape, Jean W., M. E. Stanback, M. Pamphile, M. Boncy, M. M. Deschamps, R. I. Verdier, M. E. Beaulieu, W. Blattner, B. Liautaud, and W. D. Johnson Jr. "Prevalence of HIV Infection and High Risk Activities in Haiti." *Journal of Acquired Immune Deficiency Syndromes* 3, no. 10 (1990): 995–1001.

Paris, Roland. *At War's End: Building Peace after Civil Conflict.* New York: Cambridge University Press, 2004.

———. "Human Security: Paradigm Shift or Hot Air?" *International Security* 26, no. 2 (Fall 2001): 87–102.

Parker, Richard G. "AIDS in Brazil." In *Sexuality, Politics, and AIDS in Brazil: In Another World?*, edited by Herbert Daniel and Richard Parker, 7–32. London: Falmer Press, 1993.

———. *Bodies, Pleasures, and Passions: Sexual Culture in Contemporary Brazil.* Boston: Beacon Press, 1991.

———. "Introdução." In *Políticas, Instituições, e AIDS: Enfrentando a Epidemia no Brasil*, edited by Richard G. Parker, 7–16. Rio de Janeiro: ABIA: Jorge Zahar, 1997.

———. "The Negotiation of Difference: Male Prostitution, Bisexual Behavior, and HIV Transmission in Brazil." In *Sexuality, Politics, and AIDS in Brazil: In Another World?*, edited by Herbert Daniel and Richard Parker, 85–96. London: Falmer Press, 1993.

———. "The Politics of AIDS Education in Brazil." In *Sexuality, Politics, and AIDS in Brazil: In Another World?*, edited by Herbert Daniel and Richard Parker, 115–28. London: Falmer Press, 1993.

———. "'Within Four Walls': Brazilian Sexual Culture and HIV/AIDS." In *Sexuality, Politics, and AIDS in Brazil: In Another World?*, edited by Herbert Daniel and Richard Parker, 65–84. London: Falmer Press, 1993.

Parker, Richard G., ed. *Políticas, Instituições, e AIDS: Enfrentando a Epidemia no Brasil.* Rio de Janeiro: ABIA: Jorge Zahar, 1997.

Parker, Richard, and Jane Galvão. *Quebrando o Silêncio.* Rio de Janeiro: ABIA/ Relume Dumará, 1996.

Passarelli, Carlos André. "As Patentes e os Remédios contra a AIDS: Uma Crono-logia." *Boletim ABIA* 46 (July–September 2001): 7–8.

Passarelli, Carlos, and Veriano Terto Jr. "Good Medicine: Brazil's Multifront War on AIDS." *NACLA Report on the Americas* 35, no. 5 (March/April 2002): 35–41.

Paternostro, Silvana. *In the Land of God and Man: A Latin Woman's Journey.* New York: Plume Books, 1999.

Pecheny, Mario. "Los Jóvenes, el VIH/SIDA, y los Derechos Humanos: Una Reflexión sobre las Experiencias en Argentina y en América Latina." In *SIDA: Entre el Cuidado y el Riesgo: Estudios en Población General y en Personas Afectadas*, edited by Ana Lía Kornblit et al., 413–38. Buenos Aries: Alianza Editorial, 2000.

Pecheur, Julie. "The Third Gender." OaxacaTimes.com., <http://www.oaxacatimes.com/html/third.html>. Accessed July 6, 2004.

Peragallo, Nilda. "Latino Women and AIDS Risk." *Public Health Nursing* 13, no. 3 (1996): 217–22.

Perez, F., and F. Dabis. "HIV Prevention in Latin America: Reaching Youth in Colombia." *AIDS Care* 15, no. 1 (2003): 77–87.

Pérez-Stable, Eliseo J. "Cuba's Response to the Epidemic." *American Journal of Public Health* 81, no. 5 (May 1991): 563–65.

Peterson, Susan. "Disease and National Security." *Security Studies* 12, no. 2 (Winter 2002/2003): 43–81.

Pike, Frederick B. *FDR's Good-Neighbor Policy*. Austin: University of Texas Press, 1995.

Pio Marins, José Ricard. "The Brazilian Policy on Free and Universal Access to Antiretroviral Treatment for People Living with HIV and AIDS." Powerpoint Presentation, Regional Forum of the Latin American and Caribbean Regional Health Sector Reform, Ocho Rios, St. Ann, Jamaica, February 20–22, 2002. <www.americas.health-sector-reform.org/english/jam_documpresent_eng.htm>. Accessed November 2, 2002.

Pitchenik, Arthur E., Margaret Fischl, Gordon Dickenson, Daniel M. Becker, Arthur M. Fournier, Mark T. O'Connell, Robert M. Colton, and Thomas J. Spira. "Opportunistic Infections and Kaposi's Sarcoma among Haitians: Evidence of a New Acquired Immunodeficiency State." *Annals of Internal Medicine*, March 1983, 277–84.

Price-Smith, Andrew, Steven Tauber, and Anand Bhat. "State Capacity and HIV Incidence Reduction in the Developing World: Preliminary Empirical Evidence." *Seton Hall Journal of Diplomacy and International Relations* 5, no. 2 (Summer/Fall 2002): 149–60.

Prieur, Annick. *Mema's House, Mexico City: On Transvestites, Queens, and Machos*. Chicago: University of Chicago Press, 1998.

Princeton University Microfilm Collection. Supplement no. 3, "Socioeconomic Conditions in Latin America." Roll 1, Subsection Brazil, Scholarly Resources.

Prout, Ryan. "Jail-House Rock: Cuba, AIDS, and the Incorporation of Dissent in Bengt Norborg's *Socialism or Death*." *Bulletin of Latin American Research* 18, no. 4 (1999): 423–36.

Quesada, Charo. "The Fruits of Foresight." *UNISA Latin America Report* 18, no. 1 (2002): 47–48.

———. "IDB News: Leadership, Consensus, and Technology: With Broad Support from Society, Brazil Is Improving the Life of HIV Carriers." *UNISA Latin America Report* 18, no. 1 (2002): 45–48.

Quinn, Thomas C., Fernando R. K. Zacarias, and Ronald K. St. John. "AIDS in the Americas: An Emerging Public Health Crisis." *New England Journal of Medicine*, April 13, 1989, 1007.

Ramsammy, Leslie. "Are International Pharmaceutical Companies Doing Enough to Provide Low-Cost AIDS Drugs to Developing Countries?" *International Debates*, April 2003, 123–25.

Regina Noto, Ana, José Carlos F. Galduróz, and Solange A. Nappo. *Levantamento Nacional sobre o Uso de Drogas entre Crianças e Adolescentes em Situação de Rua nas 27 Capitais Brasileiras, 2003*. São Paulo: CEBRID/Secretaria Nacional Antidrogas, 2003.

Rose, D. B., and J. S. Keystone. "AIDS in a Canadian Woman Who Had Helped
Prostitutes in Port-au-Prince." *Lancet*, September 17, 1983, 680–81.

Rosenburg, Tina. "Look at Brazil." *New York Times Sunday Magazine*, January 28,
2001, <http://www.nytimes.com/library/magazine/home/20010...>. Accessed
April 6, 2004.

Rosenfield, Tasya, and Kira Herbrand. "Part One: The AIDS Colony," <www.kfai
.org/programs/locnews/aids.htm>. Accessed February 21, 2003.

———. "Part Three: The Cure," <www.kfai.org/programs/locnews/aids.htm>.
Accessed February 14, 2003.

Russell, Asia. [Letter]. *Health Gap Global Access Project*, May 6, 2002, <http://
globaltreatmentaccess.org>. Accessed January 27, 2003.

Ryan, Cheyney. "The One Who Burns Herself for Peace." *Hypatia* 9, no. 2
(Spring 1994): 22–38.

Ryan, Frank. *Virus X: Tracking the New Killer Plagues*. New York: Little, Brown, 1997.

Sabatier, Renée. *Blaming Others: Prejudice, Race, and Worldwide AIDS*. Washington,
D.C.: Panos Institute, 1988.

Santana, Sarah, Lily Faas, and Karen Wald. "Human Immunodeficiency Virus
in Cuba: The Public Health Response of a Third World Cuba." In *AIDS: The
Politics of Survival*, edited by Nancy Krieger and Glen Margo, 167–96.
Amityville, N.Y.: Baywood, 1994.

Santillo, Henrique. "Plano Emergencial de Ação para o Setor Saúde," pp. 36–37.
Princeton University Libraries, Latin American Microfilm Collection, Supplement no. 2, "Socioeconomic Conditions in Brazil." Roll 1.

Scheper-Hughes, Nancy. "AIDS, Public Health, and Human Rights in Cuba."
Lancet, October 16, 1993, 965–67.

Schifter, Jacobo. *La Formacion de una Contracultura: Homosexualismo y SIDA en
Costa Rica*. San José, Costa Rica: Ediciones Guayacán, 1989.

Scott, Peter Dale, and Jonathan Marshall. *Cocaine Politics: Drugs, Armies, and the
CIA in Central America*. Berkeley: University of California Press, 1991.

Sell, Susan K., and Aseem Prakash. "Using Ideas Strategically: The Contest
between Business and NGO Networks in Intellectual Property Rights." *International Studies Quarterly* 48 (March 2004): 143–75.

Senderowicz, Daniela. "Towards a Discourse of Mestizaje: The Role of the Pata-
gonian Frontier in the Construction of Argentine National Identity." M.A.
thesis, History Department, Portland State University, 2001.

Sepúlveda Amor, Jaime, Mario N. Bronfman, Guillermo M. Ruiz Palacios, Estan-
islao C. Stanislawski, and José Luis Valdespino, eds. *SIDA, Ciencia y Sociedad en
México*. Mexico City: Fondo de Cultura Económica: Instituto Nacional de Salud
Pública, 1989.

Sepúlveda, Jaime. "AIDS in Mexico." *World Health*, July 1988, 18–19.

Sharif, Pamela D. "Haitians Fight Blood War against AIDS Discrimination." *Black Enterprise*, July 1990, 13.

Sherrill, Carolyn M. Somerville, and Robert W. Bailey. "What Political Science Is Missing by Not Studying AIDS." *Political Science and Politics* 25, no. 4 (December 1992): 688–93.

Shilts, Randy. *And the Band Played On: Politics, People, and the AIDS Epidemic*. New York: St. Martin's Press, 1987.

Siegal, Frederick, and Marta Siegal. *AIDS: The Medical Mystery*. New York: Grove Press, 1983.

Smallman, Shawn. *Fear and Memory in the Brazilian Army and Society, 1889–1954*. Chapel Hill: University of North Carolina Press, 2002.

————. "Shady Business: Corruption in the Brazilian Military prior to 1954." *Latin American Research Review* 32, no. 3 (Fall 1997): 39–62.

Smallman-Raynor, M. R., and A. D. Cliff. *War Epidemics: An Historical Geography of Infectious Diseases in Military Conflict and Civil Strife, 1850–2000*. New York: Oxford University Press, 2004.

Smith, Herbert L. "On the Limited Utility of KAP-Style Survey Data in the Practical Epdemiology of AIDS, with Reference to the AIDS Epidemic in Chile." *Health Transition Review* 3 (1993): 1–16.

Sontag, Susan. *AIDS and Its Metaphors*. New York: Farrar, Straus and Giroux, 1989.

Starn, Orin. "Missing the Revolution: Anthropologists and the War in Peru." In *Rereading Cultural Anthropology*, edited by G. E. Marcus, 152–80. Durham, N.C.: Duke University Press, 1992.

Stover, John, and Mario Bravo. "The Impact of AIDS on Knowledge about Condoms as a Contraceptive Method in Urban Mexico." *International Family Planning Perspectives* 17, no. 2 (June 1991): 61–64.

Summerfield, D. "Nicaragua: The Ending of the War and AIDS." *Lancet*, April 20, 1991, 967–68.

Swanson, Janice M., Ayesha E. Gill, Karen Wald, and Karen A. Swanson. "Comprehensive Care and the Sanatoria: Cuba's Response to HIV/AIDS." *Journal of the Association of Nurses in AIDS Care* 6, no. 1 (January–February 1995): 40.

Szwarcwald, Célia Landmann, Francisco Inácio Bastos, Maria Angela Pires Esteves, and Carla L. Tavares de Andrade. "A Disseminação da Epidemia da AIDS no Brasil, no Período de 1987–1996: Uma Análise Especial." *Cadernos de Saúde Pública* 16, no. 1 (2000): 7–19.

Tabet, Stephen, J. Sanchez, J. Lama, P. Goicochea, P. Campos, M. Rouillon, J. L. Cairo, L. Ueda, D. Watts, C. Celum, and K. K. Holmes. "HIV, Syphilis, and Heterosexual Bridging among Peruvian Men Who Have Sex with Men." *AIDS* 16, no. 9 (June 2002): 1271–77.

Teas, Jane. "Could AIDS Agent Be a New Variant of African Swine Fever Virus?" *Lancet*, April 23, 1983, 923.

Teixeira, Paulo Roberto. "Políticas Públicas em AIDS." In *Políticas, Instituições, e AIDS: Enfrentando a Epidemia no Brasil*, edited by Richard G. Parker, 43–68. Rio de Janeiro: ABIA: Jorge Zahar, 1997.

Teixeira, Paulo Roberto, Vera Paiva, and Emi Shimma, eds. *Tá Difícil de Engolir?* São Paulo: Nepaids, 2000.

Telles Pires Dias, Paulo Roberto, and Flavio Fonseca Nobre. "Análise dos Padrões de Difusão Especial dos Cases de AIDS por Estados Brasileiros." *Cadernos de Saúde Pública* 17, no. 5 (2001): 1174–75.

Terto, Veriano, Jr. "A AIDS e o Local de Trabalho no Brasil." In *Políticas, Instituições e AIDS: Enfrentando a Epidemia no Brasil*, edited by Richard G. Parker, 135–62. Rio de Janeiro: ABIA: Jorge Zahar, 1997.

Thomas, Patricia. *Big Shot*. New York: Public Affairs, 2001.

Timerman, Jacobo. *Prisoner without a Name, Cell without a Number*. New York: Knopf, 1981.

Torres Peña, Rigoberto, and Maria Isela Abreu. "Acerca del Programa de Prevención y Control de la Infección por el VIH/SIDA en Cuba." *Resumed*, March/April 2000, 77.

Touzé, Graciela. "Obstacles to the Development of Prevention and Public Health Policies in Argentina." *Clinical Infectious Diseases* 37 (2003): 372–75.

Ubell, Robert. "Special Report: High Tech Medicine in the Caribbean: 25 Years of Cuban Health Care." *New England Journal of Medicine*, December 8, 1983, 1468–72.

Uhlig, Mark A. "Prostitutes in Mexico Enlist in the Battle against AIDS." *New York Times*, April 10, 1991.

UNAIDS. "AIDS Epidemic Update: December 2005, Caribbean," <http://www.unaids.org/epi/2005/doc/EPIupdate2005_html_en/epi05_08_en.htm>. Accessed March 24, 2006.

———. *Integrated Plan of the UNAIDS Theme Group to Support the National Response on STD/HIV/AIDS: Brazil*. Brasilia: UNAIDS, 2001.

U.S. State Department. "U.S. President's Emergency Plan for AIDS Relief: Country Profile, Guyana," <http://www.state.gov/documents/organization/61621.pdf>. Accessed March 20, 2006.

Valdespino, José Luis, Ma. De Lourdes García, and José Antonio Izazola. "Distribución de la Epidemia del Sida." In *SIDA, Ciencia y Sociedad en México*, edited by Jaime Sepúlveda Amor, Mario N. Bronfman, Guillermo M. Ruiz Palacios, Estanislao C. Stanislawski, and José Luis Valdespino, 267–95. Mexico City: Fondo de Cultura Económica: Instituto Nacional de Salud Pública, 1989.

Valente, Marcela. "Argentina: AIDS Care Dogged by Drug Delivery Breakdowns." November 19, 2001. LexisNexis, RDS-ACC-NO 03156842.

Van Wichen, Helmien, María Jesús Largaespada, Hermen Ormel, and E. Ariel Montesdeoca. *Es Tiempo de Actuar: La Situación de HIV/SIIA en Nicaragua.* Managua: UNFPA, 1995.

Varella, Drauzio. *Estação Carandiru.* São Paulo: Companhia das Letras, 1999.

Vázquez, Priscilla. *El SIDA y el Trabajo.* Panama: CIEN, 1994.

Vieira, Jeffrey. "The Haitian Link." In *Understanding AIDS: A Comprehensive Guide,* edited by Victor Gong, 90–99. New Brunswick, N.J.: Rutgers University Press, 1985.

Voeks, Robert A. *Sacred Leaves of Candomblé: African Magic, Medicine, and Religion in Brazil.* Austin: University of Texas Press, 1997.

Wadia, Roy. "Brazil's AIDS Policy Earns Global Plaudits," <http://www.cnn.com/2001/WORLD/americas/0814/braz...>. Accessed March 1, 2004.

Walker, William O., III. *Drugs in the Western Hemisphere: An Odyssey of Cultures in Conflict.* Wilmington, Del.: Scholarly Resources, 1996.

Walsh, Ed. "Argentine AIDS Agencies Blossom, but Face Fiscal Hurdles." *Bay Area Reporter,* January 3, 2003, <www.aegis.com/news/bar/2003/BR030101.html>. Accessed April 14, 2005.

Whigham, Thomas L., and Barbara Potthast. "The Paraguayan Rosetta Stone: New Insights into the Demographics of the Paraguayan War, 1864–1870." *Latin American Research Review* 34, no. 1 (Spring 1999): 174–86.

Whipperman, Bruce. *Moon Handbooks: Oaxaca.* Emeryville, Calif.: Avalon Travel, 2001.

Whiteside, Alan, and Clem Sunter. *AIDS: The Challenge of South Africa.* Cape Town: Human & Rousseau, 2000.

Wiik, Flávio Braune. "Contact, Epidemics, and the Body as Agents of Change: A Study of AIDS among the Xokléng Indians in the State of Santa Catarina, Brazil." *Cadernos de Saúde Pública,* 17, no. 2 (2002): 397–406.

Wilson, Carter. *Hidden in the Blood: A Personal Investigation of AIDS in the Yucatán.* New York: Columbia University Press, 1995.

Winn, Peter. *Americas: The Changing Face of Latin America and the Caribbean.* Los Angeles: University of California Press, 1992.

World Bank. *Brazil—Second AIDS and STD Control Project: Project Information Document.* Report no. PID6641. Washington, D.C.: World Bank, 1998.

———. *Confronting AIDS: Public Priorities in a Global Epidemic.* Rev. ed. New York: Oxford University Press, 1999.

———. *Indigenous Peoples Development Plan: Brazil AIDS III Project.* Report no. IPP37. Washington, D.C.: World Bank, 2003.

———. *Project Appraisal Document on a Proposed Grant in the Amount of SDR 6.7 Million (US$10 Million Equivalent) to the Republic of Guyana for a HIV/AIDS Prevention and Control Project.* Washington, D.C.: World Bank, 2004.

World Bank. AIDS II. *Project Appraisal Document on a Proposed Loan in the Amount* *of US $165 Million Equivalent to the Federative Republic of Brazil for a Second AIDS and STD Control Project.* Report no. 18338-BR. Washington, D.C.: World Bank, 1998.

World Bank. AIDS III. *Project Appraisal Document on a Proposed Loan in the Amount of U.S. $100 Million to the Federative Republic of Brazil for the AIDS & STD III Project.* Report no. 25759-BR. Washington, D.C.: World Bank, 2003.

Youde, Jeremy. "Enter the Fourth Horseman: Health Security and International Relations Theory." *Whitehead Journal of Diplomacy and International Relations* 6, no. 1 (Winter–Spring 2005): 193–208.

Zapata, N., A. Mohammedan, A. Gutierrez, A. Ortega, T. Alvaredo, J. Fernandez, and R. Meza. "Perfil Epidemiologico y Seroprevalencia de la Infección VIH in Población de Comayagua con Conducta de Alta Riesgo," 23. In *1er Congreso Nacional Sobre el SIDA: La Mujer y el SIDA.* Tegucigalpa, Honduras: N.p., 1990.

282

INDEX

285

virus/SIV, 10; and sex tourism, 12; state capacity to fight, 217–18; symptoms of, 7–8; transmission of, 7–9, 11; and war, 3–4, 17, 149–51, 153–55, 157, 205, 207–8, 219. *See also specific country*

Ho, Dr. David, 8

Homophobia, 6, 14. *See also specific country*

Homosexuals, 5, 9, 13. *See also specific country*

Honduras, 146; health care, 157; history, 148; HIV discrimination, 156; HIV emergence, 151–54; HIV medication, 156, 162–63, 184; HIV policy, 156, 159; HIV rate, 3, 151–53, 155–56, 206; homosexuals, 152; and Nicaraguan contras, 151, 153–54; prostitution, 151–53; transvestites, 152; and United Nations, 155–56; and United States, 151–53, 155–56

Hong Kong, 215

Hooper, Edward, 10, 25

Ichaso, Leon, 55

India, 16, 68, 94, 123, 203

Indonesia, 122

Inter-American Development Bank, 34

Inter American Foundation of the United States, 82

International AIDS Conference in Vancouver, 91

International Monetary Fund, 88, 154

Jaffe, Harold, 26

Jamaica, 32, 34

Japan, 39, 215–16

Journal of the American Medical Association, 24

Kelly, Philip, 188

Kennedy, John, 37

Kornblit, Ana Lía, 195

Kosovo, 150

Lancet, 25

Laos, 215

Latin America: cultural unity, 4; economy, 4–5; HIV rate, 3; indigenous beliefs, 5; machismo, 5–6; perception of U.S. involvement in spread of HIV, 12–13, 29, 38–39; religion, 4–7; sexual culture, 2, 5–6; sexual identity, 6; women, 5–6. *See also specific country*

Lee, Brenda, 81

Leibowitch, Jacques, 24

Leiner, Marvin, 44, 46

Leyva, René, 120

López Saynes, Yudith, 123

Low, Nicola, 154

Lula da Silva, Luiz Inácio, 218

Lumsden, Ian, 39, 44

MacArthur Foundation, 82

Machismo, 5–6. *See also* Mexico: machismo

MacRae, John, 185

Mahuad, Jamil, 172

Malawi, 149

Malaysia, 123, 215

Malcomson, Scott, 50

Manrique, Hugo, 184

Manuel de Cespedes, Carlos, 50

Marianismo, 5

Marmo da Silva, José, 87

Martins, Timothy, 49

Maulen, Sergio, 200

Mbeki, Thabo, 15, 68

Médecins Sans Frontières (Doctors without Borders), 58, 94, 185, 211

Mejía, Max, 117

Mendoza Rivero, Dessi, 63–64

Menem Akil, Carlos Saúl, 216

Mercosul, 186, 189

Mesa, Carlos, 172

Mexico, 13, 149; Catholic Church, 117, 128–29; CENSIDA (formerly CONASIDA), 114, 129–31, 136; COESIDA, 125,

287

HEALTH LEARNING CENTER
Northwestern Memorial Hospital
Galter 3-304
Chicago, IL